Healing

IN

His Wings

Healing

IN

His Wings

DAILY DEVOTIONS FOR HEALING

ANNE B. BUCHANAN

Library of Congress Number: 00-191489

ISBN #:   Hardcover   0-7388-2834-3
         Softcover   0-7388-2835-1

Unless otherwise indicated, all Scripture quotations are taken from the *King James Version* (KJV) of the Bible.

Scripture quotations marked (NIV) are taken from the New International Version. Scripture taken from the HOLY BIBLE, NEW INTERNATIONAL VERSION®. NIV®. Copyright © 1973, 1978, 1984 by International Bible Society. Used by permission of Zondervan Publishing House. The "NIV" and "New International Version" trademarks are registered in the United States Patent and Trademark Office by International Bible Society.

Scripture quotations marked (AMP) are taken from The Amplified Bible. Scripture taken from THE AMPLIFIED BIBLE, Old Testament copyright © 1965, 1987 by the Zondervan Corporation. The Amplified New Testament copyright © 1958, 1987 by The Lockman Foundation. Used by permission.

Scripture quotations marked (NKJV) are taken from the New King James Version. Copyright © 1979, 1980, 1982 by Thomas Nelson, Inc. Used by permission. All rights reserved.

This book was printed in the United States of America.

To order additional copies of this book, contact:
Xlibris Corporation
1-888-7-XLIBRIS
www.Xlibris.com
Orders@Xlibris.com

Dedicated

To The Glory of God

Who Loves Us

And Who Heals Us

In Memory of

My mother, Elizabeth

Preface

For most of my life I did not believe that God would be interested in healing *me*. I prayed for healing, but my heart carried so many wounds that underneath was the unspoken belief that my physical problems were my punishment for all my failings. If only I were somehow better. If only I had more faith. If only . . .

Through the years I have been challenged by numerous health problems. Approaching them with fear in my heart, it never occurred to me to seek God's opinion *first* to find the path for my healing. I had not heard the message presented in these devotions and I was in deep trouble.

For the last seven years I have been on my new path to healing and every day I strengthen my relationship with God and with my Savior Jesus Christ. Aware that healing in my physical body is integrally connected with my spiritual wounds, I concentrate on giving to my Lord all the hurts and pains of the past and allowing myself to be made new. I have made many mistakes as I zigzag my way, and there are days when the evil one whispers strongly in my ear, confusing and distracting me. But I know how to re-center myself and get back on track.

I have a new reverence for God's awesome works of nature. My Heavenly Father's herbs and essential oils are some of His most wondrous little angels. Each one has His breath of life, and those who use them find that they bring divine life force into themselves.

The God who created me also created the plants, herbs, and essential oils, and I believe He did so with full *intention* – knowing exactly how our bodies worked and how these natural substances would meet our bodily needs. God's pure herbs and essential oils work within us according to His will and plan for our healing and for our health.

When I have any ailment, my first consultation is always with The Great Physician. It is to Him that I give full power and trust. I seek medical opinions when instructed by the Holy Spirit to do so, and I always remain willing to accept whatever medical treatment or drugs that the Holy Spirit directs.

I want to make it clear that this is not an anti-doctor book. It is a pro-God book. These are devotions that urge each person to look to God's Word for guidance and instruction. There is a place for medical diagnosis and treatment, especially by medical personnel who work with the Holy Spirit and who are willing to pray with their patients.

Each person takes full responsibility for his own health and must make his own personal decision about medical care. Those who are on medications need to be particularly careful. Some medications create a serious physical dependency in the natural world and to discontinue them suddenly can lead to rapid death unless God intervenes supernaturally. God's Word tells us we are not to tempt Him. Therefore, to discontinue any medication in a rush of "instant faith" would most likely be a fatal decision that would delight the evil one. Don't do it. Instead, grow your faith, pray with your medical counselors, and God will tell you exactly what changes to make and when to make them.

God has begun a good work in me and He is faithful to complete it. I stand on God's Holy Word that I am healed in the name of Jesus, and, by following God's guidance, my healing is in the process of being fully manifested. No matter what challenges I face, I stay focused on God's Word and attuned to guidance from the Holy Spirit. My life has been – and continues to be – filled with miracles which flow from God's grace and God's glorious Word.

God's Word says, "My people perish because of lack of knowledge," so through the years my journey has led me to many different programs of study. As a result, I have acquired a Ph.D. in Natural Health and I have also become an ordained minister. My mission is to share with others the good news that I missed for most of my life – that God wants His children to be well and that, when we go to The Great Physician in prayer, we are guided to God's path for our healing.

Please note that in these meditations satan's name has intentionally been printed with a small "s" except at the beginning of a sentence. Writing his name in lower case provides a visual reminder that he has been totally defeated by our Risen Savior and has only the power we choose to give him.

This book proclaims God's healing power in small daily doses, boosting our faith and reminding us of God's Holy Word and His covenant with us. It is so easy to talk about faith and quite another to navigate the path of healing with focus and purpose. I hope that all who read these meditations will be blessed by them, and I welcome any letters from readers who wish to share their testimony with me. You may send your comments to me at 1727-8A Sardis Road North, Suite 132, Charlotte, NC 28270-2402.

Please start reading with Day One no matter what day of the year that you begin these devotions. Each meditation assumes that you have read the one that preceded it, and the ideas build on each other from the beginning to the end. Proceed through the book one day at a time in the order that the devotion is presented.

At the end of the book are a few selected references to materials which you may find useful if you wish to explore further.

Before closing, I want to acknowledge and thank my three sisters – Peggy Karsnak, Nancy Bradshaw, and Sandy Griffin – for their love, support, and patience during the two years of the writing of this book. Special thanks go to Peggy for opening my heart and understanding to the message that God wants every one of His children (including me) to be well. And deepest gratitude to Nancy for the endless hours of proofreading all 365 devotions and to Sandy for her expertise and advice.

I also give a special acknowledgment to John, who is the joy of my heart – and who lifts me, encourages me, and teaches me to fly on wings of love.

Deep appreciation goes to Jim Lynn for his assistance in spreading the word to others about my book and in assisting me in making God's message heard through my own song.

Anne Buchanan
June 2000

2014
3-20-14

Day 1 ✓

I am the Lord that healeth thee. (Exodus 15:26 KJV)

Do you want to be healed? If so, there is no statement more glorious than this declaration of The Lord God Almighty, "I am Jehovah-rapha, the God who heals you." God offers you His Word, and He reaches out to touch you with His healing hand. He wants you to be well and He has a plan for your healing.

It is crucial to believe deep within your heart that God wants you to be healthy. You may have believed that illness is a part of God's plan for His children. Or you may have believed that you are being punished for some past wrongdoing. Or you may have believed that you are being taught a lesson. Read God's Word now with new eyes. Open your mind, your heart, and your soul, and see how God's will for you is revealed.

When God first created His beloved children, He placed Adam and Eve in a wondrous Garden where only goodness surrounded them. Sickness and disease did not exist. In the Garden we see the perfect expression of God's will. He wanted us to walk with Him and commune with Him in the fullness and abundance of life.

Did God's will change? Of course not. What changed was man's shift from obedience to disobedience – to eat of the fruit and to know evil. Sickness and disease occurred only when Adam chose to include evil in his world. That was a result of Adam's will and not God's. It is God's will that you be healthy.

No matter what your past has been, God wants you to be well so that you can live an abundant, vibrant life in service to Him. He has declared Himself as Jehovah-rapha, the God who heals you. Claim God's will for your health, and with joy and thanksgiving in your heart, stand on God's Word that He is healing you now.

Mighty Jehovah-rapha, You have declared that You are the God who heals me. I claim Your Word; I claim Your will; and I claim Your healing. I believe Your Word. I live Your Word. When I feel doubt, help me to remember Your Word which is Your promise and Your covenant. Help me to be ever mindful of Your voice, to listen for Your guidance, and to act on it. I am filled with Your Divine holy light and I am healed by Your power. In the name of Jesus Christ, I pray, Amen.

Day 2 ✓

And he cast out the spirits with his word, and healed all that were sick: That it might be fulfilled which was spoken by Esaias the prophet, saying, "Himself took our infirmities and bare our sicknesses." (Matthew 8:16-17 KJV)

Jesus Christ came for one purpose – to redeem us. God wanted His children to be restored and made whole according to His original plan. What we must understand is that this redemption was not just of our souls – but of our *bodies*, as well. God wanted *every* aspect of each one of His children to be redeemed. He wanted the Garden to be available to every Child of His – just as He had intended from the beginning.

The original Garden was truly heaven on earth. Through Christ, God gave us the Garden again – but in a different form. This time we were shown that even in the world of duality which we chose, with constant choices of good and evil, we could always experience the kingdom of heaven because it is within us.

Jesus took the curse upon Himself and transformed it forever. He redeemed us spiritually from our sins, our past, our patterns, and our mistakes. In addition, Matthew makes it very clear that Jesus also bore our physical sicknesses and infirmities.

Just think of that. Jesus bore your sickness. He died to redeem you – soul and *body*. Let that incredible truth sink into every cell of your body. Visualize Jesus on the Cross carrying not only your sins but also your sicknesses. Name each of your ailments, and one by one give them all to Jesus on the Cross. Take into your heart the knowing that Jesus overcame them all. He died for *you*. Now visualize your Risen Lord and accept His healing transformation in your body. Say to yourself, "Jesus took *my* infirmities and bore *my* sicknesses. In the name of Jesus I am healed." Repeat this healing truth many times during the day.

Jesus has already redeemed you, every part of you. It has already been done. All you have to do is to be ready and willing to receive the healing of the Resurrection.

Almighty Lord, thank You for loving me so much that You sent Your Son Jesus Christ to redeem me, to lift me, and to transform me. I stand on Your Holy Word when it declares that Jesus bore not only my sins but also my sicknesses. I lay each of my ailments at the foot of Calvary's Cross. Fill my soul and every cell in my body with Your eternal love. I accept my healing, Lord, and I claim it now in the name of my Savior, Christ Jesus. In gratitude and praise I pray, Amen.

Day 3

. . . there came to him a certain man, kneeling down to him, and saying, "Lord, have mercy on my son: for he is lunatic. . . . And I brought him to thy disciples and they could not cure him." . . . Then came the disciples to Jesus apart and said, "Why could not we cast him out?" And Jesus said unto them, "Because of your unbelief: for verily I say unto you, If ye have faith as a grain of mustard seed, ye shall say unto this mountain, Remove hence to yonder place; and it shall remove; and nothing shall be impossible unto you." (Matthew 17:14-20 KJV)

Here Jesus gives you the key to your healing – believe that healing is possible and then speak your belief forcefully. Believe in God's will for your healing. Trust and have faith, remembering that the *size* of your faith is not the issue. You need have only as much faith as a tiny grain of mustard seed. What is relevant, however, is the *quality* of your faith. It must be focused, concentrated, and full of intention. It must be whole. Each mustard seed is tiny, yet it is as whole as a large avocado pit.

Nothing is impossible to you. Nothing. No matter what. No matter how many medical opinions you may have received. No matter how many tests show your problems "in black and white." No matter how many symptoms you see and feel manifested in your body. No matter how big the mountain is, nothing shall be impossible unto you if you have a concentrated, tiny nugget of faith, trust, and belief.

Faith alone is not enough, however. Jesus tells you to confront the problem and then speak the outcome that you desire. You must *say* to the mountain, "Remove hence to yonder place." Words of faith are simple, few, and to the point. They allow God's Word to be fulfilled and they activate God's angels to work in your behalf. Speak to your physical ailment now. For example, say, "Heart disease, remove yourself from my body now in the name of Jesus." Focus on God's Word. Focus on your Savior Jesus Christ who died for your healing as He also died for your sins. Focus on the truth that nothing is impossible to those who believe and declare their faith boldly to Jehovah-rapha.

Dear God, it is written that nothing is impossible if I have faith. I declare my trust in You and I declare my faith in You. I claim my mustard seed faith and speak it boldly. Although my physical eyes may see the mountain of illness before me, I stand on Your Holy Word and say to all my illnesses, "Remove hence!" And so it is according to Your Word and Your Son, Christ Jesus. Thank you, God, for Your healing. In Jesus' name, I pray, Amen.

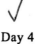

Day 4

And when the tempter came to him, he said, "If thou be the Son of God, command that these stones be made bread." But he answered and said, "It is written, 'Man shall not live by bread alone, but by every word that proceedeth out of the mouth of God.'" (Matthew 4:3-4 KJV)

Jesus is our example. He shows us the way, and He tells us how to live and how to handle the voice of evil. Here in the fourth chapter of Matthew, the devil came to Jesus three times and repeatedly tried to tempt Jesus into doing something that would separate Christ from God. Pay attention to the way that Jesus responded. He did not argue or debate with satan or give him His own personal opinions. What He said was this: "It is written . . ." Three times His reply to satan was the Word of God.

The Word of God is to be our strength and our guide. This is especially important to remember when we feel weak, overwhelmed, and defeated. Evil comes to us with whispers of temptation and most of all with whispers of doubt and fear. Satan knows that we cannot doubt God and trust God at the same time. He also knows that whenever he can get us to doubt God, he has put a wedge between God and us.

Sickness is an excellent tool for satan to use to separate us from God. If he can get us to believe that God gave us sickness, he isolates us from God's will. If he can get us to doubt God's healing power, he keeps us focused on our symptoms and our illness.

Don't let satan succeed. Follow Jesus as He reminds us to live by "every word that proceedeth out of the mouth of God." That includes not only the written Word but also daily guidance. Listen for God's voice with an open heart and He will speak to you. Ask Him to show you His path for your healing. Keep your focus on God's healing Word and God's healing power. Fill your mind and your soul with God's truth. Speak your faith until your healing is manifested in your body.

Almighty Lord, thank You for sending Your Son Jesus to teach me the way You want me to live. Thank You for reminding me to focus on Your Word. Whenever satan comes to separate me from You, help me to say always, "It is written that I shall live by every Word that proceedeth out of the mouth of God." It is written that You are the God who heals me. I claim Your healing, God. Thank You for restoring every cell, tissue, organ, and gland in my body to its proper function according to Your Divine plan. Thank You, Lord. In Jesus' name, I pray, Amen.

Day 5

. . . the God who gives life to the dead and calls things that are not as though they were.
(Romans 4:17 NIV)

In the moments when you feel despair and hopelessness that you will ever be well again, remember this passage from God's Word. Breathe deeply and allow these words to become a part of you. Feel the life of Jehovah-rapha fill every cell in your body.

Your God is the God who calls things that are not as though they were. In the beginning there was only chaos. This chaos was real, yet God saw beyond the appearance. God spoke and from the power of His Word, He manifested a new creation that was His reality. When Jesus Christ, God's Son, came to us to show us the way, He saw hurting, wounded people all around Him. The people were real, and their illnesses and difficulties were real. Yet Jesus embodied the power of Jehovah-rapha, and He manifested new life and new wholeness that was *God's* reality.

Abram knew that he and Sarah were too old to have any children; those were the facts; that was real. Yet God made a promise to Abram and even changed his name to Abraham to seal it, saying, "Abraham, you will be the father of nations." That was God's reality. God called something that was not (a mighty lineage descending from Abraham) as though it were. And it came to pass according to God's plan.

You must practice this powerful principle in your own life. You have had some illness or disease diagnosed. It is real. You look in the mirror and weary eyes look back at you. You experience your symptoms and feel the discomfort in your body. These things are real.

But now declare your faith in the God who gives life to the dead and calls things that are not as though they were. Call forth your wellness as though it were. Focus on God's reality which is beyond the appearance of your illness. Post this Scripture where you can read it and proclaim it out loud often. Let every cell in your body resonate with its truth. Claim the power of the mighty Jehovah-rapha until your healing is manifested.

Divine God, I hold on to Your Word which proclaims that You are the God who gives life to the dead and who calls things that are not as though they were. Fill me with life, Lord. I speak Your Word of health on every cell in my body so that it may manifest into being. Reveal to me those things You want me to do as I join in partnership with You for my healing. In the name of Your Son, Jesus Christ, I pray, Amen.

Day 6

And Jesus went about all Galilee, teaching in their synagogues and preaching the gospel of the kingdom and healing all manner of sickness and all manner of disease among the people. And his fame went throughout all Syria: and they brought unto him all sick people that were taken with divers diseases and torments, and those which were possessed with devils and those which were lunatic and those that had the palsy and he healed them. (Matthew 4:23-24 KJV)

Notice how often the word "all" appears in the Gospels to describe those whom Jesus healed. This tiny, easily overlooked word reinforces the limitless power of God. In this passage in Matthew we find Jesus going throughout all Galilee. And what was He doing? Two things – first, telling people His message by teaching and preaching, and second, healing the sick.

What kinds of sicknesses did the people have who came to Him? "All manner of sickness." "All manner of disease." Those with "divers (diverse) diseases and torments." "Those which were possessed with devils and those which were lunatic." "Those that had the palsy." The list doesn't leave out any kind of illness or disease whatsoever. ALL manner of disease, birth defects, mental illness.

Is there any health problem at the physical or mental level that would not be covered by this Scripture? If you had been in Galilee, would your illness have "qualified" you to be in the crowd of the sick as described by Matthew? The answer has to be yes. No illness was beyond the healing power of Jesus.

Who of the sick people was He healing? ALL of them. The Scripture says, ". . . he healed them" – period. If you had been in Galilee, you would have been healed because Matthew's description excludes no one. Jesus excluded no one. He reached out to touch every one who came to Him to be made well. Every single one.

Do you believe Jesus *could* have healed you in Galilee? Do you believe Jesus *would* have healed you in Galilee? If you do, then claim His healing now.

Almighty God, when Your Son walked on earth, He healed all who came to Him, according to Your will. There was no illness beyond His power. I come before Him today and stand in total faith. I rejoice in knowing that He has redeemed me totally – in spirit and in body – and I declare, according to Your Holy Word, that by His stripes, I am healed. In Jesus' name, I pray, Amen.

Day 7

When Jesus saw him lying there and learned that he had been in this condition for a long time, he asked him, "Do you want to get well?" (John 5:6 NIV)

Doesn't this seem to be a strange question? Who would say, "No"? Yet if you read further in this text, you will see that the man did not reply "yes" to Jesus' question. Instead, he began telling Jesus all the reasons why he hadn't been about to get into the healing waters.

People are no different today from the way they were then. Many of us may say we want to be well, and yet we are actually afraid of living. We put on a brave front, and we create an outward appearance of "normalcy" even though inside we are afraid, lonely, and wounded. The truth is that sickness provides a hiding place that seems safe to us. It may provide a reason to withdraw from others; or it may give us a reason to ask for support and for loving care that we aren't able to ask for when we are healthy; or it may provide a physical focus so that we don't have to deal with our emotional and spiritual issues. Oddly enough, in these and in many other ways, feeling sick actually serves some purpose for us.

Jesus came to heal us totally. He came to heal our spirits and He came to heal our bodies. When He looked at the man lying at the pool at Bethsaida, Jesus knew He could heal him. But He knew that the man must want to be well and must want to change his old patterns.

As Christians, we are used to saying to Jesus, "I believe You have saved my soul and, therefore, I do not fear death to the body." Now we must learn to say, "I also believe You have redeemed my body from illness, and, therefore, I do not fear *life* to the body in full service to You."

Look into your heart now. Search out all the possible reasons why being ill serves some purpose for you. List them on paper and bring them into the light. Then decide if you are ready to live without them. If so, offer them to God. Destroy the list and tell satan, "It is written that Christ Jesus bore all my sicknesses and all my infirmities. The victory has been won. You must leave my body now. I claim my healing. Hallelujah."

Yes, Jehovah-rapha, I want to be well. Yes. Remove from me all blocks to my spiritual, mental, emotional, and physical healing. Cleanse me of all old hurts, wounds, and patterns which separate me from You. Take my fears and my doubts. I choose to live, to be well, and to serve You. In Jesus' name, I pray, Amen.

Day 8

Now faith is the substance of things hoped for, the evidence of things not seen. (Hebrews 11:1 KJV)

As human beings, we like to say, "Seeing is believing." However, God's truth, the *real* truth, is that believing is seeing. God asks you to believe before you see. When you feel ill, your symptoms parade before you and seem to scream that they are your true reality. Yes, they do exist. However, what you must understand is that there is a reality *beyond* your symptoms and *beyond* your illness.

You must grasp at the core of your being that your ailments have their source in the father of lies. The evil one wants you to focus on the appearance of your situation and buy into it. He wants you to believe that God made you sick, and he wants to keep you from using God's remedies for healing. Don't be deceived by the evil one. Turn to God's Holy Word. We are told here in Hebrews about faith. What is faith? It is *substance.* It is something that is very real. It is *evidence.* How ironic that faith is its own proof.

This is a very difficult concept for us to grasp because we live in a world of machines that can see into our bodies, and we are bombarded by tests that produce official-looking reports. Yes, all these things exist. Yes, they give us information.

However, remember that the conclusions that are drawn from them are based entirely on elements from the physical realm. God's Word tells us that there is another dimension beyond the physical – and that it is even more powerful. It is substantial and it is evidence. Evidence of what? Of the things that are unseen.

All of the most important things of life are unseen. The Lord God Almighty Himself is unseen. Science will never find Him under a microscope or with a test of any kind. Love is unseen. Science will never find it with an MRI scan or in a blood test. The Holy Spirit is unseen. Science will never find it with surgery or EKGs or ultrasound.

Believe in God's Holy Word. Look with your heart for truths that are unseen by the eyes. Accept the substance and evidence of faith.

Lord God, strengthen my faith. Teach me to walk with You, ever growing in my trust, knowing that You guide me always. Help me to look with eyes of faith beyond my symptoms that I can see and beyond conclusions drawn from my medical tests. I stand on Your Word, God, and proclaim You as Jehovah-rapha, the God who heals me. Show me each step I need to take in order to be well. In the name of Jesus Christ, I pray, Amen.

Day 9

The Lord said to Moses and Aaron: " . . . I have heard the complaints of these grumbling Israelites. So tell them, 'As surely as I live, declares the Lord, I will do to you the very things I heard you say: In this desert your bodies will fall – every one of you twenty years old or more who was counted in the census and who has grumbled against me. Not one of you will enter the land I swore with uplifted hand to make your home, except Caleb . . . and Joshua.' " (Numbers 14:26-28 NIV)

"*I will do to you the very things you say,*" says God Almighty. Can you understand the staggering meaning of that statement? God plainly tells you that He will fulfill your inner beliefs which are revealed in the words that you speak. He allows you to determine your life; He allows your free will to establish what happens to you. God creates with His Word and He has established that you do the same.

In Numbers, the Israelites were grumbling against Moses and Aaron, saying, "If only we had died in Egypt! Or in this desert! Why is the Lord bringing us to this land only to let us fall by the sword? Our wives and children will be taken as plunder. Wouldn't it be better for us to go back to Egypt" (Numbers 14:2-3)? Even though they had witnessed miraculous signs in Egypt and in the desert, that wasn't enough for them. Instead, they were loudly proclaiming all the details of their problems. Their words revealed their lack of faith that God would keep His Word and would deliver them to the home He had promised.

What about you? Do you pray, "Lord, please heal me" and then turn around and repeatedly say to everyone, "I'm a heart patient"? If so, God says to you, "Then I will give you what you say – you are a heart patient." Or do you say, "I've been praying and following the guidance I hear, I'm just not getting any better"? If so, God says to you, "Then I will give you what you say – you are not getting any better." Each one of these "ordinary" statements betrays a lack of faith that the victory over your illness has already been won by Jesus Christ.

Guard the words you speak, and make sure they are ones that you want God to fulfill for you.

Dear Jehovah-rapha, I have not understood that You have declared that You will do to me the very things that You hear me speak from my heart. From this moment on I will speak those things that are in alignment with Your Word. I will pray the solutions I seek instead of the problems I see. I will declare the end result that I desire and will stand firm in my faith until my healing is fully manifested. In Jesus' name, I pray, Amen.

Day 10

Finally, be strong in the Lord and in his mighty power. Put on the full armor of God so that you can take your stand against the devil's schemes. For our struggle is not against flesh and blood, but against the rulers, against the authorities, against the powers of this dark world and against the spiritual forces of evil in the heavenly realms. Therefore, put on the full armor of God, so that when the day of evil comes, you may be able to stand your ground, and after you have done everything, to stand. Stand firm then, with the belt of truth buckled around your waist, with the breastplate of righteousness in place, and with your feet fitted with the readiness that comes from the gospel of peace. In addition to all this, take up the shield of faith, with which you can extinguish all the flaming arrows of the evil one. Take the helmet of salvation and the sword of the Spirit, which is the word of God. (Ephesians 6:10-17 NIV)

Jesus was not hesitant to name satan as His foe. Nor were Jesus' disciples and followers of the early church. Paul, who wrote these words in Ephesians, knew very vividly the power of satan in his life, for he, himself, had been one of those who had once persecuted Jesus' followers. Warning us of the forces of evil, he exhorts us to "be strong in the Lord and in his mighty power," and then he tells us how to do it – through truth, righteousness, readiness, faith, and the Word of God.

One of the ways that satan attacks us is through sicknesses and diseases. Protect yourself not only by following God's guidelines for healthy living but also by putting on your spiritual armor. Buckle on the belt of God's truth – by claiming that your God Jehovah-rapha wants you to be well. Wear the breast-plate of righteousness – by examining and releasing resentments you are holding toward other people.

Fit your feet with readiness – by going into action and following God's guidance for your healing. Take up the shield of faith – by believing that God can and is healing you. Put on the helmet of salvation – by understanding that you are saved in soul and in body. Take up the sword of the Spirit – by immersing yourself in the Word of God. Resist the devil. Be strong in the Lord. Rest in His power. Claim the full authority of God in your life. Allow God to heal you.

Almighty God, I put on Your mighty armor and I take my stand against the devil's schemes. In the name of Your Son Jesus Christ, I command the devil to leave me and my body. I stand firm, armed with Your truth, readiness, righteousness, faith, salvation, and Holy Word. I boldly proclaim that I am redeemed and healed. In Jesus' name, I pray, Amen.

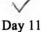

Day 11

. . . and on either side of the river, was there the tree of life, which bare twelve manner of fruits, and yielded her fruit every month: and the leaves of the tree were for the healing of the nations. (Revelation 22:2 KJV)

Here, in this description of the New Jerusalem, we see the tree of life, just as it is described in Genesis 2:9 as being in the Garden of Eden. It is interesting that from the beginning of all time (Genesis 1:29) to the end of all time God has given a special place to the plant kingdom in the health of His children.

The more we learn about the function of the human body and the more we learn about herbs, the more we see how herbs and plants fit perfectly in the plan of human health. Science will never understand fully the value of herbs and plants to human health because it disregards all factors that cannot be measured, tested, or seen. Herbs can be analyzed under a microscope, but they are much more than the sum of their chemical components.

Herbs and plants have in them the breath of life of God and the energy of God. Because science ignores this very real truth, it sometimes draws conclusions that are either misleading or incomplete.

There are thousands and thousands of healing herbs and health-giving plants on our planet. These natural substances have been used since the beginning of time for our great benefit.

It is tragic that most Americans today are afraid to use God's remedies for healing because they mistakenly believe that what we humans have synthetically created is far better than what The Great Physician has created. Too many of us have forgotten that our scientific endeavors should flow from the revelation knowledge and guidance of God and should complement rather than replace God's own remedies.

God has provided for us and for our healing in glorious abundant profusion. Learn about herbs and plants. Listen for God to speak to you. Then follow His guidance.

Wonderful Creator, thank You for the awesome abundance of herbs and plants which You have given me. Help me learn about them, Lord, and to use them in the way and for the purpose that You intended for my health and for my healing. Show me the herbs and plants and other natural remedies which You want me to use. I will do my part at the physical level just as I trust You to work Your healing power at the Divine level. Guide my path and every decision, no matter how small. In Jesus' name, Amen.

Day 12

Now Naaman . . . had leprosy. . . . Naaman went [to] the door of Elisha's house. Elisha sent a messenger to say to him, "Go, wash yourself seven times in the Jordan, and your flesh will be restored and you will be cleansed." But Naaman went away angry and said, "I thought that he would surely come out to me and stand and call on the name of the Lord his God, wave his hand over the spot and cure me of my leprosy. Are not Abana and Pharpar, the rivers of Damascus, better than any of the waters of Israel? Couldn't I wash in them and be cleansed?" So he turned and went off in a rage. (2 Kings 5:1, 9-12 NIV)

How interesting that Naaman refused his healing because it didn't take the form that he thought it should take. When Elisha told him to go wash seven times in the river Jordan he was furious because he knew that the Jordan was a very muddy, dirty-looking river. How could those waters possibly cleanse and heal him?

So his arrogance made him choose to keep the leprosy for a while longer. Eventually he reconsidered, washed himself as he was instructed, and was healed.

Too often we react just as Naaman did. We decide what our course of healing "should" look like. Usually, it follows the general pattern of feeling sick, going to a doctor, and then taking medication, having treatments, or undergoing surgery. If there is a problem along the way, we go from one doctor to another until we are given the "cure" that looks like the one in our thoughts.

God requires that He be our Great Physician and primary consultant. It may turn out that the path that God wants us to take matches the one we have in mind.

On the other hand, it may be that God's Divine will is something totally different from what we have considered previously. It may even, as in Naaman's case, defy logic and reason. Washing seven times in a dirty river in order to be cleansed and healed seems ridiculous and stupid. Think of all the diseases you could get in a dirty river!

Don't sell God short. Don't throw away your healing by insisting that it be done your way. Trust Jehovah-rapha, who wants to heal you.

Almighty God, save me from being arrogant and stubborn. Give me an open mind so that I can be receptive to Your voice. I vow to consult You at every step along my path to my healing and to follow Your commands to me, no matter what they are or how unusual they seem. You are my Great Physician and Healer. In Jesus' name, Amen.

Day 13

Praise the Lord, O my soul; all my inmost being, praise his holy name. Praise the Lord, O my soul, and forget not all his benefits – who forgives all your sins and heals all your diseases, who redeems your life from the pit and crowns you with love and compassion, who satisfies your desires with good things so that your youth is renewed like the eagle's. The Lord works righteousness and justice for all the oppressed. (Psalm 103:1-6 NIV)

In a beautiful song of praise, David summarizes the great goodness of God. He lists six of the most extraordinary "benefits" provided by God that could ever be given. Let's take a look at the first three:

1. God forgives all your sins.
2. God heals all your diseases.
3. God redeems your life from the pit.

God wants you just as He created you in the beginning. Take a moment to absorb this list of blessings into your soul, mind, and body. One by one make each blessing come to life for you.

Visualize all your sins. All of them. Bundle them up with a contrite heart, and place them at the feet of the Lord Your God. See Him raise His hand and wash them clean. Let your gaze move to the Cross. See your Lord Jesus Christ hanging there for the redemption of your sins. Let that sacrifice fill your soul with awe and gratitude.

Now visualize all your diseases. Every single one. Gather them together and give them to Your Lord Jesus Christ. See Him stretch out His arms and take them up. Hear Him ask you, "Do you want to be well?" Answer Him with the truth from your heart. Hear Him say to you, "I have borne every one of these ailments and conditions on the Cross for you. Now go your way and be healed."

Next visualize yourself in the bottom of a pit of despair, anger, sorrow, frustration, loneliness, and fear. See God's hand reach down to you and gently lift you up onto high ground. Feel the joy of God's saving grace fill you up.

O Gracious God, You grant me so many blessings. Thank You for forgiving all my sins. Thank You for healing all my diseases. And thank You for redeeming my life from the pit. I accept these gifts with awe and gratitude. I seek to hear Your voice and to follow Your path for my healing according to Your perfect will. Guide me, Heavenly Father. I am listening and I will obey. And, Lord, help me to be a faithful witness to others of Your magnificent glory. In Jesus' name, I pray, Amen.

Day 14

Praise the Lord, O my soul; all my inmost being, praise his holy name. Praise the Lord, O my soul, and forget not all his benefits – who forgives all your sins and heals all your diseases, who redeems your life from the pit and crowns you with love and compassion, who satisfies your desires with good things so that your youth is renewed like the eagle's. The Lord works righteousness and justice for all the oppressed. (Psalm 103:1-6 NIV)

Now we turn to the last three benefits provided by God that are listed by the psalmist David. Again we focus on each item in the list to make it come to life and to absorb it deeply within us.

4. God crowns you with love and compassion.
5. God satisfies your desires with good things so that your youth is renewed like the eagle's.
6. God works righteousness and justice for all the oppressed.

Visualize the immensity of God's love and compassion for you. It is the essence of who He is – love. See God's love streaming down from the heavens and crowning your head with its brilliant light. Interwoven with His love is His tender compassion for you. Let yourself *feel* this Divine love and compassion touching your soul and bathing every cell in your body. See each cell relaxing and then functioning just as God ordains.

Visualize the true desires of your heart and see God's satisfying each one with good things. Let your mind comprehend the Divine truth that God is the source of all the good things in your life. And how is the presence of good things manifested? God transforms you; He transforms your internal vigor in soul and in body.

Visualize all the things that oppress you and keep you locked in the prison of your fears and your doubts. Now see the Lord your God flinging open the doors, taking all the burdens that oppress you, and setting you free. Run with a joyful heart to the Lord God, your deliverer and healer.

Dearest Heavenly Father, thank You for crowning me with love and compassion. Thank You for satisfying my desires with good things so that my youth is renewed like the eagle's. Thank You for working righteousness and justice in my life and for setting me free from all that oppresses me. You shower me constantly with abundant blessings, and I am filled with awe and gratitude for all that You do for me. You are the source of my healing and I praise Your Holy name. To You I give all glory and honor. In Jesus' name, I pray, Amen.

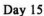

Day 15

But he was wounded for our transgressions, he was bruised for our iniquities: the chastise-
ment of our peace was upon him; and with his stripes we are healed. (Isaiah 53:5 KJV)

Here is the prophecy that summarizes Jesus' mission. He was bruised for our iniquities and by His stripes we are healed. He came to save us from our sins and He came to bear our illnesses.

Isaiah was given revelation knowledge that was and is God's truth. He was an instrument to tell the people of God's promise. "I will reclaim you," God is saying to His people. "I will reclaim you. Body and soul, mind and emotions, every single part of you, I will reclaim."

Jesus' mission has never been a surprise to those who read the Holy Scriptures. Over and over again God proclaimed it. When Jesus came, He taught it to His disciples. Before He ascended into heaven, He passed it on to all those who would follow Him.

Imagine for a moment that horrendous day when Jesus stood before Pilate with His arms bound. Barrabas was released and then "Pilate took Jesus and had him flogged" (John 19:1). "They spit on him, and took the staff and struck him on the head again and again" (Matthew 27:30).

Make these words come alive in your mind so that you can comprehend that redemption was not just a spiritual event. See each blow fall on Jesus' body. Feel each blow as it lands. Jesus bore the assaults on His physical body because He was taking them for you. For *you.* Blow after blow fell on Him. Why? Because "by His stripes we are healed."

With each blow *you* are healed. Lay an ailment at the feet of Jesus. Wham! Jesus has overcome it.

Lay another health condition at His feet. Wham! Jesus has overcome it. And another and another and another. Jesus has overcome them all.

By His stripes you are healed.

Heavenly Father, I come with tears in my eyes for the overwhelming sacrifice of Your Son
Jesus Christ who died for my sins. Mine. And who bore my infirmities on the Cross.
Mine. I can barely comprehend this magnificent gift of salvation and redemption. By the
stripes of Your Son Jesus Christ, I am healed. I declare my faith in Your Holy Word, and I
stand on it until my healing is manifested in my body. With a heart filled with gratitude, I
humbly pray in the name of Jesus, my Savior and my Redeemer, Amen.

Day 16

"I will give you the keys of the kingdom of heaven; whatever you bind on earth will be bound in heaven, and whatever you loose on earth will be loosed in heaven." (Matthew 16:19 NIV)

Many people skip pass this statement of Jesus, even though it is so important that it appears twice. In fact, Jesus tells us what He is saying is so vital that He considers it to be *the keys of the kingdom of heaven*. "Whatever you bind on earth will be bound in heaven, and whatever you loose on earth will be loosed in heaven." One more time we are told that our lives are largely the result of our own free will and not God's will. When our life is going well, we like to take credit for our hard work. But when difficulties come, Christians are quick to point the finger at God and say that it's "God's will."

Jesus is reminding us that God gave us dominion over the earth and that He gave us free will. He is telling us that we had better take responsibility for our actions – especially our words. When we feel sick, we can either bind God from helping us or we can bind satan from hurting us further. We can either loose the power of God's Word in our lives or we can loose further attacks of satan. The choice is ours.

We do it all by our words. If you say, "I feel terrible and I'm getting worse," then you bind God and His angels (because it is written that God gives you what you say). If you say, "satan, you cannot stay in my body; you are defeated; I am healed according to God's Word," then you bind satan instead. If you say "I have liver disease. I probably don't have but six months to live," then you loose satan to destroy your body. If you say, "I stand on God's Word; it is written that Jehovah-rapha is the God who heals me; it is written to ask believing that I have already received it without doubt in my heart; it is written that nothing is impossible with God," then you loose God and all His angels to raise you up.

Every single word you speak – *every single one* – is heard by God and also by satan. Whom do you want working to fulfill your words? God asks you to choose Him and, therefore, to choose life.

Jehovah-rapha, I have been holding the keys of the kingdom in my hands and haven't understood how to use them. Now I know, Lord, and I will speak words of healing and victory to loose Your mighty power in my life. I now bind satan and will guard my tongue so that I do not speak negatively to loose his destructive force. You are the God who heals me. In Jesus' name, I pray, Amen.

Day 17

I will lift up mine eyes unto the hills, from whence cometh my help. My help cometh from the Lord, which made heaven and earth. He will not suffer thy foot to be moved; he that keepeth thee will not slumber. Behold, he that keepeth Israel shall neither slumber nor sleep. The Lord is thy keeper: the Lord is thy shade upon thy right hand. The sun shall not smite thee by day, nor the moon by night. The Lord shall preserve thee from all evil: he shall preserve thy soul. The Lord shall preserve thy going out and thy coming in from this time forth, and even for evermore. (Psalm 121:1-8 KJV)

Read this Psalm out loud three times in a row to let its message of comfort, protection, and peace sink deeply into your soul. As you speak the words, the vibration of your vocal cords will send an energy of healing to every cell in your body. You are speaking God's Word. You are proclaiming God's truth. You are declaring God's presence in every aspect of your life.

Your help comes from the Lord, who made not only the heaven and the earth, but who also made you. God made every cell in your body. Is there anyone else who knows more about what you need for your healing than the Lord God, your deliverer? All answers of perfect truth are to be found in Him.

God neither slumbers nor sleeps. He never leaves you, never abandons you. He is never too busy or too distracted. Day or night, whenever you turn to God asking for help in your physical distress, He is there. Is there anyone else who is able to provide this kind of perpetual, constant, everlasting care and attention? All needs of eternal love are to be found in Him.

God preserves you from *all* evil. He is your complete safety and always reigns victoriously over attacks of the evil one. Is there anyone else who can shelter you from satan? All protection from all enemies is to be found in Him.

Rest now in the everlasting arms of love and healing of your Heavenly Father.

Wonderful Jehovah-rapha, I lift up my eyes to You, who made heaven and earth and me. I know You are my keeper and You do not slumber or sleep. You watch over me faithfully and lovingly and protect me from all evil. Preserve my going out and my coming in from this time forth and forevermore. In the name of Your Son, Jesus Christ, my Savior and my Redeemer, I pray, Amen.

Day 18

And ye shall know the truth, and the truth shall make you free. (John 8:32 KJV)

God has always wanted us to be free. From the very beginning He gave us free will so that we would enter into relationship with Him voluntarily out of our desire to do so and for no other reason. When we disobeyed Him and ruined the plan, Our Heavenly Father sent Jesus to reclaim us and to remove the bonds of the evil one. Jesus set us free, and He told us how to remain free – to live in the truth. Satan cannot tolerate the truth because the truth is God manifested.

The truth is especially crucial to our healing. Since sickness itself is a tool of the father of lies, we are especially vulnerable to deceptive appearances when we feel ill. The truth is often difficult to accept and often it is impossible to "prove." Many times "facts" seem real, yet they are only partly so. In court, we are asked to tell "the truth, the whole truth, and nothing but the truth." Yet with illness we are deceived into looking at the physical level only and that is not the *whole* truth. To see the *whole* truth we must look to things unseen, and we are called to depend on God's faith rather than man's scientific "facts."

To be free from sickness we must know the truth about it. And what is that truth? That its source is the evil one. That it has been borne on the Cross by Jesus Christ. That it is not part of God's will for us. That God does not want us to be enslaved by it. That God wants us to be free from it.

The Holy Spirit was sent to us as a beacon of truth, and, therefore, it has a vital role to play in our healing. Take your health questions to God. One by one place your questions at the feet of Jesus, and then ask the Holy Spirit to reveal to you the Divine answers. Be very specific in your questions. Make most of them answerable with either yes or no – because in the beginning it is easier to "hear" a short response than a long one. After each question be quiet and listen. You will know the truth, and the truth shall make you free by being the tool for your healing.

Gracious God, I walk gladly into the sunshine of Your truth, goodness, and mercy. It is through Your love and Your compassion that I am healed. Keep me always centered in Your perfect truth, which sets me free from the bondage of the father of lies and which keeps me grounded in Your healing love. Your truth lights my way and directs the path for my healing that You have selected for me. In Jesus' name, I pray, Amen.

Day 19

The heavens declare the glory of God; the skies proclaim the work of his hands. (Psalm 19:1 NIV)

Looking up into the sky can fill you with wonder and awe. Tonight gaze into the heavens and breathe deeply. Let yourself feel the immensity of space, and allow your spirit to expand outward until it touches the stars.

Know that, as enormous as the universe is, you are important to God. You are His special child and He loves you. While you are basking in the wonder of the heavens, connect with God's healing energy.

Visualize the stars twinkling with God's love, and see them shrink to form a beam of tiny sparkles streaming down from the heavens into the top of your head. Watch them dance through your blood stream and your nervous system to every part of your body until a tiny star shines in every one of your trillions of cells. Allow them to remain there radiating God's healing light within you.

During the day, take time to be appreciative of the beauty of nature wherever you find it. You may discover it in a park down the street or in a violet on your dining room table or in a brave little weed poking its head through a crack in a cement walkway. God has been extravagant in the display of His majesty and glory as expressed in the natural world around you. Look for it and connect to it.

Nature changes people. It is interesting that most people who take herbs over a period of time find that they undergo a spiritual renewal as well as a physical healing. The herb is much more than the sum of its chemical components. Like us, it carries Divine life and purpose, and, when we eat the herb, we absorb that life energy. That is one of the reasons that God's remedies for healing are so different from synthetic, lifeless remedies of man.

Don't forget to include God's remedies from nature among your options for healing. Offer your health questions to God; then quieten your soul and listen for His guidance. Let God determine what is right for you and what your choice should be.

God of glory, the heavens do, indeed, declare Your glory, and the skies proclaim the work of Your hands. Your works of nature abound around me and I am filled with awe and wonder. Help me to value and protect your creations. Teach me especially how to use your herbs in my healing process. I will obey your guidance in their use for my recovery. In Jesus' name, I pray, Amen.

Day 20

Jesus saith unto him, "I am the way, the truth, and the life." (John 14:6 KJV)

When Moses wanted to know what name to use for God, God told him, "I AM who I AM" (which is translated "Yahweh" or "Jehovah"). God is the great "I AM," and He gave special importance to those words and whatever followed them.

As the Son of God, Jesus also knew of the importance of "I am." He knew that, when we use those words, we define ourselves. Watch how Jesus defines Himself. "I am the bread of life." "I am the light of the world." "I am the good shepherd." "I am the resurrection and the life." "I am the true vine." "I am the way, the truth, and the life."

What about you? Notice how often you define yourself by your illnesses and your state of health. "I am anemic." "I am a diabetic." "I am tired." "I am sick." None of these definitions of yourself as a sick person is who you are in God's eyes. Like all words that we speak, each of these statements has energy and life – and our souls and bodies take in the words and believe them.

We perpetuate and live our definitions of ourselves at every level of our being. When we define ourselves by our ailments, satan is delighted. He gains great power when we become so enmeshed with our illnesses that we no longer see ourselves whole and healthy. Our very language keeps us bound to our diseases.

Stop speaking satan's deceptions and start speaking God's truth. Notice how often you use "I am" followed by some indication of your poor health. Change your words from "I am . . ." to "I feel . . . ." Say, "I feel sick" or "I feel tired." Better yet say, "I may feel sick at the moment, but I stand on God's Word that 'by His stripes I am healed.'" Describe health conditions as something you are experiencing at the present time. For example, "I am experiencing anemia." Don't give your illness your power by reinforcing it with your words.

Instead, declare boldly, "I am a child of God." "By His stripes, I am healed." Stand firm on the Word of God. Use the powerful words "I am" in ways that reflect God's will and God's vision for you.

Dear Heavenly Father, help me to choose my words with care. Let not only the meditations of my heart but the words of my mouth declare Your vision of me. Thank you for guiding me every moment of every day. Thank You, Jehovah-rapha, for being the God who heals me. In Jesus' name I pray, Amen.

Day 21

Be strong and of a good courage, fear not, nor be afraid of them: for the Lord thy God, he it is that doth go with thee; he will not fail thee, nor forsake thee. (Deuteronomy 31:6 KJV)

Fear is your worst enemy. It is never from God; therefore, when you are filled with fear, you are in a place of separation from your Heavenly Father. Fear is satan's tool. Since it comes from the father of lies, you can be sure that it is always based on falsehood and deception.

Despite satan's best efforts to overcome us, God is more powerful than satan, and God is perfectly faithful to us. He knows how devastating illness can be, so He covenants with us that He, The Lord God Almighty, has the power to make His own plan prevail. No matter what the author of disease has done and no matter what sickness may befall us, Jehovah-rapha is there, healing and restoring us. Through any disease we can say, "Fear not, for the Lord our God, He it is that goes with us."

We need not fear as we undergo any medical treatment. Spirit-led doctors are wonderful and can be useful partners in our recovery process when God sends us to them. If we go for any other reason, we are operating from fear and we are outside the plans that God has for us. If we are sitting in the doctor's office, let it be because God told us to go – and not because "everybody" thinks we should. If we are undergoing a particular surgery or treatment, let it be because God told us to do so – and not because we were told by a doctor that we "have" to have it. Let God lead every step of the way and decide with finality all questions that arise in our healing process.

When God is your partner *and you are sure of it,* fear actually seems ridiculous. When God is your partner *and you are standing on God's Word,* there is no room in your heart to be afraid. When God is your partner *and you are filled with faith,* you know that you are safe. You know that you are God's beloved child and that He will never fail you or forsake you.

Almighty God, help me to be strong and of good courage. I give You grateful thanks for revealing Yourself as the great Jehovah-rapha, the mighty God who heals me. I give grateful thanks that You are above all sickness and disease. Your message is always, "Fear not, for I am with you." You are my shield and my salvation, my refuge and my strength. You go with me always and You have promised never to fail or forsake me. In the name of Your Son, Jesus Christ, I pray, Amen.

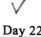

Day 22

For ye shall go out with joy, and be led forth with peace: the mountains and the hills shall break forth before you into singing, and all the trees of the field shall clap their hands. (Isaiah 55:12 KJV).

What a delightful image it is for the hills to break forth singing and the trees to clap their hands! See that in your mind's eye. You can't help but smile.

Isaiah speaks to us of joy and of peace. When we feel ill, we often have little of either of those emotions, yet both are critical to our recovery. Healing isn't just about mending a broken bone or lowering a fever or balancing hormones. It doesn't occur only at the physical level. Healing is a total experience of the complete person, and, therefore, it operates at all levels – body, mind, emotions, and soul.

One area that we seem to ignore is our emotional health. Most of us carry wounds throughout much of our lives unless we do the work that is necessary to release them. These wounds create a spiritual drag and provide an environment at the physical level for disease to manifest. Anger – resentment – blame – grief – guilt – fear – all these are old, buried, unresolved emotions that take a heavy toll on our health.

Our language is filled with phrases that acknowledge our understanding of the relevance of our emotional health to our physical health. We speak of being "eaten up with guilt," "dying of loneliness," being "brokenhearted with grief," and being "scared to death."

In order to be well, we must be willing to let go of old hurts. Are you ready to be well emotionally as well as physically? Are you ready to put away your resentment and anger once and for all? Are you ready to stop being a martyr and lay down your guilt once and for all? Are you ready to stop hiding in your grief once and for all?

God wants you to live – singing with the hills and clapping your hands with the trees. And His Holy Word tells you that in addition to covering you with joy, your Heavenly Father wishes to lead you to His peace.

Dear Father, I have many old hurts that are painful to carry and yet strangely comfortable. They have been a good hiding place, given me excuses for taking my pain out on others, and even allowed me to manipulate and control others. God, I give them all to You. Whatever You want me to do to confront these emotional scars, tell me and I will do it. I want to be totally well and whole before You so that I can go out with joy and be led forth with peace. In Jesus' name I pray, Amen.

Day 23

My son, attend to my words; incline thine ear unto my sayings. Let them not depart from thine eyes; keep them in the midst of thine heart. For they are life unto those that find them, and health to all their flesh. (Proverbs 4:20-22 KJV)

These three verses in Proverbs sum up the most important steps for being healed. Let's take a look at the first sentence: "My son, attend to my words; incline thine ear unto my sayings."

Attend means "to give heed to." God is saying, "Pay attention. Give heed." To what? "To my words." God tells us, "Listen to what I have to tell you." How? By studying His Word written in the Holy Scriptures and by listening to His voice as He gives you revelation knowledge.

If you want healing, then search out the Scriptures that speak of God's will on the subject. Fill your mind and your heart and your soul with those Scriptures. You will find many of them in this little book, but there are hundreds more.

Certain Scriptures will touch your heart more than others. Write them down on little note cards and post them around the house – on your bathroom mirror, on the refrigerator door, on the end table next to your favorite chair.

Another way to fill your mind and spirit with the Word of God is to get some audiotapes of the New Testament. Play them when you are in the car; play them while you are doing housework; play them when you are taking some quiet time to rest and relax.

You may also want to make your own tape of the Scriptures that are especially powerful for you. Listening to your own voice speaking God's Words of healing and love can be very empowering.

Begin to memorize healing verses, and say them to yourself as often as possible during the day. Incline your ear to the sayings of the Lord. God wants your full attention as though you were straining to hear something being whispered to you. God has many answers for you in His Word. Be diligent and faithful to find them.

Wonderful Jehovah-rapha, how grateful I am to have Your Holy Scriptures to lift me and strengthen me. Give me the discipline to incline my ears more often to Your sayings. Help me to develop habits of immersing myself in Your Word and to hear Your Holy voice. In the name of Jesus Christ, my Redeemer and my Savior, I pray, Amen.

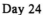

Day 24

But those who hope in the Lord will renew their strength. They will soar on wings like eagles; they will run and not grow weary, they will walk and not be faint. (Isaiah 40:31 NIV)

Read this Scripture out loud and then shout, "Hallelujah!" Let every word sink deeply into your heart and soul. "Those who hope in the Lord will renew their strength. They will soar on wings like eagles; they will run and not grow weary, they will walk and not be faint."

The Lord God Almighty created you in His image with the tenderest love and care. He loves you. He loves *you* and calls you by name. Think of the person you love most in the world, and then try to comprehend that your love pales in comparison to the depth of the love that Your Heavenly Creator has for you.

Out of that love, He offers His strength, His power, and His healing. Let yourself relax for a moment and connect with this awesome power of God. If you have some inspiring music, play it now. Get in a comfortable position and close your eyes. Open your heart and your soul to God, and feel the connection of your spirit to His. Welcome His Holy presence into your body, and feel its warmth and power pouring strength and healing into each cell.

Now in your mind's eye, see yourself totally well. See yourself serving God in vigor, in joy, and in humility. Ask God to show you the purpose He has for you to fulfill.

Let God speak to you, and give thanks for the information you are given. Ask for God's protection and for God's help so that you will be able to serve Him and glorify His name according to His plan.

Wonderful Jehovah-rapha, I confess my faith in You. Lord and Creator, renew my strength. Help me to soar on wings like eagles, to run and not grow weary, to walk and not be faint. You are the God who heals me. You are my strength and my salvation. Help me, God, in the times when I become discouraged and when I focus on the appearance of my illness and infirmities. Keep me grounded in Your truth and in Your Word. Lift me up, God. Guide me every minute of every day, and help me to stay faithful to the path You want me to follow for my life and for my healing. Thank You for Your Son, Christ Jesus, who died on the Cross for my sins and for my infirmities. By His stripes I am healed. Through His sacrifice I have been redeemed. Thank You, God. Thank You. In the name of Jesus Christ, my Savior and my Redeemer, I pray, Amen.

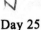

Day 25

Therefore I tell you, whatever you ask for in prayer, believe that you have received it, and it will be yours. (Mark 11:24 NIV)

Jesus has had His triumphal entry into Jerusalem, hearing the people shout, "Hosanna! Blessed is He who comes in the name of the Lord!" That night He and His disciples went to Bethany. The next morning they were hungry and looked around for something to eat. Jesus saw a fig tree and went up to it for some figs.

Now even though it was not the growing season for figs, fruit usually stays on the tree for several months afterward until a new growing season arrives, producing more fruit. On this particular tree, however, Jesus found nothing but leaves, so He says to the tree, "May no one ever eat fruit from you again." The disciples heard Him say this to the tree but they didn't really understand what He meant. (Scholars tell us that the tree was a symbol of the fruitlessness of Israel and of the rejection that Jesus would soon experience.)

The next day they passed by the fig tree. Peter says, "Look! The tree that You cursed is withered!" Peter is shocked that it has happened so quickly. At this point Jesus says, "Have faith in God. I tell you the truth, if anyone says to this mountain, 'Go, throw yourself into the sea,' and *does not doubt in his heart but believes that what he says will happen,* it will be done for him. Therefore I tell you, whatever you ask for in prayer, believe that you have received it, and it will be yours."

Believe with *no* doubt in your heart. And believe that you have *already* received it. You must believe *before* you see the manifestation of what you want. You must believe even though the appearance says that nothing has changed. You must believe even though the appearance seems to be getting worse.

With that kind of belief you can tell a mountain to throw itself into the sea, and it will be done for you. Notice *you* don't have to "make" it happen. It will be done for you. God will do it for you. What is required is your unshakable faith.

Heavenly Father, I want to be a tree that always bears fruit – Your fruit. There are times when my faith is strong and I stand firmly on Your Holy Word. I confess, though, that there are other times when I let fear overtake me, and I falter. Help me, Lord. I turn to You. Strengthen me so that I do not doubt but instead believe that what I say will happen. Help me to guard the words of my mouth as well as the thoughts in my mind. I believe You are healing me now. In Jesus' name, I pray, Amen.

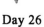

Day 26

Then Jesus looked up and said, "Father, I thank you that you have heard me. I knew that you always hear me, but I said this for the benefit of the people standing here, that they may believe that you sent me." When he had said this, Jesus called in a loud voice, "Lazarus, come out!" (John 11:41-43 NIV)

This is a powerful example for us in the way we are to pray for our healing. Lazarus, a dear friend of Jesus, has died, and Jesus arrives at his tomb after he has been buried for three days.

Notice what Jesus says when He prays. He doesn't beg God to heal Lazarus. What He does is to *thank God* for hearing him. Jesus says to God, "I know you always hear me, but I'm saying this for the benefit of the people standing here." And because this is recorded in the Holy Scripture, Jesus was saying it for your benefit, too.

Notice that Jesus thanks God *in advance* for fulfilling His request. God hasn't done anything yet, and Lazarus' healing has not yet been manifested – but Jesus is saying "thank you" anyway.

That is what you must do. Are you waiting for your healing to manifest itself before you thank God for it? The gratitude must come first – before the manifestation. Why is this so important? Because the thanks are based on faith and belief that God is indeed Jehovah-rapha.

If you are waiting for the manifestation to happen first, then you are, in fact, living in doubt that your healing with occur. You may be *saying* "I believe" with your mouth, but you are *living* "I'll believe it when I see it" in your heart.

Jesus' faith was unshakable; examine your own. What do you really believe? Lay your doubts at the feet of Jesus. Look to the Cross and then to the glory of the Resurrection, and say, "Thank you."

Mighty Jehovah-rapha, thank You for healing me. I trust You, God, with all my heart. You are The Great Physician and nothing is beyond Your power. There is no place for the evil one in my body or in my soul. Your loving Son Jesus Christ has shed His precious blood for my complete redemption and salvation. He bore my sins on the Cross and He bore my infirmities there also. I have been completely and totally redeemed at every level of my being. Thank You, God. Show me if there is anything I need to do at the physical level to join in partnership with You for the manifestation of my healing. I am willing to obey whatever You tell me to do. In the name of Your Son Jesus Christ, my Redeemer and my Savior, I pray, Amen.

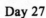

Day 27

Do you not know that your body is a temple of the Holy Spirit, who is in you, whom you have received from God? You are not your own; you were bought at a price. Therefore honor God with your body. (1 Corinthians 6:19-20 NIV)

Here Paul reminds us that our bodies are holy. God designed our bodies and breathed into us the breath of life. How different our actions would be if we could keep focused on the fact that our bodies are temples. Every item we eat is really a prayer and an offering to God. Think about that the next time you open your mouth to eat.

The choice is ours whether to fill our temple with wholesome food that nourishes, builds, and fortifies our body or whether to trash it with unhealthy foods filled with toxins, antibiotics, hormones, and empty calories. We are offered more and more items that are called food but are either genetically altered, artificial, or chemically treated. We are sadly mistaken if we think that we can improve on God the Creator when it comes to our nourishment. We fill our bodies with junk, get sick, and then blame God by saying it was His will that we became ill.

Satan is the one who works to get us off the track by misleading us into making poor choices. He gets us to believe we can deceive our bodies with fake food and synthetic vitamins. How easy it is for him to get us to defile the temple.

Food is not the only area of concern when we look at the issue of keeping our temple. We honor our temple by giving it the proper exercise. We honor our temple by keeping it clean. We honor our temple by following God's laws for appropriate sexual behavior. (It was on this particular point that Paul was writing to the people of Corinth.)

The Lord is in *our* holy temple. The Lord dwells in us. He has always been there. When we were lost, He sent His Son to redeem us – soul and body. We have indeed been bought with a great price. Therefore, honor God with your body – with every substance you eat and with every movement you make. When you do so, you join in partnership with God to create health not only in your soul but also in your body.

Lord God, my body is Your temple. Often I find it hard to do the things I know I ought to do. My life seems so hectic, and I let the "busy-ness" of life interfere with keeping my temple holy and healthy. Give me strength each day to follow Your instructions for healthy eating and healthy living. Help me to stay in partnership with You in honoring my body as Your holy temple. In Jesus' name, I pray, Amen.

Day 28

And Jesus came and spake unto them, saying, "All power is given unto me in heaven and in earth. Go ye therefore, and teach all nations, baptizing them in the name of the Father, and of the Son, and of the Holy Ghost: Teaching them to observe all things whatsoever I have commanded you; and, lo, I am with you alway, even unto the end of the world." (Matthew 28:18-20 KJV)

Here is The Great Commission with which most of us are familiar, although there are certain elements that are often overlooked. First, Jesus says that *all* power is given to Him in heaven and in earth. That means that no power is greater and that nothing can subdue Him. Jesus overcame *everything*, including satan and including the weapons that satan uses to attack people.

Next, what does Jesus tell His followers to do? Go into *all* the world and teach. Teach what? Teach *all nations* "to observe *all* things whatsoever I have commanded you." And what did Jesus command? He repeatedly and consistently gave His disciples and followers a dual mission – to preach the gospel and to heal the sick. He always paired the two instructions in His message.

First, He sent His followers to tell people to love God, to love each other as themselves, to forgive each other, and to repent of their sins. He repeatedly told them to tell everyone the good news that God loves each one of them. Second, He said, "And heal them."

In Mark 16:14-20 we see an expanded version of The Great Commission, in which Jesus declares that healing the sick will be a sign of those who believe in Him. Why? Because illness and disease are the result of satan's handiwork. Therefore *overcoming* sickness is a sign of Jesus' victory over the evil one's attempt to weaken and destroy God's people.

Accept The Great Commission of Jesus in its entirety. Jesus says, "I am with you always." Always. He never leaves you. His power which encompasses *all* power in heaven and earth is available to you right this minute. Accept it with thanksgiving, humility, and gratitude.

Heavenly Father, I accept the Great Commission of Your Son Jesus Christ. I will tell everyone the good news. And I will share with others Your message of healing as well. I know that You have taken my sins and washed me clean. I now open my heart, mind, soul, and body to receive God's love, grace, and healing power. By the stripes of Your Son, I am healed. In Jesus' name, I pray, Amen.

Day 29

And there was delivered unto him the book of the prophet Esaias. And when he had opened the book, he found the place where it was written, "The Spirit of the Lord is upon me, because he hath anointed me to preach the gospel to the poor; he hath sent me to heal the brokenhearted, to preach deliverance to the captives, and recovering of sight to the blind, to set at liberty them that are bruised." . . . This day is this scripture fulfilled in your ears. (Luke 4:17-18, 21 KJV)

Physical illnesses and infirmities are obvious to those who have them. What is not so obvious are the emotional wounds. In order to be well, we have to understand the connection between our emotional and our physical health.

Jesus was very aware of the connection. He knew the effect of guilt and shame not only on a person's soul but also on his body. When someone came to Him who was sick, He often said to him *first,* "Your sins are forgiven" and *then* told the lame to walk and the blind to see. Jesus came to set us at liberty. He came to heal the brokenhearted and to preach deliverance to the captives.

People who become ill often have an underlying anger or grief or fear. True healing cannot occur until these wounds are acknowledged and healed. Sometimes these hurts are buried very, very deeply because they are so painful.

How do you reach them? Tell God that you want to be healed in mind and spirit as well as in body. Ask Him to reveal to you those things that you need to know in order to release old emotions that are holding you captive. Do not fear the pain of the process because in the end it hurts far less than allowing your internal programming to be destructive to you and others.

One technique that you might try is to ask Jesus to walk with you into a particular memory that is painful. Hold His hand, and feel His support and His love as you bring this hurtful memory into the transforming presence of the Savior. Ask Jesus to heal this memory and to release you from its power over you. Day by day, week by week, you can find healing of your emotional wounds one at a time.

Merciful God, You have always wanted me to be free. I have become trapped by many memories and old programming from the past. Give me the courage and the strength to face these hurts and to let them go. Cleanse me, Lord, so that I may live according to Your purpose for me. In the name of Jesus Christ, my Savior and my Redeemer, I pray, Amen.

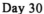

Day 30

Our mouths were filled with laughter, our tongues with songs of joy. Then it was said among the nations, "The Lord has done great things for them." The Lord has done great things for us, and we are filled with joy. (Psalm 126:2-3 NIV)

When you laugh, physiological changes occur in the body, promoting healing. Your pituitary gland releases substances called endorphins, which have a pain-relief action that is very strong. Tears often stream from your eyes, giving them a cleansing bath. Muscles in your head and abdomen contract and your lower jaw actually vibrates. Your arteries tense and then relax. Your vocal cords contract making the music of laughter – as varied in sound as loud guffaws to soft titters to an up-and-down roller coaster.

Your heart rate increases, and the extra blood flow sends more oxygen to all the cells of your body. Your lungs expand and your diaphragm is activated. The nervous system triggers the adrenal glands to release adrenaline, which raises your energy level and lifts your spirits. Your leg muscles relax, and, if you laugh hard enough, you end up sitting down because you are literally too weak to stand.

Laughter has been described as "internal jogging" because it is so beneficial to all the organs, glands, and cells of the body. Norman Cousins developed a debilitating collagen disease and created a healing program of laughter. In case after case, people with arthritis, depression, and numerous other diseases have been helped tremendously by the simple act of laughing throughout their day.

No matter how serious the health challenge before you, remember the truth that the Lord God Almighty loves you and wants you well. Remember that nothing is too hard for God. Remember that no power – and that includes satan – is stronger that Jehovah-rapha.

Accept these truths totally and you will be filled with praise which naturally bubbles out in the form of joy. And joy turns into laughter. Declare like the Psalmist, "The Lord has done great things for me, my mouth is filled with laughter, and my tongue is filled with songs of joy."

Wonderful Jehovah-rapha, thank You for the miracle of laughter. Thank You for all the healing actions it has in my body. Help me to see the humor in my life and to spend time every day laughing out loud and singing songs of joy. Lord, you have done so many great things for me, and I am filled with gratitude, happiness, and joy. Thank You, God, for healing me. In the name of Your Son, Jesus Christ, I pray, Amen.

Day 31

Trust in the Lord, and do good; so shalt thou dwell in the land, and verily thou shalt be fed. (Psalm 37:3 KJV)

The bottom line is always trust. It is the foundation on which everything stands. All things flow from it.

Do you trust God enough to put Him first in your life? Do you trust God enough to let Him make all your health care decisions? Do you trust God enough to go to Him in prayer before you follow any earthly advice about your health?

Stop and think what this means. When most people feel sick, they usually do one of two things. They either try to ignore it and pretend that it will go away – or they go to the doctor. In neither case have they turned to God *first*. Trust is always based on giving God the supreme authority in your life.

What do you do if you trust God wholeheartedly? You go to Him in prayer. Tell Him your concern. Describe exactly what you have noticed. That isn't for His benefit. He knows better than you do what the condition of every cell in your body is – and you have trillions of them. He even knows the exact count of each hair on your head. The reason that you need to describe what you have noticed is to increase your awareness of your body and how it is working. The more you can notice small, subtle changes in your body and attend to them, the more you can prevent serious illnesses from developing through neglect.

Ask God for healing. Ask Him if He wants you to work at the physical level in any way. Ask Him to tell you exactly what He wants you to do. Then be quiet and listen. Give yourself a generous amount of time to be still and to hear God's voice. If you are having a hard time "hearing" anything, ask God to speak more clearly. Ask Him to send the Holy Spirit with revelation knowledge to you. Trust that God loves you, will guide you, and will feed you with His Word.

Almighty Lord, You know my struggles with trust. I think I trust You, and then I find myself doing things and following advice from people when I haven't asked You what Your opinion is and what Your instruction is. Forgive me, Lord. Feed me with Your love and healing grace. In Jesus' name, I pray, Amen.

Day 32

Then they came to Jericho. As Jesus and his disciples, together with a large crowd, were leaving the city, a blind man, Bartimaeus (that is, the son of Timaeus), was sitting by the roadside begging. When he heard that it was Jesus of Nazareth, he began to shout, "Jesus, Son of David, have mercy on me!" Many rebuked him and told him to be quiet, but he shouted all the more, "Son of David, have mercy on me!" Jesus stopped and said, "Call him." So they called to the blind man, "Cheer up! On your feet! He's calling you." Throwing his cloak aside, he jumped to his feet and came to Jesus. "What do you want me to do for you?" Jesus asked him. The blind man said, "Rabbi, I want to see." "Go," said Jesus, "your faith has healed you." Immediately he received his sight and followed Jesus along the road. (Mark 10:46-52 NIV)

Jesus asks a blind man what appears to be a strange question. He asks, "What do you want me to do for you?" Why would He ask that? Surely He knows the man wants his sight to be restored. Jesus asks the question so that the man will clarify his intention, will verbalize his intention, and will focus on his intention.

Intention is critical. It is the truth that lies underneath our actions. We *say* many things. But it is our *actions* that reveal our true intention. When we want to be well, we may say that we will change our diet to conform to God's health laws, but we continue to have daily meals of burgers, fries, soft drinks, and synthetic vitamins. We have to get down to the bedrock of intent. Is our intent really to be well? Or is it to keep on living as long as we can doing what we are currently doing?

In the blind man's case, notice how persistent he had been in getting Jesus' attention. He kept calling out, even though those around him told him to be quiet. Jesus understood and valued persistence. Giving the man His complete focus, He now wanted to know the man's true intent. Notice the man answered quickly and without hesitation, "Teacher, I want to see." The man was willing to be taught, to be shown what to do. "Go, your faith has healed you," Jesus said.

See Jesus turning to you and asking, "What do you want me to do for you?" Answer Him with honesty, willingness, intention, and faith. Believe that He will respond.

Merciful God, I clarify my intent. I want to be well. I am willing to fulfill my part in following Your plan. Teach me, Father. Thank You for healing me. In the name of Your Son, Jesus Christ, my Redeemer, I pray, Amen.

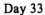

Day 33

There is a way that seems right to a man, but in the end it leads to death. (Proverbs 14:12 NIV)

Human beings have limited knowledge, wisdom, and understanding. Despite the fact that we actually know so little, we often forget we are not God. We declare science to be built on facts that are absolute and conveniently forget how over the years scientific "facts" have changed as our knowledge has changed. In *Confessions of a Medical Heretic* Dr. Robert Mendelsohn writes that modern medicine is "neither an art nor a science" but that its foundation depends on patients' trust and faith in it.

Most people do not know that Hippocrates, the father of medicine, gave only herbs to his patients, refusing to prescribe drugs as other doctors did. He knew that drugs (which are really poisons) might seem "right to a man" by relieving symptoms, but often in the end "lead to death." On the other hand, he knew that herbs are concentrated foods and nourish the body to help it overcome the basic problem of the illness.

We get off the track when we separate our learning from our belief in God. As we engage in scientific exploration, our endeavors should be in partnership with God. When that is the case, we are constantly in alignment with Divine outcome and Divine will, and our human creations will be beneficial. When we pretend that God has no place in science, however, we become easily led by the evil one into reckless arrogance. What seems to be logical, ultimately leads to death.

God gave us intelligence, and He wants us to learn about the human body so that we may help in the healing process when there is illness. There is a time and place for drugs, surgery, and other medical treatments. However, we must be very careful when we alter God's design for life and health so that we do not find ourselves on a path leading to untimely death. Look to God's herbs, essential oils, and healing substances, and learn about them. Then learn about the things that the mind of man has devised. But, first and foremost, pray for guidance, and follow the course God desires for you and your healing.

Almighty God, I pray for those scientists who are filled with Your Holy Spirit and who are working to benefit all people. When I have medical tests and am told that certain results will happen unless I have certain treatments, remind me, God, to seek Your guidance after hearing these opinions. Help me to make my decisions based on Your truth rather than on my fear. Show me Your way and I will follow it. In Jesus' name, I pray, Amen.

Day 34

But when he asks, he must believe and not doubt, because he who doubts is like a wave of the sea, blown and tossed by the wind. That man should not think he will receive anything from the Lord; he is a double-minded man, unstable in all he does. (James 1:6-8 NIV)

James was the half-brother of Jesus, and he well knew the pitfalls of doubt. Doubt can tie you into knots of indecision and render you impotent and paralyzed with fear. James describes it so well, "He who doubts is like a wave of the sea, blown and tossed by the wind." Doubting saps your strength, depresses your immune system, and makes you vulnerable to disease. As the tool of the devil, doubt cannot exist where there is faith in action. If you are being tormented by doubt about some decision in your life, you have fallen victim to satan's seductive whispers. Unfortunately, it often happens that you find yourself in uncertainty because you did not ask God for guidance at the very beginning of your difficulty. You just forged ahead using your own judgment and found yourself deeper in trouble.

There are times you may have asked for God's help, yet you missed the point that James emphasizes. You must ask *believing.* "Therefore I tell you," Jesus said, "whatever you ask for in prayer, believe that you have received it, and it will be yours" (Mark 11:24). However, this is possible if you ask only for those things which it is written that God promises.

It is written that Jehovah-rapha is the God who heals you. It is written that Christ Jesus bore your infirmities on the Cross. Therefore, pray for your healing, believing that it is happening. If you ask to be healed, yet are not really sure whether it is God's will that you be well or not, then your doubt controls you. James is very blunt about the results you can expect. "That man should not think he will receive anything from the Lord."

Don't let satan destroy your life and your relationship with God through doubt. Trust God with your life and with all your decisions.

Almighty God, I give You all my doubts and declare my faith in You and in Your Holy Word. Let me not be double-minded, but clearly focused on You and You alone. Thank You for Your guidance in my life. In Jesus' name, I pray, Amen.

Day 35

Let the words of my mouth, and the meditation of my heart, be acceptable in thy sight, O Lord, my strength, and my redeemer. (Psalm 19:14 KJV)

Do the words that come out of your mouth describe the life you want to live? Imagine that a tape recorder were running and retaining every single comment, word, and thought. Does that thought make you cringe a little? Well, the fact is that there is such a recording – a heavenly recording. And some day there will be an accounting.

There is another recording happening which is producing an immediate earthly accounting. This is occurring in your body. Each cell hears everything you say and will accept what you say and think as the truth. It will conform to your words just as you speak them or think them.

We shape our world with our words. The Holy Scripture tells us repeatedly how vital and how powerful the Word of God is. Our own words have great power as well. If we constantly language negative thoughts, we create a negative world around us. This is as true with regard to our health as it is for other areas of our lives.

Listen to yourself today. Do you find yourself saying things such as, "I'll never get well"? Or "This pain in my back is killing me." Do these words describe the life that you really want for yourself? If not, as soon as they slip out of your mouth, say, "Cancel that." Say it out loud if at all appropriate. If not, say it silently.

Then rephrase the sentence and say the revised words out loud. For example, "The despair I feel is coming from the father of lies. Jehovah-rapha, I trust You as You lead me on the path of my healing."

When are the words of our mouth acceptable offerings to God? When they are in alignment with His will and His purpose for us. When they are words of truth. When they are filled with praise and thanksgiving for His blessings. Monitor your words and thoughts one day at a time. Make the changes you need.

Send your words out as little messengers of God's light so that they create an atmosphere of love and faith around you.

Gracious Father, let the words of my mouth and the meditation of my heart be acceptable in thy sight, O Lord, my strength, and my redeemer. When my words are acceptable to You, then I know that they are in alignment with Your will and Your purpose for my life. Thank You for giving me an awareness of my words and of their power. In the name of Your Son, Jesus Christ, I pray, Amen.

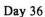

Day 36

Again Jesus said, "Peace be with you! As the Father has sent me, I am sending you." And with that he breathed on them and said, "Receive the Holy Spirit." (John 20:21-22 NIV)

Would you have liked to have been standing there before Jesus so that He could breathe on you, too? What would that have meant to you? Just think – to be standing before Jesus, to have Him breathe on you, and to receive the Holy Spirit directly from Him. What an incredible experience!

What if you could *really* experience the breath of Jesus today? Well, you can. The reason is due to the awesome fact that molecules of the air that Jesus breathed are still in the air today. Scientists have calculated detailed mathematical computations based on atmospheric pressure today and in Jesus' time, the amount of air that we breathe, the wind currents, and the amount of oxygen used by plants or dissolved in the ocean. They have determined that there are probably 1.6 million molecules of air that Jesus breathed in every liter of air that we breathe in the United States today. Surely *one* of those molecules is from the very breath described here in John 20:22.

Jesus told us, "Surely I am with you always, to the very end of the age" (Matthew 28:20). We have understood those words to refer to His abiding with us spiritually, but isn't it awesome that science reveals that Jesus is also with us at the *physical* level to the very end of the age?

Re-read chapters 20 and 21 of the Gospel of John, pondering in a new way the accounts of Jesus' activity after His resurrection. Get in a comfortable position, sitting or lying down. Let your breath become slow and deep. Now breathe in fully, expanding all your lungs from the bottom first and then all the way to the top. As you do so, hear Jesus tell you, "Receive the Holy Spirit." Release your breath and receive the peace of Christ. Offer your life in willing service to go where you are sent.

Almighty God, today I attempt to comprehend the miracle of breathing and to fathom the probability that at this very moment I am breathing in the very same oxygen molecule that Jesus breathed after His resurrection. I stand before Your Son and hear Him say to me, "Peace be with you! As the Father has sent me, I am sending you." I feel His breath on me and I hear Him say, "Receive the Holy Spirit." I accept Your peace and I accept Your healing. I am willing to go wherever You send me to fulfill Your purpose for my life. I do all these things in the name of Christ Jesus, my Savior and my Redeemer, Amen.

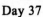

Day 37

Thy word is a lamp unto my feet and a light unto my path. (Psalm 119:105 KJV)

The first thing that God created was light. How do we keep His light shining brightly in our lives? By following His Holy Word, which is truly the lamp unto our feet and the light unto our paths. God's Word is available in The Holy Scriptures, and it is also revealed when He speaks to us directly.

When you are ill or injured, you need the illumination of God's Word to keep you grounded in God's truth for you. It is easy to be swept up in the appearance of your condition and to be swayed by the well-meaning advice of others. This is the time to turn to God's Word. Read it, breathe it, swim in it! Seek out the revelation of God's will in the Garden of Eden, in heaven, and in the ministry of His Son Jesus Christ. Pay attention to the life and words of Jesus. He referred often to God's Holy Word, saying, "It is written, it is written, it is written."

Repeat the Word to yourself many times each day. It is written, "I am the God who heals thee." It is written, "By your faith, you are healed." It is written, "Himself took our infirmities and bore our sicknesses." It is written, "If ye have faith as a grain of mustard seed, ye shall say unto this mountain, 'Remove hence to yonder place;' and it shall remove; and nothing shall be impossible to you." It is written, "And great multitudes followed him and he healed them all." It is written, "Praise the Lord, O my soul, and forget not all his benefits – who forgives *all* your sins and heals *all* your diseases."

Sometimes there are passages that you may not understand. Don't spin in your confusion because satan is particularly eager for you to discard the Scriptures as your guidepost. Do your best to understand and then turn your frustration over to God. Ask for revelation knowledge to clear your mind and your heart, to light your way, and to bring you to God's truth.

Almighty and merciful Father, thank You for Your wonderful Holy Word. It is indeed a lamp unto my feet and a light unto my path. It is my best and truest source of inspiration. It gives me examples of real people in real situations who kept the faith and remained steadfastly obedient to You. It shows me how You shed Your love and Your power over Your children in countless acts of mercy and grace. Thank You, Lord, for this great gift of Your Word which I cherish in my heart. In Jesus' name, I pray, Amen.

Day 38

From inside the fish Jonah prayed to the Lord his God. He said: "In my distress I called to the Lord, and he answered me. From the depths of the grave I called for help, and you listened to my cry. . . . But you brought my life up from the pit, O Lord my God. When my life was ebbing away, I remembered you, Lord, and my prayer rose to you, to your holy temple. . . . But I, with a song of thanksgiving, will sacrifice to you. What I have vowed I will make good. Salvation comes from the Lord." (Jonah 2:1-2, 6, 9 NIV)

If you are experiencing serious illness, you understand Jonah. This is particularly true if you have a disease which modern medicine pronounces incurable because it is easy for despair to set in. The words, "no cure, no cure, no cure" echo in your head like a broken record. Treatment options offered are often a double-edged sword; while appearing to slow one health problem, they often lead in the end to creating another. So there you are, deep in the belly of the giant fish just like Jonah.

What did Jonah do? He calls to God, saying, "You heard me and You answered me, God." *Past* tense. Remember *that he is still in the belly of the fish!* The appearance is that he is still trapped and that his situation is hopeless. Yet Jonah then sings a song of thanksgiving! Even though it looks as though he is still doomed, here he is loudly thanking God for saving him. He trusts God completely, so much so that he sees his deliverance as *already* accomplished. It is only *after* he does these things that he is saved from the fish.

Be like Jonah. Call on Jehovah-rapha. Know that He hears you and that He answers you. Find music of thanksgiving and praise and sing along with it every day. Believe in the innermost parts of your heart that God is delivering you *now* – not sometime in the future, but right now. Jehovah is the God of your salvation, and He is faithful and will not let you down.

Almighty Father, I long to be like Jonah. There are many times when I feel trapped by medical "facts" and I feel my courage slipping away. In my distress I call to You, O Lord. From the depths of the grave I call for help. Bring my life up from the pit of my despair. There are times when I feel my life is ebbing away like Jonah's. I raise my prayer to you, Lord. Thank you, God. Thank You for delivering me. You are my salvation, saving my soul and my body. I claim Your Divine will for my life. I claim Your healing grace. In the name of Your Son, Jesus Christ, I pray, Amen.

Why do you call me, "Lord, Lord" and do not do what I say? I will show you what he is like who comes to me and hears my words and puts them into practice. He is like a man building a house, who dug down deep and laid the foundation on rock. When a flood came, the torrent struck that house but could not shake it, because it was well built. But the one who hears my words and does not put them into practice is like a man who built a house on the ground without a foundation. The moment the torrent struck that house, it collapsed and its destruction was complete. (Luke 6:46-49 NIV)

Saying the words of belief is not enough. It is easy to "talk the talk." The hard part is to "walk the walk." Jesus illustrates very clearly the importance of putting His words into practice. Saying that you put your faith and trust in God and in Christ Jesus means nothing if you are not willing to *live* your faith and trust every day.

We all know this is true intellectually, and most of us think we do live our faith. Yet when we feel sick, these words of Jesus become particularly relevant. Feeling sick makes us particularly vulnerable. Our ability to function is at a low ebb because we are often weak, and it is hard to think clearly. The evil one whispers in our ear, and we become filled with fear.

We soon are faced with our moment of truth. Do we put the words of Jesus into action – or not? What are Jesus' words? "Love the Lord with all your soul." "Seek and you shall find." "Whatever you ask for in prayer, believe that you have received it, and it will be yours."

When you feel sick, do you turn first to God for instruction about what you should do? Or do you turn first to humans? Do you follow God's instructions for each step of your treatment and healing? Or do you unquestioningly follow the treatment plans of humans?

How often it is that we follow our own course until something goes wrong and then, when we find we have built a house without a foundation, we call on God to save us. Jesus asks us to build our house on Him from the beginning. Are you really willing to turn your life over to God?

Wonderful Jehovah-rapha, teach me to trust You and to build my house only on You and Your Son Jesus Christ, my Redeemer and Savior. You are the foundation that will never fail me. I trust You completely and I will follow You every step of the way along Your path to my healing. In Jesus' name, I pray, Amen.

Day 40

And He replied to him, "You shall love the Lord your God with all your heart and with all your soul and with all your mind (intellect). This is the great (most important, principal) and first commandment. And a second is like it: You shall love your neighbor as [you do] yourself. These two commandments sum up and upon them depend all the Law and the Prophets." (Matthew 22:37-40 AMP)

Two times in Matthew we hear Jesus tell people to love their neighbors as they love themselves. Generally, we interpret this as a warning against being selfish and self-centered. It is.

Yet, it is more than that. We must fully grasp that we must love ourselves before we can truly love others. Loving others is really about being filled to the brim with God's love *inside ourselves* so that it bubbles up joyfully from us and flows over everyone we meet, naturally and without effort. It comes from our own fullness.

Too often we misguidedly focus on everyone else. And we fail to follow this commandment which Jesus says is so important that on it all the law depends. What laws are Jesus talking about? God's laws. And one of them is God's law of health: we have to take care of ourselves.

How do you know if you are obeying this commandment? You eat foods God intended you to eat for your health and nourishment. You make time to move and exercise your body. You get proper rest. You seek God's advice about His plan for the recovery and maintenance of your health. You learn about God's natural remedies and herbs which He provided in such profusion for your healing. You laugh, play, and spread God's joy to all you meet.

By doing these things you join with God as a partner in your healing. And you model to others what Jesus' commandment is all about.

Almighty God, I know that You love me. Help me to love myself in the way that Your Son commanded me. A lot of time I feel guilty, God, when I think about loving myself and taking the time to focus on meeting my needs. But I am beginning to understand that doing so allows Your Love to fill me up and flow through me. Thank You for sending Your Son to heal me and to show me the way to love myself and to love my neighbors. Keep me on Your path, Father. Into Your loving care I place my life. In Jesus' name, I pray, Amen.

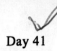

Day 41

Do not be anxious about anything, but in everything, by prayer and petition, with thanks-giving, present your requests to God. And the peace of God, which transcends all under-standing, will guard your hearts and your minds in Christ Jesus. (Philippians 4:6-7 NIV)

Worry depletes you and undermines your faith. When you are filled with worry, you are not standing fully in God's light; instead, the shadow of satan is on you, eroding you with fear. To acknowledge this can be frightening, espe-cially when you have a health problem, because there seems to be an endless string of worries. Each new symptom creates a new concern that something else is going wrong. And always looms the largest fear that, if you take the wrong action, you will suffer a disastrous result such as blindness, crippling, or per-haps death. The largest anxiety is often the sense that your own body is out of control and that you feel helpless.

All of these fears and beliefs will keep you sick. What is the solution? Go to God in prayer with every problem, every question, and every decision you have. Don't assume any particular answer or any particular action. Be sure to give God the final authority over each tiny decision in your healing process. And be prepared to be surprised by what God tells you. Trust that the Holy Spirit will give you revelation knowledge.

If you feel fear, ask for help in releasing it and replacing it with trust. However, notice whether you are constantly going to God from a position of fear. Understand that having an attitude of gratitude is essential. As Paul says, "Present your requests to God *with thanksgiving.*"

Thank God for all the properly functioning parts of your body. Thank Him for guiding you to the right information about the underlying reason for your body's becoming so unbalanced as to be subject to the health condition you are experiencing. Thank God for being with you every step of the way, for guiding each decision, and for healing you.

What is the result of following this procedure in handling worry? The peace of God which passes all understanding. Peace in your heart. Peace in your soul. Peace in every cell in your body. And what better environment is there for healing?

Wonderful Jehovah-rapha, I come to You in gratitude for the miracle of my body, which is Your Holy temple. I give You all my worries about my health. Guide me, Lord, in the steps You want me to take today to join in partnership with You for my healing. In Jesus' name, I pray, Amen.

Day 42

I assure you, most solemnly I tell you, if anyone steadfastly believes in Me, he will himself be able to do the things that I do; and he will do even greater things than these, because I go to the Father. (John 14:12 AMP)

Let's look at the New International Version of this Scripture: "I tell you the truth, anyone who has faith in me will do what I have been doing. He will do even greater things than these, because I am going to the Father."

Most Christians say they believe Jesus and what He taught. Nevertheless, this Scripture usually makes most people take a deep breath and have second thoughts. Jesus very plainly says that any person who believes in Him can do the things that He does. Not only that – but we are told we can do *greater* things than Jesus did because we will have His help as He sits at the right hand of the Father.

His statement was so preposterous that He wanted to make sure we knew He wasn't joking. "Most solemnly I tell you," The Amplified Bible reads. "I tell you the truth," the New International Version reads. "Verily, verily," says the King James Version. Christ wanted us to understand that, just as the Father was the source of all the works that He (Jesus) did, the Father is the source of all works that *we* do.

Jesus tells us here that the Father will continue to do His mighty works – using us just as He used His Son. God wanted His Son to teach, preach, and heal. Jesus did the works and the will of the Father. And Jesus taught His followers to do the same thing. God wants *us* to teach, preach, and heal. He wants you to be saved. He wants you to be healed. And He wants you to pass it on. Pass it on.

Jesus promises that we can pass it on in a way even greater than He passed it on when He was on earth. Why? Because we have His support as He has joined the Father. This is Christ's promise. Believe Him. And act on your belief.

Dear Heavenly Father, thank You for Your mighty works. Thank You for letting Your saving grace flow to me and around me. I accept Your Word and I ask to serve You and to glorify You in everything that I do. Holy Father, thank You for healing my spirit and healing my body. Help me to be an example to all who see me of Your will in action. Help me, Lord Jesus, to do the will of the Father and to be a vessel for His mighty works. In the name of the Father, Son, and Holy Spirit, I pray, Amen.

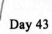

And He Who searches the hearts of men knows what is in the mind of the [Holy] Spirit [what His intent is], because the Spirit intercedes and pleads [before God] in behalf of the saints according to and in harmony with God's will. We are assured and know that [God being a partner in their labor] all things work together and are [fitting into a plan] for good to and for those who love God and are called according to [His] design and purpose. (Romans 8:27-28 AMP)

This statement of Paul that "all things work together for good" is often used to convince people that everything that happens to them is an act of God's will. The consequence of that belief is that people do not resist satan and his destructive acts but actually declare them to be some mysterious act of God.

This confusion comes from removing the sentence from its context. Note that Paul is talking about the effects of intercessory prayer. Prayers are being offered *in harmony with God's will.* Nothing is being prayed for that is *not* according to God's will. We are now assured that, *whenever God is a partner,* all things work together for good for those who love Him. Wow! Now it all makes sense.

Do things happen to people that were *not* intended for their good? Absolutely, yes. Satan is not working for your good. Satan is trying to destroy you. Attributing every event in your life to God is to deny satan's existence. It is written that satan creeps around like a lion looking for prey. Some of the easiest pickings are those who believe that everything that happens in their life is planned by God. God has made it clear that people can *choose* between good and evil, between Him and the devil. You have that choice a thousand times a day and so does everyone else.

The good news is that evil cannot win when we choose to follow the Lord God Almighty. The battle is the Lord's and Jesus has overcome satan. No matter what way that satan attacks you, no matter what illness or accident may befall you, the victory over it has already been won by Jesus Christ. God can create good out of any situation, no matter how badly it may have begun. Claim God as your partner and trust Him completely with your life.

Father, You know the healing that I need. I ask the Holy Spirit to intercede for me in harmony with Your Divine will. I am assured that, when You are my partner, all things coming from You work together for my good. Thank You, Father, for healing me. In Jesus' name, Amen.

Day 44

The Lord said to Moses, "Take the staff, and you and your brother Aaron gather the assembly together. Speak to that rock before their eyes and it will pour out its water. You will bring water out of the rock for the community so they and their livestock can drink." So Moses took the staff from the Lord's presence, just as he commanded him. He and Aaron gathered the assembly together in front of the rock and Moses said to them, "Listen, you rebels, must we bring you water out of this rock?" Then Moses raised his arm and struck the rock twice with his staff. Water gushed out, and the community and their livestock drank. But the Lord said to Moses and Aaron, "Because you did not trust in me enough to honor me as holy in the sight of the Israelites, you will not bring this community into the land I give them." (Numbers 20:7-12 NIV)

The Israelites are wandering in the desert, tired and thirsty. To release water trapped in the veins and crevices beneath the surface, Moses was accustomed to give a hard blow to a rock of limestone with a heavy stick. There was nothing extraordinary at all about hitting a rock to get water; that was the way you were *supposed* to do it. But God didn't want Moses to get water the conventional way. He told Moses to gather the Israelites together and to *speak* to the rock to bring water out of it. Moses followed only part of God's instructions because he didn't have enough faith to wait after he spoke to the rock for the water to begin flowing. He hit the rock anyway. For that lack of trust, he suffered the consequence of dying before he reached the Promised Land.

God's thoughts are not our thoughts and God's ways are not our ways. Our minds are infinitesimal when compared to the vastness of the Almighty. Nevertheless, we ironically place our faith in a "science" that declares as its foundation that it will consider no input from God whatsoever. We give medical opinions equal – and often heavier – weight than God's instructions. We often suffer consequences as devastating as that which Moses experienced. Moses did not follow the instructions of the Lord, and he paid a high price for his lack of faith and his lack of obedience. Pray with your health care advisors and also on your own. Learn from the experience of Moses and live.

Wonderful Jehovah-rapha, let me learn from Moses. I seek Your guidance in every step in my healing process. I trust You to tell me exactly what You want me to do, and I will do it – no matter how unconventional it might be. I honor You as Holy, and I thank You for my healing. In Jesus' name, I pray, Amen.

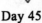

Day 45

Great is the Lord and most worthy of praise; his greatness no one can fathom. One generation will commend your works to another; they will tell of your mighty acts. They will speak of the glorious splendor of your majesty, and I will meditate on your wonderful works. They will tell of the power of your awesome works, and I will proclaim your great deeds. They will celebrate your abundant goodness and joyfully sing of your righteousness. (Psalm 145:3-7 NIV)

Notice the connection between God's works and His Words. The Almighty created through His Words. He declared His intention and He spoke us into being. Actions followed the intention and the words, and the result was mighty works reflecting the majesty of Jehovah.

Often God instructed His people to follow His example. Moses was to *speak* to the rock to get it to produce water (Numbers 20:7-12). Joshua was to *shout* and the walls would come tumbling down (Joshua 6:15-20). Other actions and works would follow, but first was the intention and the spoken word.

Jesus continued the example of His Father by commanding authority through His Word. He *spoke* to the wind and the waves, and they were quietened. He *spoke* to disease and it left people's bodies. He *spoke* to dead bodies and they were filled with life once more. Mighty and glorious works followed after the proclamation of intention and the Word.

Likewise, Jesus told us to follow His example. Therefore, speak to your illness and infirmity, and enforce God's Word on it. Command the evil one to leave you, and ask the Holy Spirit to fill you with Divine love in every cell of your body and at every level of your being. Having spoken your intention and having enforced God's Word on your illness, you now are called to action to follow the will of God. Ask for guidance for today. Do not be misled into thinking that God's plan for you today is necessarily the same plan for you tomorrow. Each day is a new one and you may be led to a new approach. Thank God constantly for healing you. Allow the Lord God Almighty to demonstrate His greatness and majesty in your life.

Almighty Lord, I praise You and tell all of Your mighty acts in my life. I meditate on Your wonderful works. You bless me with abundant goodness and I joyfully sing of your righteousness. I speak to my illness and enforce Your Word upon it. I command every cell in my body to align with Your Divine will. It is written, "I am the God who heals you." And so it is. In Jesus' name, I pray, Amen.

Day 46

After this the Lord appointed seventy-two others and sent them two by two ahead of him to every town and place where he was about to go. He told them, "The harvest is plentiful, but the workers are few. . . . Heal the sick who are there and tell them, 'The kingdom of God is near you.'" (Luke 10:1-2, 8-9 NIV)

Here we see Jesus setting up His church; we see His church in action. And what does this church look like? What are the people doing? The picture we see is an interesting one because Jesus' church isn't a church of buildings. It isn't a church led by ministers with theological degrees. It is simply people going out two by two. They were given two specific things to do: to heal and to preach the gospel. Here again is the dual mission. Heal and preach. Heal and preach.

Seventy-two people. What kind of people? Scripture doesn't indicate that there was anything particularly remarkable about these first missionaries. There is no mention of their being well-educated or their having degrees or their having medical training. They were apparently "ordinary" people who were sent to preach and to heal.

This is the way the church was to act and to look. Jesus put healing on the same level as preaching. Where there was one there was always the other. The two actions work in tandem with each other. Healing and preaching make a complete unit because it takes both of them to meet people's complete needs. Jesus came to make us whole. He came to do the perfect will of the Father and to redeem us to God's original intent for us.

Jesus sits today at the right hand of the Father and *still* desires to make us whole. He went to the Cross to atone for our sins *and* our sicknesses. What is required is that we believe that this is so. Lift up your eyes to your Savior and believe.

Dear Gracious God, thank You for showing me the way. Help me to understand in the deepest parts of my soul and in the innermost places of my mind that You sent Your precious Son to atone for me completely – for my soul and for my body. Help me to visualize my Savior Jesus sending out those seventy-two ordinary people to preach the gospel and to heal the sick. Just ordinary people, God, like me. As You work Your mighty healing in my body and my soul, help me to be an instrument for the healing of others, God. Help me to join with those whom Jesus sent out then and sends out now to do His work. Thank You, God, for Your many blessings in my life. In Jesus' name, I pray, Amen.

Day 47

But the Counselor, the Holy Spirit, whom the Father will send in my name, will teach you all things and will remind you of everything I have said to you. (John 14:26 NIV)

Jesus said, "The Holy Spirit will teach you all things." *All* things. "And [he] will remind you of everything I have said to you." *Everything.*

What were those things? To love God with all our soul. To love one another. To heal the sick. To forgive one another. To carry out His instructions. To follow Him.

Jesus is saying that the Holy Spirit is going to help to continue His own work by reminding us constantly of everything He has said. One thing that Jesus said over and over again was that all things were possible. He beseeched those who were willing to hear Him not to be deceived by the appearance of things but to stand on faith and to believe that nothing is impossible. Jesus asked God to send us the Holy Spirit to remind us of this.

Sickness itself is a tool of the father of lies; so, when we are ill, we are especially vulnerable to deceptive appearances and to "facts" that seem real but are not. It is a major relief to know that we have been given a strong guide in the Holy Spirit to help us to find God's truth.

When we feel sick, we have an especially deep need for the Holy Spirit because the decisions we have to make are often literally life-and-death decisions. And there is no one single decision to be made. Instead, there are hundreds of them as each day passes.

Just exactly how can the Holy Spirit guide us when we feel sick? He can reveal to us the precise things we need to do for our healing at the exact moment that we ask. As our bodies heal and change, the revelation knowledge that the Holy Spirit imparts will change. Therefore, the knowledge that we receive at one particular moment may be different from instructions we were given an hour or a day before.

How wonderful to know that, when we are filled with the Holy Spirit, we are transformed, we are changed, and we are healed.

Almighty God, send Your Holy Spirit to teach me, instruct me, and guide me. I am willing to listen. I want to make decisions today that are part of Your will for my recovery, God, and I am so grateful that You gave the Holy Spirit to me to help me choose wisely. Thank You, God, for all Your many blessings. In the name of the Father, Son, and Holy Spirit, I pray, Amen.

Day 48

. . . he (Peter) said to them, "Men of Israel, why does this surprise you? Why do you stare at us as if by our own power or godliness we had made this man walk? The God of Abraham, Isaac and Jacob, the God of our fathers, has glorified his servant Jesus. . . . By faith in the name of Jesus, this man whom you see and know was made strong. It is Jesus' name and the faith that comes through him that has given this complete healing to him, as you can all see." (Acts 3:12-13, 16 NIV)

Peter's question is one we need to ponder. Why *does* healing surprise you? From the first moment of our creation, we were made whole, well, and without sickness. Our willfulness caused us to know evil and to know disease – yet God never changed His desire, and He reminds us in His Word that He is the God who heals us. Present tense. Now. Today.

God never wanted us to have lives subject to evil, so He sent His Son to overcome the power of the evil one. Yet here we are two thousand years later, just like the people in this story – still surprised by the power of God's healing hand. How sad God must be that we have not comprehended what has already been done for us. Jesus has died for us – for our sins and for our health. The Word proclaims it. "Himself took our infirmities and bore our sicknesses." Peter proclaims it. "It is Jesus' name and the faith that comes through him that has given this complete healing to him." Hallelujah! It is written.

Stop being surprised. The members of the early church *expected* healing because they knew it was integral to Jesus' mission. Expect *your* healing. Read the entire chapter of Acts 3. Give the Word your attention. Give Jesus your attention.

Jesus told everyone that they must believe. Do it. It is the unbelievers who should be surprised, not the believers. Declare the Word several times a day, saying, "By faith in the name of Jesus, I am made strong. It is Jesus' name and the faith that comes through Him that gives me complete healing."

Dear God, I confess that for too long I have been among those who are surprised by Your healing. No more, God, no more. I accept Your Son Jesus Christ as my Savior, my Healer, and my Teacher. By faith in the name of Jesus, I am made strong. It is Jesus' name and the faith that comes through Him that gives me complete healing. I thank You, Jehovah-rapha, for my healing. Help me to be a witness for You and to be an instrument for the healing of others. In the name of Jesus Christ, I pray, Amen.

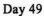

Day 49

And Jesus knew their thoughts, and said unto them, "Every kingdom divided against itself is brought to desolation; and every city or house divided against itself shall not stand." (Matthew 12:25 KJV)

All too often when we feel sick, we become divided against ourselves. Fighting "the disease" often ends up with our fighting parts of our own bodies. We even use terms of warfare when we talk about illness and the process to deal with it; for example, we speak of heart "attacks" as though our heart is attacking us. How satan loves to get us to view our own body as the enemy! When we spend our time fighting ourselves, we have little time or energy left to fight him.

Our body is never the enemy. It is a holy temple. God designed it to survive and to heal itself; it is handling the situation in the best way possible. Whenever we look at the cause at the physical level, we generally find that the body part is not the culprit. For example, a gallbladder "attack" is the cry of an organ overwhelmed by years of improper eating. Cancer cells are our own cells, whose growth has gone wild and out of the pattern God designed for them, and they multiply because our immune system is too depleted to remove them appropriately.

What we need is to become whole again with all our cells functioning as the Creator intended that they do. For those cells that are out of control or are malfunctioning, seek transformation of them so that they come into Divine alignment.

Visualize God's holy light streaming down from heaven and flowing into the top of your head, through every part of your body, and down to the soles of your feet. See it flooding every cell, transforming and re-balancing each one. See all cells in your body working in perfect harmony with each other. See any cell which cannot accept this Divine pattern simply being removed by the cells which do accept and radiate Divine light. Visualize your God-filled cells enforcing Divine alignment in whatever way is appropriate. Remember that when all cells are functioning in a vibrant manner, deviant cells are removed along with inappropriate viruses, bacteria, and parasites. See every cell in your body through the Creator's eyes in its perfect wholeness – and rejoice.

Dear Gracious Lord, help me to stop fighting myself. Bring me into full unity with You. Transform every cell in my body so that it is filled with Your Divine love, light, and health. Thank You, O Jehovah-rapha, for touching me with Your healing hand. In Jesus' name, I pray, Amen.

Day 50

When Pharaoh let the people go, God did not lead them on the road through the Philistine country, though that was shorter. . . . So God led the people around by the desert road toward the Red Sea. . . . By day the Lord went ahead of them in a pillar of cloud to guide them on their way and by night in a pillar of fire to give them light, so that they could travel by day or night. Neither the pillar of cloud by day nor the pillar of fire by night left its place in front of the people. Then the Lord said to Moses, "Tell the Israelites to turn back and encamp near Pi Hahiroth, between Migdol and the sea." (Exodus13:17-18, 21-22, Exodus 14:1-2 NIV)

Imagine that you are one of the tired, frightened group of Israelites. You have been in captivity in Egypt and after a terrible sequence of events you have been allowed to leave that country. You are fleeing for your life, being lead by Moses. Ahead of you, you see a pillar of cloud in the day and a pillar of fire in the night, which you believe is the Lord your God.

Moses has told you that you and all the other Israelites will follow the instructions of the Lord God Almighty exactly as they are given. Once on the road, you realize that you are not being led down the shortest, most direct path. You feel a little nervous, but you press on. Eventually, however, you become very alarmed because God has led you into what appears to be a trap. You can see nothing but the sea in front of you, and you know that the Egyptians are close behind, racing to catch up and to kill you.

Just as the Israelites so many years ago, we, too, are called to trust the Lord our God. God's path to your healing may not be what looks like the straightest path. It may not be what would be the "normal" treatment. On the surface, it may look like a trap, literally a dead-end road.

Do not allow your fear and the fears of others to set your course of recovery. Go to God in prayer – both alone and with your health care advisors. Listen to His voice. And once you receive your guidance, trust God. He will not fail you. When you least expect it, the Red Sea will part, and you will walk to safety and healing.

Lord God Almighty, You are my leader and my deliverer. Teach me to follow You faithfully and to trust You with my life. You can see so much more than I can and I will walk the path You want me to follow. Part the sea for me, Lord. Thank You for healing me. In the name of Your Son, Jesus Christ, I pray, Amen.

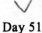

Day 51

As the Father has loved me, so have I loved you. Now remain in my love. If you obey my commands, you will remain in my love, just as I have obeyed my Father's commands and remain in his love. I have told you this so that my joy may be in you and that your joy may be complete. My command is this: Love each other as I have loved you. (John 15:9-12 NIV)

Jesus hands us the key to heaven and it is love. Love forms an eternal chain and it is meaningful only when it is given away. Jesus tells us that, just as God loves Him, He loves us. Once again, He always shows us the perfect example. He was given great love, and He passes it on.

We are told to pass it on – "love each other as I have loved you." How do we do that? By the paradoxical method of remaining in the love of God and the love of Christ. By staying in it, we can pass it on.

And what are the benefits of basking in this holy love and then of passing it on? Joy. Sheer, unadulterated joy! "I have told you this so that my joy may be in you and that your joy may be complete." Think of what it means to you for your joy to be *complete*. Totally, absolutely complete.

It is impossible to find lasting healing without receiving the love of God and without learning to remain in that love. Why? Because all negative emotions drain the body, mind, and soul of energy and you need that energy both to heal and to be well. It is impossible to *remain* in God's love while simultaneously holding onto great bitterness toward other people.

Jesus tells us what to do. "Obey my commands," He said. Live love, spread love, manifest love. Use your prayers to strengthen yourself, your friends, and your family in love.

Also use your prayers to lift someone you don't even know but who is lonely, sick, afraid, and who feels unloved and unlovable. God knows who needs your prayer most, so offer your prayers to God in his behalf.

As you receive love and let it flow from you, you create a great tree of life to the glory of your heavenly Father. And you will know joy.

Loving Father, I am awed by Your overwhelming love which blesses me in so many ways. Help me to obey the commands of Your Son Jesus Christ and to remain in His love. Help me to spread this love to others. I pray not only for my friends and family whom I love dearly, but I also pray in behalf of those who feel alone and unloved. In Jesus' name, I pray, Amen.

Day 52

Let us not become weary in doing good, for at the proper time, we will reap a harvest if we do not give up. (Galatians 6:9 NIV)

If Paul lived today and wanted to convey this message, he would probably say, "Hang in there! Don't give up, no matter what."

Have you been praying for your healing and it hasn't happened yet? Don't give up. Are you following Divine guidance for each step of your healing and you aren't well yet? Don't give up. Are you tired of waiting on the Lord? Don't give up. Say it out loud three times: "I will not give up. I will not give up. I will not give up."

At the proper time you will reap the harvest if you do not give up. If you are basing your belief that you are being healed on seeing improvements in your symptoms, you are way off track. Faith is steadfast belief in what is *still unseen.*

Remain firm in your belief that it is God's will that you be well. Remain firm in your belief that God is not the author of your infirmity. Remain firm in your belief that Jehovah-rapha is healing you and that it will be manifested at the proper time if you do not give up.

Satan wants you to quit. He will use as many delaying tactics as he can, and he will especially create lots of opportunity for doubts to creep in. Whenever he can get you to think, "maybe I won't be healed" or "since I don't see anything happening, maybe it really *is* God's will that I not get well," the evil one is claiming a victory.

Never forget that the battle is the Lord's. Jesus Christ came to earth and gave this life for you. He took your infirmities to the Cross and your sins as well. It has already been done. Claim the victory of Jesus Christ. Read the Holy Scripture, and notice how often Jesus told someone, "Your faith has made you whole." Over and over and over again He said it.

Don't lose faith. Hand over your fears to God. Claim the victory that Jesus Christ won for *you.*

Wonderful Jehovah-rapha, give me strength. Help me not to become weary in doing good and not to become weary in waiting for You to work Your healing in me. I believe You are Jehovah-rapha, who heals me. I trust that at the proper time I will reap a harvest of recovery if I do not give up. In the name of Your Son, Jesus Christ my Savior and my Redeemer, I pray, Amen.

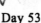

Day 53

The God who made the world and everything in it is the Lord of heaven and earth and does not live in temples built by hands. And he is not served by human hands, as if he needed anything, because he himself gives all men life and breath and everything else. From one man he made every nation of men, that they should inhabit the whole earth; and he determined the times set for them and the exact places where they should live. God did this so that men would seek him and perhaps reach out for him and find him, though he is not far from each one of us. For in him we live and move and have our being. As some of your own poets have said, "We are his offspring." (Acts 17:24-28 NIV).

Seek. Reach. Find. God lives in each one of us. We are His Holy temple. When something happens within your body, remember that you are a holy temple, hallowed and special. God lives within you and He is there at this very moment.

Seek the experience of God within you. Reach for it and you will find it. God says He is always available to us. Always. We know what it means to have the experience of God within spiritually. But what does it mean at the physical level? It means to be able to allow the energy of God to fill every cell in your body and to restore it to health.

Jesus was very aware of the Divine energy within His body. He knew when the bleeding woman touched Him even though a large crowd of people was pressing in on Him. Follow Jesus' example and allow God's Divine energy to fill you. In the often frantic, hurried lifestyle that we lead, we close ourselves off from this energy and, like plants without water, we droop from lack of Divine nourishment. This isn't God's fault, but our own.

We are God's offspring. We are His children. Set aside time after your meditation to allow the Holy Spirit to fill you with Divine healing energy. Take "one-minute Holy Spirit breaks" during the day for the same purpose. Give grateful thanks to God for healing you.

Dear God, You created me and put me in this time and this place on this earth. In You I live and move and have my being. I am Your child. I am hurting, Father, and I seek You and reach out to You. You promise in Your Holy Word that if I seek and if I reach, I will find You. I am Your Holy temple. Flood me with Your healing light. Thank You for touching me with Your healing hand. Thank You, Lord. In Jesus' name, I pray, Amen.

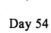

Day 54

Now a man crippled from birth was being carried to the temple gate called Beautiful, where he was put every day to beg from those going into the temple courts. When he saw Peter and John about to enter, he asked them for money. Peter looked straight at him, as did John. Then Peter said, "Look at us!" So the man gave them his attention, expecting to get something from them. Then Peter said, "Silver or gold I do not have, but what I have I give you. In the name of Jesus Christ of Nazareth, walk." Taking him by the right hand, he helped him up, and instantly the man's feet and ankles became strong. He jumped to his feet and began to walk. (Acts 3:2-8 NIV).

What is the church supposed to be like? In Acts you see the early church at work. Jesus had trained His disciples, and He had given them two instructions: to preach the gospel and to heal the sick.

Here in this story Peter and John, as they go about fulfilling the mission that Jesus gave them, encounter a man who has been crippled from birth. Let's put that man in today's world. Imagine the size of the medical report on him. See in your mind all the scientific data showing that this man would never walk. Hear in your mind the words, "I'm sorry but nothing can be done."

The man asked Peter and John for money. Peter told him, "Give me your attention – your full attention." The man did so, expecting to receive something. However, never in his wildest imagination did he expect to receive what he got – a complete healing.

Peter said, "What I have, I give you." What was it that he had? He had the Word ("it is written"), he had Jesus' example, he had Jesus' mission ("go ye . . . and heal"), he had the power of the Holy Spirit, and he had faith. Peter didn't have anything you don't have! You must understand that and believe it in the very core of your being.

Give God your full attention, and expect to receive His love, blessings, and healing. Declare positive words of your faith daily. In the name of Jesus Christ of Nazareth, your Redeemer, walk in health.

Dear God, thank you for showing me how the first followers of your Son Jesus Christ fulfilled the mission to heal the sick. Sometimes I doubt that what was true two thousand years ago is true now. Help me to look to You and Your Son and to give my full attention to Your gift of healing. Let me focus in expectation and belief. I gratefully receive Your healing and Your blessings so that I may glorify Your holy name. In the name of Jesus Christ, my Redeemer, I pray, Amen.

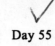

Finally, brethren, whatsoever things are true, whatsoever things are honest, whatsoever things are just, whatsoever things are pure, whatsoever things are lovely, whatsoever things are of good report; if there be any virtue, and if there be any praise, think on these things. Those things, which ye have both learned, and received, and heard, and seen in me, do; and the God of peace shall be with you. (Philippians 4:8-9 KJV)

Whatever you spend your time thinking about reveals the condition of your innermost heart and soul. That is a rather frightening thought, isn't it? Particularly when we apply it to our health.

Do you spend your day thinking about God's truth – that He wants you to be well? Do you spend your day repeating God's healing promises? Do you spend your day giving thanks to God for healing you? Do you spend your day listening for the Holy Spirit to reveal to you what the next step in your healing is to be? Do you spend your day creating pictures in your mind of yourself living whole and healthy? Do you spend your day repeating to God your trust that He will show you a way to healing that leads to life and not to a wheelchair?

Or do you spend your day listening to the father of lies tell you that God's will is to bring sickness on earth and that healing is for heaven? Do you spend your day following the advice of family, friends, and medical personnel without having received Divine guidance and instructions first? Do you spend your day thinking about this pain or that discomfort? Do you spend your day creating pictures in your mind of yourself getting worse? Do you spend your day preparing for degeneration in your condition because it has been predicted for your illness?

Whatever you think defines who you really are and what you will become. Think on positive things and join with your Creator to bring them into reality. Here we are talking about thinking with intention. This is positive thinking *based on the Word of God;* it is not wishful thinking which attempts to override human doubt. God's positive Word increases your faith, and it is your faith which makes you whole.

Almighty God, fill me with Your positive Word. I choose to listen to You and fill my mind with positive thoughts, with hymns of praise, and with Your Holy Scriptures. Create in me a new heart, Jehovah-rapha. I glorify You and focus my thoughts on the truth of Your Word that You are my healer. In the name of Christ Jesus, my Redeemer, I pray, Amen.

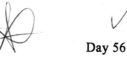

Day 56

My son, attend to my words; incline thine ear unto my sayings. Let them not depart from thine eyes; keep them in the midst of thine heart. For they are life unto those that find them, and health to all their flesh. (Proverbs 4:20-22 KJV)

God's Word is filled with empowerment for His people. It is filled with promises that God makes to us. In order for those promises to be fulfilled we must attend to God's Words, and we must focus completely on them. "Keep your eyes on Me," God says to us. Gaze steadfastly on Him. Follow unswervingly God's will for you. Keep God's Word and God's promises deep within your heart.

Remember that it is those things that are deep within your heart which will be fulfilled. God has promised us that He will give us the desires of our heart. If we have our symptoms buried there instead of God's Word, we will surely reap what we sow.

Examine what is in the midst of your heart now. Oddly enough, being ill often carries benefits with it. One of those is receiving more support and love than when you are well. Are you reluctant to ask your friends and family for attention when you are well and strong? Read the Scriptures which teach about asking, and learn to request the support you need.

Another benefit is that illness is a hiding place from the world. Are you afraid of living? Do you feel you have failed to accomplish anything of value? Do you feel disconnected from the flow of life around you and that you don't fit in it or belong? Know that all these feelings and beliefs originate from the father of lies.

The truth is that you are a child of God and consequently have great value. God constantly asks you to choose life. He wants you to live in joy and in fulfillment of His purpose for you.

Examining these beliefs buried in your innermost heart can be painful. Acknowledge them, give them to God for cleansing and healing, and feel God's forgiveness heal you. Let go of these old patterns that trap you, and keep only God's Word in the midst of your heart.

Almighty God, I clear away all my old beliefs and allow my innermost heart to be washed by the blood of Your Son Christ Jesus. I focus only on Your Word and Your will for my life. I absorb Your Holy Scriptures into the midst of my heart, for I know that they are life to me and health to my body. In Jesus' name, I pray, Amen.

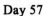

Day 57

I will sing to the Lord all my life; I will sing praise to my God as long as I live. May my meditation be pleasing to him, as I rejoice in the Lord. (Psalm 104:33-34 NIV)

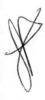

Sing praises to the Lord! For how long? All your life. As long as you live. God is the source of every good thing and is worthy to be worshipped and praised.

This Psalm also speaks of meditation. "May my meditation be pleasing to Him." When you pray, you talk to God. Of course, God already knows what your needs are, and He already knows what is in your heart. Nevertheless, prayer is a concrete act of seeking God and choosing to move close to Him. Prayer also clarifies for your own benefit exactly what the desires of your heart are, and it provides a mechanism for you to crystallize your thoughts and emotions.

Meditation moves a step further. Prayer is one half of the circle of communication with God. Meditation is the other half. It is the half in which you listen to what God has to say. It is your time for silence, your time for hearing the Holy Spirit speak to you. Since it is a vital part of your healing process, be sure that you set aside additional time for meditation every day after your prayer time. Formulate in your prayers questions you may have about your recovery. Ask specific questions about decisions you must make about herbs to use, medications to take, health professionals to visit, or treatments to undergo.

Don't assume any answers. Allow God to work in His own way. For example, if your back hurts, don't assume you should go to a chiropractor. Take it to the Lord first in prayer and then in meditation so He can reveal His answer to you.

You may be surprised at many of the answers you receive if you remain open to God's truth. Quieten your mind and your heart, and wait for the Holy Spirit to speak to you, revealing God's path for your recovery.

Dear Heavenly Father, I will sing to You all my life. I will sing praise to You as long as I live. May my meditation be pleasing to You always, Lord. Keep me open to hear Your will for me. I know You want me to be well but I don't know what my part in the process is supposed to be. Reveal that through my meditation, O Lord. Help me to drop all my assumptions, and let me hear Your voice and only Your voice. Thank You for Your eternal love and healing. In the name of Your Son, Jesus Christ, my Savior and my Redeemer, I pray, Amen.

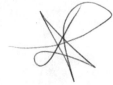

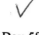

Day 58

He delivereth and rescueth, and he worketh signs and wonders in heaven and in earth, who hath delivered Daniel from the power of the lions. (Daniel 6:27 KJV)

Taken captive by the Babylonians, Daniel came to be held in high esteem by several kings of that nation. King Belshazzar described Daniel this way: "I have heard of you, that the Spirit of the holy God is in you and that light and understanding and superior wisdom are found in you" (Daniel 5:44). After Belshazzar was killed, Darius became the new king. Many of the people under King Darius were jealous of Daniel and tricked Darius into making a law forbidding any person from praying to anyone except the king for thirty days.

Despite the new law, Daniel opened his windows, got down on his knees, and prayed to Jehovah three times a day just as he had always done. He was then brought before the king, who was forced to uphold his new law. Daniel was taken to a den of lions, and a stone was laid against the mouth of the cave. The king was so upset that he didn't get any sleep that night. The next morning he raced to the lion's den. Standing outside, he called, "Daniel! Daniel, servant of the living God! Is your God, whom you serve continually, able to deliver you from the lions?" To his relief, Daniel answered from within the den, "My God has sent His angel and has shut the lions' mouths so that they have not hurt me, because I was found innocent and blameless before Him" (Daniel 6:22). And Daniel was released.

Daniel was in a tight spot in the lions' den. If you feel sick, you are in a tight spot, too. The enemy sought to devour Daniel, and the enemy seeks to devour your body and your energy. But your God is a Savior and Deliverer. He works signs and wonders. He works His will in the heavens, and He works the same will here on earth if we will let Him. Saving you from your health problem is no harder than saving Daniel from the hungry lions. Allow Jehovah-rapha to work His wonders in your life. Trust Him and give thanks for your deliverance.

Almighty Lord, how grateful I am for this wonderful story of Daniel which gives me an example of faith and trust in the most difficult circumstance. Thank You for sending Your Son to bear my sins and infirmities on the Cross so that I may be found innocent in Your sight. Send Your angels to be with me, to protect me, and to guide me. I acknowledge You as my Lord and Deliverer. In the name of Your Son, Jesus Christ, my Redeemer, I pray, Amen.

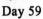

Day 59

The effectual fervent prayer of a righteous man availeth much. (James 5:16 KJV)

We want our prayers to "avail much," but exactly how *do* we pray effectively for our healing? First, acknowledge the sovereignty of God, who has made us so awesomely. Second, name your ailment or health situation. If you have never asked for healing for this particular condition, then do so. If you have already asked, do not ask again. Praying isn't begging, whimpering, and pleading repeatedly for the same thing. Instead, trust that you have been heard, and offer prayers of thanksgiving.

Third, affirm your belief that Jesus carried to the Cross not only your sins but also the particular health condition that you have named. Jesus has already released you, and it is extremely important that you claim this atonement. What you are asking for is the manifestation of that healing in your body. Fourth, in your prayer enforce God's Word on your body, and speak with authority to the parts which are out of balance. Visualize each cell in perfect alignment and functioning exactly as the Creator intended it to operate. Command every cell, gland, or organ to operate in harmony with God's Divine plan. Call on the name of Jesus, and ask Him to cast out satan and his influence from every cell of your body.

Fifth, ask for God's guidance for the steps you need to take in order to facilitate your healing. Ask Him to reveal to you the things you need to do in the natural realm to support your body in repairing and rebuilding itself. Last, declare your belief in your healing. Ask God to support you and your faith as your healing is made manifest. Stand on God's Word. Speak God's Word numerous times during the day.

Almighty God, Your Word tells me that great power is released when I come to You in prayer. How grateful I am that You are my God who is approachable, who knows me by name, and who cares about me personally. You are Jehovah-rapha, my Creator and my healer. I now name my health condition. I stand on Your Word which declares that Your Son Jesus Christ bore my diseases and infirmities on the Cross. In the name of Your Son Jesus, I command satan to leave my body, and I command all the cells, tissues, organs, and glands to function according to Your Divine plan. Heavenly Father, I humbly ask for Your guidance, showing me what You want me to do to work in full partnership with You for my complete healing. In Jesus' name, I pray, Amen.

Day 60

Peace I leave with you, my peace I give unto you: not as the world giveth, give I unto you. Let not your heart be troubled, neither let it be afraid. (John 14:27 KJV)

How often the message of God's Word tells us not to be afraid. Fear does not come from God. Fear is the work of the devil, and it separates us from God because love and fear cannot operate simultaneously.

God is perfect Love. Jesus, the Son of God, is also perfect Love. Jesus trusted God so totally that there was no room in Him for fear. Whether confronted with satan, bad weather, multitudes of needy people, or a betrayer's kiss, Jesus remained at peace, centered in the love of God.

Jesus calls you to Him and asks you to trust Him. "I give you my peace," He said. "Don't be afraid." The devil knows all our weaknesses and he especially knows our fears. Most of us are driven by some fear. It may be the fear of loneliness, of being unloved, of being unworthy, of being poor, of being abused, of being rejected, or of being abandoned.

Deep in our hearts, a surprising number of us are afraid of being healthy. If we feel sick, we have an excuse to fail. If we feel sick, we have a reason to protect ourselves from a dangerous world. If we feel sick, we have "permission" to ask for kindness from others. As long as we receive these hidden benefits from illness, our fears of being well are triggered, and the true desire of our heart is really to be sick. We must first ask for healing of these fears so that we have a unity of purpose and intent for healing. We have to end satan's hold on us through our fears.

Choosing to live in faith instead of in fear would seem to be an easy choice, but it is not. Jesus knows how much courage it takes to let go of fear. He tells us He will help us and that He has His precious peace to give us. Tell Him your fears. Hand them over to Him ten times a day or a hundred times a day or a thousand times a day until those fears are no longer a part of you. Accept the peace of Christ in your heart.

Almighty God, I want to be clear in my heart as I claim Your healing. I release to You all my fears. Take them now. Remove them from me and remove their hold over me. Free me from the evil one and throw the demons of fear out of me. Holy Father, enfold me in Your loving, protective arms. Surround me with Your strength, Your healing light, and the peace of Your Son, Jesus Christ, my Redeemer. In the name of the Father, Son, and Holy Spirit, I pray, Amen.

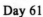

Day 61

And God said, "Behold, I have given you every herb bearing seed, which is upon the face of all the earth, and every tree, in the which is the fruit of a tree yielding seed; to you it shall be for meat." (Genesis 1:29 KJV)

In the first chapter of Genesis God has created us, His beloved children, and now He needs to get us started on the right track. He has two initial things to say. The first is that we are to have dominion over the earth. The second instruction is largely overlooked and ignored. The bottom line is: eat plants for food.

What? Yes, that means fruits and vegetables. The essential nature of plants is for our health and nutrition, and we cannot be healthy without them because God ordained this from the first moment of our creation.

Many people today "don't like" vegetables and consider a little iceberg lettuce in a hamburger and their French-fried potatoes to be their vegetables for the day. Our government once even declared ketchup to be a vegetable. Children are often allowed to fill up on snacks loaded with sugar, and, consequently, they aren't hungry at mealtime for nutritious food. Even more sadly, we have allowed our lives to become so hectic and frantically filled with activities that we don't have time to prepare healthy meals. The more stressed we are, the less time we take to prepare what we know is nutritious for our bodies.

Take a look at your own meals. Food was so important that God told you from the very beginning what to eat. How many fruits and vegetables do you include in your daily diet? Are some of them eaten raw? Plants are filled with enzymes to aid in digestion but heat destroys these substances. How many of your vegetables are overcooked, saturated with pesticides, and covered with butter and salt?

What you eat has a major role in the state of your health because your cells depend on the nutrients you give them. How ridiculous to willfully disregard God's instructions and then blame Him when your body breaks down and you feel ill.

Take responsibility for your health. Ask forgiveness for abusing your body, and then eat the right foods to support its healing.

Almighty Creator God, thank You for this marvelous earth. You have given me a vast array of plants to eat for food and a multitude of herbs to use not only for food but also to help my body heal when it is sick. I seek to learn more about Your plants and herbs so that I will be a good steward over all these many gifts. With grateful thanks, in Jesus' name, I pray, Amen.

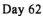

Day 62

Jesus left there and went along the Sea of Galilee. Then he went up on a mountainside and sat down. Great crowds came to him, bringing the lame, the blind, the crippled, the mute and many others, and laid them at his feet; and he healed them. The people were amazed when they saw the mute speaking, the crippled made well, the lame walking and the blind seeing. And they praised the God of Israel. (Matthew 15:29-31 NIV)

Allow this Scripture to come alive. Imagine yourself sitting outside your home near the Sea of Galilee. The sun shines brightly but you hardly feel its heat because you are worried about your health. In your mind you are thinking about your symptoms, and you are wrestling with indecision. You don't know what to do and you feel frightened. Allow yourself to be immersed in your situation.

You hear a lot of noise and see a man going up into the mountains with a great crowd of people following Him. "Is it the man from Nazareth?" you wonder. "Is it the man they call Jesus?" Someone runs by, and you call out to him, asking him your question. He turns briefly and with a great smile, says, "Yes, it's Jesus. Come on. Hurry!"

You get up and join the crowd going to the mountainside. "I am just one person in a great crowd," you think as you find a place to sit down. "There is no way I can get close to Him. Why, there are so many people here, He will never even see me, much less heal me."

Close your eyes, and feel the hopelessness wash over you, that feeling you have felt so often lately. Your mind wanders to the "if-onlys" and "what-ifs" and "whys," and you are lost for quite awhile in your own little world of despair.

Suddenly you feel a presence and a warmth around you. You open your eyes and see Jesus standing in front of you. He squats down and gazes into your eyes with the most compassionate and loving look you have ever seen. He reaches out and takes your hand in His. "Do you want to be well?" He asks you. Give Him your answer. He is as real now as He has ever been.

Heavenly Father, Your Son is the risen Christ, who died for my sins and my infirmities. It gives me great comfort to know from Your Holy Scripture that great crowds came to Him, bringing their sick, and that He healed them all. Just as He touched them, I know that He touches me. By His stripes, I am healed. Guide me always, Father. Show me the path that You want me to take for the full manifestation of my healing, and I will follow it. In Jesus' name, I pray, Amen.

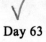

Day 63

Jesus replied, "I tell you the truth, if you have faith and do not doubt, not only can you do what was done to the fig tree, but also you can say to this mountain, 'Go, throw yourself into the sea,' and it will be done. If you believe, you will receive whatever you ask for in prayer." (Matthew 21:21-22 NIV)

Jesus was constantly stressing the importance of belief. Faith is the foundation of everything, He tells us.

Having *partial* faith is not sufficient. Have you noticed how people have a way of having faith in God up to a point? Then they are controlled by their belief in the world around them and of what "facts" appear to be. They succumb to doubt that faith really can overcome everything.

Take a look at the story in Matthew 21. Jesus has gone to a fig tree which should have had fruit on it. He found it bare and told it that it would never bear again. The tree withered immediately in this account. His disciples were amazed! Still more shocking was what Jesus told them – that if they had faith and did not doubt, not only could they do what was done to the fig tree but also they could do anything.

Do you hear Jesus telling this to you today? He says to you that, if you follow His example, you can do not only what He does but also even greater things (John 14:12). Be careful not to be deceived by the evil one into believing that these words of Jesus applied to some special gift that was given only to the twelve disciples.

When you ask for healing, ask knowing that it is the will of God that you be well. Ask believing. Ask without any doubt in your mind.

The presence of doubt means that the evil one is working somewhere in your vulnerable places. Root it out. Tell the devil he must leave you.

Let your faith be complete and whole as you stand in the presence of Jehovah-rapha. Ask knowing not only that you *will* receive what you have asked for, but also that you have *already* received it.

Almighty God, Your Son Jesus Christ is Your perfect example. He shows me the way. He tells me to believe with all my heart and soul. He tells me to have faith and not to doubt. That is hard sometimes, God. The medical reports seem clear, and I am tempted to see them as the only reality. Help my unbelief, Father. I lay my doubts at Your feet. I say to the mountain of my illness, "Leave my body," and I stand on Your Word that it will be done. Strengthen me as I fulfill Your will and Your purpose for my life and as I walk the path to recovery that You desire me to walk. In the name of Your Son, Jesus Christ, my Redeemer, I pray, Amen.

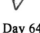

Day 64

They came to Bethsaida, and some people brought a blind man and begged Jesus to touch him. He took the blind man by the hand and led him outside the village. When he had spit on the man's eyes and put his hands on him, Jesus asked, "Do you see anything?" He looked up and said, "I see people; they look like trees walking around." Once more Jesus put his hands on the man's eyes. Then his eyes were opened, his sight was restored, and he saw everything clearly. (Mark 8:22-25 NIV)

How interesting to read in the Holy Scriptures that it took two attempts on Jesus' part before the blind man at Bethsaida was healed. Was there some momentary problem with Jesus' healing ability? Of course not. We are repeatedly told that Jesus healed every single person who came to Him and that He did this in accordance with God's will for all to be healed.

This account sends us an important message: our healing may come in stages, as a result of gradual changes. While the two stages of the process related here in Mark happened within minutes of each other, our own process may take weeks or months or even years. Even though speed is enormously important to most of us, it means little to God. Just as it was then, it is our Heavenly Father who determines the right path to recovery for each one of us.

The fact is that God is in charge of our healing only if we allow it. When we give God control, He will determine exactly how and when our healing is to occur. Often there are certain things we must do (such as to forgive someone who hurt us), and, if we do not do those things, God cannot heal us.

Believing that God desires us to be well does not give us an excuse to *demand* healing from Him. Prayer is a request. In it you confess your faith in God's Word that He is Jehovah-rapha, and it must be followed by listening and obeying. Examine your heart, and make sure that you are willing to follow God's method and God's timetable for you. Then stand on the Word, and offer your thanksgiving and praise for your recovery.

Dear God, forgive me for being impatient. I am tired of feeling sick and looking at this long list of symptoms that I have. I profess my trust in You, and I steadfastly believe that Your timetable for my recovery is perfect for me. Show me what I can do to participate in this healing process, and lead me from the temptations of the evil one to sabotage it. Thank You, Lord, for healing me. In Jesus' name, I pray, Amen.

Day 65

"Have faith in God," Jesus answered. "I tell you the truth, if anyone says to this mountain, 'Go, throw yourself into the sea,' and does not doubt in his heart but believes that what he says will happen, it will be done for him." (Mark 11:22-23 NIV)

Here Jesus reveals the way to activate faith in your life. First, face your problem squarely, and speak the solution firmly and succinctly. Second, do not allow doubt to distract you from focusing on that goal. Third, believe that *what you say* will happen.

Decide whether you want your words to manifest just as you say them. Too often we pray one thing and spend the rest of the day saying something else. For example, suppose you have migraine headaches. Medical tests reveal nothing and you frequently have attacks. One morning you pray, "God, please heal me of my migraines. " Thirty minutes after you offer your prayer, your head begins to hurt, and you say to your wife, "I feel another migraine starting up. My head is beginning to throb. It's already getting worse. I'll bet it'll be killing me before the day is out." You say the same thing to several colleagues at work – and sure enough you have a terrible headache. Then you come home and pray, "Lord, I really want to be healed of these migraines." And so it goes. Day after day you pray the same prayer, and day after day you voice your statements of doom.

Imagine the difference if you were to spend your day saying, "In the name of Jesus I am healed. Pain, you have no place in my body for I am redeemed." God values words; He creates with His Word; and He expects you to respect your own words because they are the seeds that you are planting. Here He tells you that *you can have what you say.* Instead, too often you keep "telling it like it is," which really means that you keep describing the problem. This reveals an underlying lack of faith in the innermost places of your heart, and it is fertile ground for satan to keep you sick and separated from God's benefits. Jesus taught you to pray the solution. Do it now with your song of thanksgiving and allow Jehovah-rapha to guide you on His healing path.

Almighty God, help me to say what I believe and to believe what I say. I know that doubt comes from the evil one. I bind satan in the name of Jesus, and I command all the cells of my body to function according to Your Holy plan and design. By the stripes of Your Son Jesus Christ I am healed. Reveal to me anything I need to do to participate in my healing process. In Jesus' name, I pray, Amen.

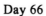

Day 66

Because you are my help, I sing in the shadow of your wings. My soul clings to you; your right hand upholds me. (Psalm 63:7-8 NIV)

Isn't this a wonderful picture? See yourself in the shadow of God's wings. Visualize your soul clinging to Him, and see God's right hand holding you up. The Lord God Almighty is your deliverer, your strength, and your healer. He wants you to be well. He offers you His love as a beloved child, and He smiles at you with tenderest care and affection.

Over and over again David fills his psalms with words of praise and tells of the strength of the Lord. Feast your eyes on these verses. Let your soul be filled with the promise of God's Holy Word.

This poor man called, and the Lord heard him; he saved him out of all his troubles. The angel of the Lord encamps around those who fear him, and he delivers them. (Psalm 34:6-7 NIV)

But you are a shield around me, O Lord; you bestow glory on me and lift up my head. To the Lord I cry aloud, and he answers me from his holy hill. (Psalm 3:3-4 NIV)

Blessed is he who has regard for the weak; the Lord delivers him in times of trouble. The Lord will protect him and preserve his life; he will bless him in the land and not surrender him to the desire of his foes. The Lord will sustain him on his sickbed and restore him from his bed of illness. (Psalm 41:1-3 NIV)

Fill your soul with these positive words from the Holy Scripture. Take time today to read these verses out loud and to absorb their meaning deeply within your heart.

Wonderful Jehovah-rapha, You are my strength. With You I know that I can overcome every obstacle that the evil one may put in my path. I call on Your strength, and, as You instructed me, I take dominion over my life. Because You are my help, I sing in the shadow of your wings. My soul clings to You; Your right hand upholds me. Guide me, God. Lead me in the path You want me to follow for my healing. In Jesus' name, I pray, Amen.

Day 67

There was an estate nearby that belonged to Publius, the chief official of the island. He welcomed us to his home and for three days entertained us hospitably. His father was sick in bed, suffering from fever and dysentery. Paul went in to see him and, after prayer, placed his hands on him and healed him. When this had happened, the rest of the sick on the island came and were cured. (Acts 28:7-9 NIV)

Isn't it regrettable that some people have turned the laying on of hands into a performance, complete with fake "cures"? Satan never ceases to work to get control, and he is delighted that laying on of hands is now perceived by many people as a kind of bogus hocus-pocus.

The laying on of hands is real. Jesus did it. He taught His disciples to do it. And He told them to teach others. In the Great Commission described in Mark 16:14-20, Jesus rebuked his followers for their lack of faith. Then He told them to go into all the world, preach the good news, teach others what they had been taught, and place their hands on sick people so they would get well.

Here we see Paul doing exactly that – following Jesus' instructions, laying his hands on the sick, and healing them. This was done by the followers in the early church, and then was done less and less until it is rarely found in the church today.

Paul was not one of Jesus' disciples. He was called after Jesus had ascended into heaven. In this story he is on the island of Malta where, by prayer and the laying on of hands, he heals a man sick with a fever and dysentery. The word of this healing spread and then everybody else on the island who was sick came to him. Every single one of them was healed and again we find no exceptions.

The truth is that you are no different from Paul. You have your own strengths, weaknesses, and talents, but Jesus' commission is as valid for you as it was for Paul. It is not a requirement that someone lay hands on you in order for you to be healed, but it is one way that has been given to you as a method for healing. Ask Jehovah-rapha if it is to be part of your path to healing.

Almighty God, thank You for the example of Paul. I am filled with humble awe at his willingness to follow the commands of Your Son Jesus Christ. Teach me that faith, O Lord, so that I, too, can be an instrument of healing for others. Thank You for healing me, Jehovah-rapha, and showering Your blessings upon me. In the name of Your Son, Jesus Christ, I pray, Amen.

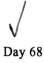

Day 68

Enter his gates with thanksgiving and his courts with praise; give thanks to him and praise his name. (Psalm 100:4 NIV)

Give thanks to the Lord, for he is good; his love endures forever. . . . Let them give thanks to the Lord for his unfailing love and his wonderful deeds for men. Let them sacrifice thank offerings and tell of his works with songs of joy. (Psalm 107:1, 21-22 NIV)

Be joyful always; pray continually; give thanks in all circumstances, for this God's will for you in Christ Jesus. (1 Thessalonians 5:16-18 NIV)

Flooding your soul and mind and body with words and thoughts of thanksgiving accelerates your healing process. When you are focused on thanksgiving, you are concentrating on the positive elements in your life, you are increasing your awareness of the improvement in your health, and you are strengthening the immune function of your body.

Notice that Paul connects joy, prayer, and thanksgiving. He exhorts the Thessalonians to give thanks in *all* circumstances. No matter how bad things look, find something worthy of gratitude, and praise God for it. Offer your thanks with joy. Offer your thanks in *continual* prayer; that is, pray prayers of gratitude without ceasing.

The evil one wants you to focus on the negative. He wants you to focus on all the things that you have done wrong and all the mistakes that you have made. He wants you to focus on your weaknesses, your failures, and your inadequacies. He wants you to focus on your aches and pains and medical predictions of gloom.

Don't allow satan to take control over you. Christ Jesus defeated the evil one and rose victorious. Stand up in your faith, and claim the victory and power that was won for you.

Each day create a thank-offering for Jehovah-rapha, the God who heals you. Today you can make each application of essential oils and each swallow of herbs a special thank-offering to God, and tomorrow you can take a walk of gratitude. Select something each day and offer it to the Lord in thanksgiving and praise.

Wonderful Jehovah-rapha, thank You, thank You, thank You. I joyfully give thanks for Your many blessings and for Your constant love. I offer my thank offerings humbly to You, and I proclaim my willingness to work in partnership with You for my healing. In the name of Your Son, Jesus Christ, I pray, Amen.

Day 69

May the God who gives endurance and encouragement give you a spirit of unity among yourselves as you follow Christ Jesus, so that with one heart and mouth you may glorify the God and Father of our Lord Jesus Christ. Accept one another, then, just as Christ accepted you, in order to bring praise to God. (Romans 15:5-7 NIV)

Receiving encouragement from other believers makes an enormous difference in your recovery from illness and disease. When you join together with others in a spirit of unity and with an attitude of expectancy for healing, you are lifted up in an environment of faith and trust in Jehovah-rapha.

Paul exhorts the Christians in Rome to stand together, especially during their tough times. He reminds them that God gives them endurance and encouragement. These are important words to remember in times of illness because that is also a difficult time filled with challenges. Rely on God for your strength – and your endurance. Sometimes healing comes swiftly, but often it comes as a result of our walking God's path faithfully, persistently, and determinedly. We are called to obedience and to total trust – even when the appearance doesn't seem to be indicative of our recovery. We must stay in constant communication with the Lord to make sure that we are doing everything we are supposed to do. And then we must believe.

Seek out people who share your belief that Jehovah-rapha is the God who heals us. Find people who believe that Jesus Christ died on the Cross for our complete salvation, that He died not only for our sins but that He also carried our infirmities to the Cross. Join in unity with these believers. Ask them to pray for you and to help you remain positive and faithful. Then join them in prayers for the recovery of others who seek healing.

Wonderful Jehovah-rapha, give me endurance and encouragement. Carry me through the tough spots and teach me always to trust You. Lead me, Lord, to people who believe as I do that You want Your children to be well and that it is Your will that Your children be healed. Lead me to people who believe that Your Son carried our infirmities to the Cross as well as our sins. I seek those believers with whom I may have a spirit of unity as I follow Christ Jesus, so that with one heart and mouth we may glorify You. I praise You, Lord, and I thank You for my healing. In the name of Your Son, Jesus Christ, my Savior and my Redeemer, I pray, Amen.

Day 70

Cast your cares on the Lord and he will sustain you; he will never let the righteous fall. (Psalm 55:22 NIV)

God will never let you down. Most people say they believe this is true, yet they really don't. How can you tell if you believe it? By the amount of peace in your soul.

Being ill is different from other problems of life because a wrong decision – or series of decisions – can cost us our lives, and, if that happens, all the other issues which we thought were so important simply end. Too often we permit all decisions about our treatment and recovery to be made solely by humans – either ourselves or others. Then when we get deeply into a treatment process, we ask for God's help and prayers from our church members.

Psalm 55 exhorts us to get our priorities straight. Cast your cares on the Lord. Turn to God *first*. Ask at each step along the way what you should do. At the first symptom or at the first sign that something is different in your body, ask God for guidance. Ask, ask, ask. It is written that, if we ask, we will receive.

God will sustain us because God wants us to be well. He sent His Son to die on the Cross to save us at every level of our being – to save our souls and to save our bodies from attacks of the evil one.

We have to do our part. We have to be righteous, to place the Lord God Almighty first in our lives and first in our decisions. When we do that, we will experience great inner peace. There will be no terrible struggles of indecision because we *know* that we are doing what God wants us to do. We have cast our cares on God and He carries them easily. He sustains us, holds us up, and supports us.

As He led the Israelites in a pillar of cloud by day and a pillar of fire in the night, so He leads us every second of our lives, never abandoning us, always blazing the trail ahead of us. All we must do is to trust Him and to follow Him.

Wonderful Jehovah-rapha, I cast my cares on You. Hold me, Lord; sustain me especially when I feel tired and scared. I know You don't let the righteous fall, but, God, I often feel unworthy instead of righteous. I know these feelings are from the evil one because You have created me in Your image and I am to come boldly before You as Your beloved child. I give You my worries and I trust You with my life. Thank You for guiding me and for healing me. In the name of Your Son, Jesus Christ, Amen.

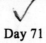

Day 71

When you sit to dine with a ruler, note well what is before you, and put a knife to your throat if you are given to gluttony. Do not crave his delicacies, for that food is deceptive. (Proverbs 23:1-3 NIV)

People haven't changed much since the days when Proverbs was written. Look at some of the primary health problems in our country – obesity, diabetes, hemorrhoids, varicose veins, heart attacks, cancer, peptic ulcer, hiatal hernia, appendicitis, and gallstones, just to name a few. There is a nutritional component to each of these ailments, and we must take responsibility for the willful choices we are making in our diets. Too much salt, too much sugar, too few vegetables, too little pure water, too little fiber. To make poor choices and then to blame God for the result by calling our illness His will is unfair, to say the least.

Most of us don't know how to make the shift from unhealthy foods to healthy ones. We have in our mind that we will have to eat food that looks like grass and tastes like hay – and we decide that we would rather be dead than eat *that!* Unfortunately, many people end up sacrificing their lives because they believe that lie of the evil one. Begin gradually and take one step at a time. Start by drinking pure water, one-half ounce for each pound of body weight. Add one vegetable to your diet every three days until you are eating at least four (preferably more) vegetables a day. Let at least one of them be raw and steam the others lightly. Make the extra effort to get organic produce because, when you feel sick, you need to remove the toxic load from your liver. To keep the same food amounts on your plate as you add more vegetables, simply reduce the portion sizes of the other items. Now add fresh fruit to your diet in the same gradual manner. Use it for snacks instead of soft drinks, cookies, and candy bars. Next, reduce the meat that you are eating to only once per day. Shift to hormone-and antibiotic-free chicken, turkey, and fish. Add more beans to your diet.

Be sure you ask for guidance whether these nutrition guidelines are appropriate and healthy for you to follow – rather than making assumptions according to man-made rules. Let the Holy Spirit be your daily guide. As you make changes in your diet and feel the difference in your body and health, give grateful thanks to God for healing you.

Almighty God, I really like certain foods that I know are not healthy and I need Your help in making a commitment to follow Your will for my diet instead of listening to the evil one. Help me to make the changes I need to make, God. In Jesus' name, I pray, Amen.

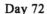

Day 72

Pleasant words are as an honeycomb, sweet to the soul and health to the bones. (Proverbs 16:24 KJV)

Words have great power. God's Holy Word is the ultimate Word and the ultimate power. "In the beginning was the Word, and the Word was with God, and the Word was God" (John 1:1). Words are important because they reveal our inner condition. They are a reflection of what we are thinking and what we are feeling inside. Jesus told us, "The things that come out of the mouth come from the heart," so these are the things that make us either clean or unclean (Matthew 15:18).

Pleasant words, positive words, agreeable words all affect us. They are "sweet to the soul" because they put us in greater harmony with the God of love and compassion and kindness. They bring us closer to Him. Each word is a seed and pleasant words will bear sweet fruit.

This verse in Proverbs reminds us that positive thoughts and words have a major impact on our health. They are "health to the bones" which is a way to describe health all the way through our body to the cells in our innermost core. Words are understood by the cells in our bodies, and these cells take our words literally, just as we think or say them.

For example, when we use expressions such as "I'd die for a soft drink!" or "That joke just kills me!" our bodies take the words at face value. When we say, "I am a diabetic" or "I have heart disease," our bodies actually work to fulfill the meaning of those words.

Be mindful of your words today – both spoken and unspoken. Just for today let them be positive words to assist and accelerate your healing. If negative words pop out, say immediately, "Cancel that," and then make a positive statement instead.

Continue developing this habit until you have transformed your speech and your thoughts. This brings you into partnership with God, pleases Him, and facilitates your healing.

Heavenly Father, today I will be mindful of every word I think and every word I say. I know the power of words, and I seek to use that power for Your glory, for the benefit of others, and for my own good. I stand on Your Holy Word. I affirm Your Word which declares, "I am the God who heals thee." I proclaim the Word of Jesus Christ who said, "Your faith has made you well." Today I will let the words of my mouth and the meditations of my heart be positive, uplifting, and acceptable in Thy sight. In the name of Your Son, Jesus Christ, my Savior and my Redeemer, Amen.

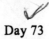

Day 73

Stand up and praise the Lord your God, who is from everlasting to everlasting. Blessed be your glorious name, and may it be exalted above all blessing and praise. You alone are the Lord. You made the heavens, even the highest heavens, and all their starry host, the earth and all that is on it, the seas and all that is in them. You give life to everything, and the multitudes of heaven worship you. (Nehemiah 9:5-6 NIV)

The Lord God Jehovah gave life to everything. The heavens, the earth, you – and even the germs, bacteria, and viruses that we so love to hate.

We seem to spend our time focused on killing viruses and bacteria. Yet illness can't take hold within us unless the environment exists for it to grow. Contrary to popular belief, disease isn't due as much to the existence of germs in our bodies as it is to the fact that conditions in us are optimal for those germs to grow and multiply. For example, at this very moment you probably have the strep virus in your body, yet you probably do not have strep throat. Why? Because your immune system is working effectively enough to keep the strep virus from causing any problem for you. Most illness and disease work that way.

During the Middle Ages a great plague swept Europe and killed over one-third of the population. What about the other two-thirds? They were exposed to the same viruses and bacteria. What was different about the ones who survived? Interestingly, there developed a band of thieves who went among the sick, dying, and dead, stealing objects of value from the bodies, and they didn't die. When they were captured, they were forced to reveal their secret. They had covered themselves with a blend of essential oils – including cloves, cinnamon, eucalyptus, and rosemary – that raised their immune levels so that they did not succumb to the disease.

Let your focus be on those things which give life because this brings you into alignment with God's own life force. Learn how the systems of your body function, what nutrients you need to support those systems, what is the best source of those nutrients, and how you can strengthen all those parts of your body which are weak. Seek the Holy Spirit's counsel and then act on the guidance that is given to you.

Almighty God, You are the maker of all life. Help me to glorify You by learning how I can strengthen my own body. Send me teachers, Lord, and I will learn. I promise to act on my knowledge, according to the guidance from the Holy Spirit. Thank You. In Jesus' name, I pray, Amen.

Day 74

A man in the crowd answered, "Teacher, I brought you my son, who is possessed by a spirit that has robbed him of speech. Whenever it seizes him, it throws him to the ground. He foams at the mouth, gnashes his teeth and becomes rigid. I asked your disciples to drive out the spirit, but they could not." . . . When the spirit saw Jesus, it immediately threw the boy into a convulsion. He fell to the ground and rolled around, foaming at the mouth. Jesus asked the boy's father, "How long has he been like this?" "From childhood," he answered. "It has often thrown him into fire or water to kill him. But if you can do anything, take pity on us and help us." "'If you can'?" said Jesus. "Everything is possible for him who believes." Immediately the boy's father exclaimed. "I do believe; help me overcome my unbelief!" When Jesus saw that a crowd was running to the scene, he rebuked the evil spirit. "You deaf and mute spirit," he said, "I command you, come out of him and never enter him again." The spirit shrieked, convulsed him violently and came out. The boy looked so much like a corpse that many said, "He's dead." But Jesus took him by the hand and lifted him to his feet and he stood up. (Mark 9:17-18, 20-27 NIV)

A father, desperate for healing for his son, turns to Jesus for help after the disciples have failed. He utters words of complete doubt when he asks, "Help him, *if you can.*" Not even "if you *will*" but "if you *can.*"

Look at Jesus' response. <u>First</u>, he repeats the man's question. "<u>If you can?</u>" as though it were incredulous even to raise such a doubt. "Everything is possible to him who believes," He says. Imagine the look of compassion and love that he gives this distraught father. The man looks back at Jesus and the words pour from his heart. "I do believe; help me overcome my unbelief!"

When we feel sick, there are often times when we relate to the father in this story. We feel bad, we have prayed for healing, yet we still see the sickness in our body. In the turmoil of our doubt, we see only the outward appearance of things. Hand your doubts to the Lord and ask for His help, believing that He will give it. <u>Receive His healing touch.</u>

Almighty God, it is written that everything is possible for him who believes. I believe, Lord; help thou my unbelief. When satan comes with whispers of doubt, help me to banish him from my sight by saying, "I command you to leave!" I stand firm on Your Holy Word, Father. Thank You for healing me. In the name of Christ Jesus, my Savior and Redeemer, I pray, Amen.

Day 75

So then faith cometh by hearing, and hearing by the word of God. (Romans 10:17 KJV)

My soul is weary with sorrow; strengthen me according to your word. (Psalm 119:28 NIV)

For this cause also thank we God without ceasing, because, when ye received the word of God which ye heard of us, ye received it not as the word of men, but as it is in truth, the word of God, which effectually worketh also in you that believe. (1 Thessalonians 2:13 KJV)

Faith comes by hearing, and hearing by the Word of God. If we want to build the faith that makes us whole, we must immerse ourselves in God's Word and absorb it into our minds and hearts. This requires a commitment of time on a daily basis so that we may be filled at every level of our being with God's glorious good news.

Examine the habits of your life. Do you find ways to integrate God's Word into your daily living patterns? There are several simple techniques to do this. For example, each week select a particular verse of Scripture that uplifts you and write it on a couple of note cards. Then post these note cards in places where you will see them frequently – on the refrigerator door or the bathroom mirror or the television remote control! Every time your eyes see the card, make sure that you read the message with intent and focus.

Another way to incorporate the Word into your life is to get some audio-cassettes of the Psalms or the New Testament or the entire Bible. Play these cassettes in the car while you are commuting to work or running errands or driving children to their activities. You can put the cassettes in a Walkman and listen while you are taking a walk or doing your exercise. You will be surprised at how much listening time you will have.

When the Word is a part of you, then it can work effectively in you and through you so that you will be a glorious witness to others.

Wonderful Jehovah-rapha, thank You for Your Holy Word. I know I need to hear Your Word so that I can continue to increase my faith. Reveal to me creative ways to make time for filling my soul with Your Word. Let Your Word work effectually in me, and let me be a joyous witness of Your love and care and healing power. In the name of Your Son, Jesus Christ, I pray, Amen.

Day 76

For I came down from heaven not to do mine own will, but the will of him that sent me. (John 6:38 KJV)

Healing has to be the will of God because Jesus tells us clearly that He came to do only the will of our heavenly Father. Sent to us by the Almighty, Jesus' purpose was ordained at the time of Adam and Eve's transgression and was prophesied by Isaiah. He came to redeem our sins and bear our infirmities on the Cross. He healed everyone who came to Him and who wanted to be well.

Are you ready to come to Jesus? Do you want to be well? Before you blurt out a "yes," imagine for a moment the full implication of your answer. Infirmities often provide a hiding place for us. We often don't have to take full responsibility for the details of life when we feel sick. Other people often give us more attention and support when we feel ill than they do when we are well. We even can get away with being irritable and difficult, letting our buried anger bubble out over those around us.

Take time to make a full internal inventory. Do it on paper. Write down all the disadvantages of feeling sick. That is the easy part and your answers will probably come quickly. Now write down the benefits you receive by being ill – those quiet, subtle things that hide, protect, and shield you from engaging fully with life and with other people. Give yourself several days to do this. Pray to the Holy Spirit to reveal to you what you need to know. If you feel bold, ask a trusted friend to help you.

Once you have both lists, decide whether you are willing to give them to God and to His Son. You cannot give up one list and keep the other. You either relinquish them both or hold onto them both.

If you are sure you are ready to give them to God, imagine Jesus is walking down the road. He sees you, He stops, and He holds out His arms to you. He tells you, "I have come down from heaven, not to do my will, but the will of Him who sent me. You are set free from your infirmity." Stand on the Word that it is God's will for you to be made whole, and well. Thank you!

Gracious God, through Your Holy Word I know that Jesus healed everyone who came to Him for healing. No one was turned away. No one was passed by. I stand on the road, Father. I come before You. I trust Your Holy Word that You can heal me. I trust Your Holy Word that You are healing me. With gratitude and thanksgiving, in Jesus' name, I pray, Amen.

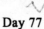

And he that sat upon the throne said, "Behold, I make all things new." And he said unto me, "Write: for these words are true and faithful." And he said unto me, "It is done. I am Alpha and Omega, the beginning and the end. I will give unto him that is athirst of the fountain of the water of life freely. He that overcometh shall inherit all things; and I will be his God, and he shall be my son." (Revelation 21:5-7 KJV)

Take a moment to focus on the words, "Behold, I make all things new." This includes not just our spiritual self, but our physical self as well. The design of our bodies when they are functioning healthily is the continual making anew.

God's Divine plan provided that most cells in our body have a fairly short life span. Blood, muscles, organs, and even bones – all are constantly being made and remade as old cells die and new cells are born. Where that pattern has not been interrupted, we create new healthy cells over and over again.

The sacrifice of Jesus Christ makes available to us the fountain of the water of life freely. Spiritually (and most importantly, of course) that means eternal life. However, since Jesus bore our infirmities on the Cross, it also means that renewal is available to our holy temples while we are still here on earth. Life through the blood of Jesus Christ means health to our bodies physically. Ask Jesus Christ to transform each cell that is sick so that a new, healthy cell is created in its place.

"He that overcometh shall inherit all things." There's that little word "all" again. Naturally, the most important inheritances are spiritual. Yet once again we cannot discount our physical body, which is our temple of the Holy Spirit.

This body is God's creation. We are to overcome the power of satan and to remove his influence from us both spiritually and in his manifestations physically. We will then be fully God's child as He intended, and we can claim Divine renewal in every cell of our being.

Thank you, God, for making me new. I am grateful to know not only that nothing is beyond Your power but also that you want me to be renewed in spirit and in mind and in body. I stand on Your Word which was written and which You have proclaimed to be true and faithful. I speak to every cell in my body and command each one to be made new, according to Your Holy Word. In the name of Jesus Christ, I command each cell to function according to Your Holy design and purpose. Thank you, God, for healing me. In Jesus' name, I pray, Amen.

Day 78

Now when Jesus was born in Bethlehem of Judea, . . . behold, there came wise men from the east to Jerusalem, saying, "Where is he that is born King of the Jews? For we have seen his star in the east and are come to worship him. ". . . And when they were come into the house, they saw the young child with Mary his mother, and fell down, and worshipped him: and when they had opened their treasures, they presented unto him gifts; gold, and frankincense and myrrh. (Matthew 2:1-2, 11 KJV)

What gifts would you take to a king? The three wise men believed they were looking for a child who had been born to be a king, and they wanted to bring Him treasures that reflected their feeling of awe. Consider their selections. Not one of the three gifts was made by man. No ornate jewelry. No luxurious clothes. No art objects. No toys.

All three gifts for the Son of God were made by God. They were all items found in nature. Everyone understands gold and recognizes it as a precious metal of great value. What about frankincense? It is a fragrant gum resin and essential oil that was used for various healing purposes. It was considered to be a holy oil because it had the effect of increasing a person's spiritual connection and awareness. Its many uses at that time included helping physical problems we now associate with the immune system. Like frankincense, myrrh was also considered to assist in creating spiritual awareness. In both oil and herb form, myrrh was also extremely useful for healing because it has strong antiseptic, anti-bacterial, and anti-viral actions.

Like the wise men, we, too, worship our Lord and Savior. As we seek to connect spiritually with Him, we, too, can use herbal treasures God gave us in the beginning when He created our universe. God wants us to be well, so He filled nature with many plants, essential oils, and herbs for our healing. He gave them to us in abundance because He knew our need for them would be great. Our responsibility is to learn about them, to use them wisely according to His purpose and in accordance with His guidance, and to value them as precious gifts from our heavenly Father.

Most Glorious Creator, thank You for the profusion of herbs which You have given to me. You have blessed me with an array of Your healing herbs, essential oils, and natural substances that is so vast that I can hardly comprehend it. Teach me about Your healing remedies, O God. Guide me so that I may learn about them and may use them wisely according to Your will, purpose, and guidance. In Jesus' name, I pray, Amen.

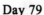

Day 79

And great multitudes followed him and he healed them all. (Matthew 12:15 KJV)

Here again Jesus healed them *all*. He healed everyone in the great multitudes. No illness is excluded and no person is excluded. We so often hear people and ministers say that it is "God's will" that a certain individual be sick. Sometimes there is the suggestion that sickness makes people strong or noble. Sometimes there is the suggestion that the illness is meant to teach us a lesson. Sometimes sickness is believed to be a way that God punishes people who have been "bad."

Keep your focus on the places where God's will is clear – first, in heaven where His will is kept perfectly and, second, in the Garden where he first placed His beloved creation, a perfectly healthy Adam and Eve.

There is a third example of God's perfect will in action and that is found in the life and mission of His Son, Jesus Christ. "I do nothing of myself," Jesus said in John 8:28. If it were not God's will that ALL be healed, Jesus would not have healed everyone.

Surely, he would have said to some, "I'm sorry but God is trying to teach you an important lesson and I cannot violate the will of the Father. So I can't heal you but I will pray that you understand the lesson so that you can recover." He would have had to say that on many, many occasions, and certainly it would have been reported at least *once* in the Scriptures.

No matter what translation you read, you will never find Jesus refusing to heal. Never. Notice how consistently Jesus healed them *all*. Since Jesus was always acting on the will of God and since Jesus healed them *all*, it must be the will of God for all to be healed. That includes you. Let this truth sink deep into the core of your being. Close your eyes and see yourself standing in the multitude. Now see yourself walking up to Jesus. See Him look at you, smile, and heal you with His touch.

Dear God, thank You for the example of Your Son, Jesus Christ, who came to carry out Your will. Thank You for His example of healing Your children over and over and over again. I come before You, God, as one of Your children. I declare Your will for my healing as revealed in the Holy Scriptures. I stand before You in trust and acceptance for Your personal love for me. Help me to walk always according to Your perfect will. Show me Your path for my healing. In the name of Jesus Christ, I pray, Amen.

Day 80

Then Jesus told him, "Because you have seen me, you have believed; blessed are those who have not seen and yet have believed." (John 20:29 NIV)

Do you realize that Jesus is talking directly to you? He knows your name and He is standing before you. He is looking directly into your eyes and He is speaking these words.

Let the incredible awesomeness of this truth sink deep into your soul. We often make rationalizations that "things" are different for us because we live now and Jesus lived then. Maybe all the healings of Jesus was just for two thousand years ago so that people would understand that Jesus was really Divine. Maybe the healings were just part of a sign for that particular time. Maybe we shouldn't expect them to be relevant for us two millennia later.

But what about Jesus' statement that "I say unto you, He that believeth on me, the works that I do shall he do also; and *greater works* than these shall he do; because I go unto my Father" (John 14:12). We are supposed to be doing even greater works than Jesus did because we have His help and the help of the Holy Spirit.

Let go of the idea that the twenty-first century is somehow different. Jesus stands before you now. Reach out for His hand. Feel His love, peace, and healing flow into your soul, into your heart, and into every cell in your body. Hear Him say directly to you, "Blessed are you – who have not seen and have yet believed."

Wonderful Jehovah-rapha, there are times when my faith seems to waiver. Strengthen me, Lord. Help me to immerse myself in Your Word and especially in the words of Your Son, Jesus Christ. Jesus was clear in telling me to believe in Him and in You, God. I believe, Lord. Help my unbelief, especially as it relates to the awesome healing You are performing in my life. Help me to stop watching for my symptoms to change before I allow belief in my healing to take firm root in my heart. Help me to believe before I see. I didn't live two thousand years ago when Your Son Christ Jesus walked in Galilee. Just as I must believe in Him even though I have not seen Him, I must believe in my healing even when I have not seen it. I stand on Your Word, God, and I covenant to do everything You want me to do in partnership with You for my healing. In the name of Your Son, Jesus Christ, my Savior and my Redeemer, I pray, Amen.

Resist him [the devil], standing firm in the faith, because you know that your brothers throughout the world are undergoing the same kind of sufferings. (1 Peter 5:9 NIV)

People rarely want to talk about the devil these days. It isn't very "politically correct." Jesus, on the other hand, was not hesitant to talk about satan, the evil one. He knew that we can't resist what we don't acknowledge. When He taught us to pray the Lord's Prayer, He told us to ask God to "deliver us from the evil one" (Matthew 6:13). Those words warn us strongly of the threat at hand.

Jesus confronted the devil and resisted him vigorously. Of course, Jesus' whole purpose in coming was to overcome the devil and to redeem us, soul and body. Therefore, we can't be Christians and keep our heads in the sand by talking only about love without ever acknowledging the existence and activity of satan.

Sickness itself is the devil's handiwork to begin with. So when we feel sick, we are already vulnerable. We must be bold in our resistance. We must declare with the authority of Jesus Christ that sickness cannot stay within us any more than satan himself cannot stay within us.

Sickness makes us an easy target of attacks of the evil one. We often experience fear – fear of knowing the right choice for our healing, fear of making changes in our lives, fear of the future. Remember that all fears are seeds of the evil one and resist him. Allowing fear to rule us gives satan our power and often results in satan's talking us out of our healing.

God plants only love, faith, and strength. Jesus has defeated satan and has borne all your sicknesses and sins for you. It is already done. Thank God and claim His power. Stand firm in your faith. Assert your dominion over your body and banish satan from it. Boldly claim the healing of Jehovah-rapha in the name of Christ Jesus.

Almighty God, Your Precious Son, Jesus Christ, taught me to pray, "Deliver me from the evil one." Deliver me, God. Often I feel afraid, and I know that those feelings are not from You but that they are seeds of the evil one. Help me, God, to stand firm in my faith. Help me to resist satan. Help me to be bold. Make me strong, firm, and steadfast. Let me be a living example of Your power, Your mercy, and Your love. Thank You, Father, for Your healing grace. In Jesus' name, I pray, Amen.

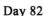

Day 82

Ah Lord God! Behold, thou hast made the heaven and the earth by thy great power and stretched out arm, and there is nothing too hard for thee. . . . "Behold, I am the Lord, the God of all flesh: is there any thing too hard for me?" (Jeremiah 32:17, 27 KJV)

Nothing is too hard for God, the great I AM. Nothing. Just by stretching out His arm and speaking the Word, God created the heavens and the earth. He is mighty and awesome – yet He knows your name and He cares about you personally. You. Right here. Right now.

"Behold, I am the Lord, the God of all flesh: is there anything too hard for me?" What is God saying? He tells you that He is the God of all flesh. He created your flesh; He designed your body; He breathed life into each cell; He created the pattern for each cell to function perfectly. Your flesh belongs to God, and it is special and important because it was designed as the temple of the Holy Spirit. If you abuse your temple, you show disrespect for the Holy Spirit. You succumb to the temptations of the evil one, and you set up an environment where disease can grow and flourish.

God wants you to know that He is the God of every aspect of your humanness; that includes not only your soul but also your body and your mind and your emotions. No matter what circumstances you find yourself in, there is nothing too difficult for God.

No matter how the evil one has affected your body, God is stronger and more powerful, and nothing is too hard for Him to overcome. If disease has taken hold in your body, it is not too hard for God to overcome it. If an accident has injured you, it is not too hard for God to overcome it.

God wants you to answer the question that He asks. "Is anything too hard for me?" What do you *really* believe?

Dear God, You ask me a question: "Is anything too hard for me?" You know the doubts I have in my heart. I wouldn't do some of the things I do if I truly believed that the answer could be "no" for my particular health condition. And I wouldn't have some of the fears I have. Just for today I choose to answer "No, Lord, nothing is too hard for You." And just for today I will bring every action I do into alignment with that belief. I ask for Your guidance; I will listen for Your instructions; and I will allow You to work Your healing wonders on me. In the name of Your Son, Jesus Christ, my Savior and Redeemer, I pray, Amen.

Day 83

. . . the God who gives life to the dead and calls things that are not as though they were. (Romans 4:17 NIV)

What does it mean to call things that are not as though they were? You start with the absence of something, and you speak that "missing something" until it is manifested. When you feel sick, it means that you have illness and disease in your body. What you are missing is health. So you use the principle Jesus taught of having the focused, concentrated faith of a mustard seed – and you speak health and wellness as though it *were* in your body.

Are you one of those people who says, "I call it like I see it"? If you do that with your health, then your health will always be just exactly the way you keep seeing it. If you declare yourself to be a cancer victim, then so it is and so it will be. If you declare yourself to be a diabetic, then so it is and so it will be. If you declare yourself to be disabled by a stroke, then so it is and so it will be.

As long as you are focused on the way "things are" and the way they appear to be, you are being deceived by satan that God's reality does not exist. God is the essence of "things unseen" rather than things seen.

Isn't speaking "what is not" just playing pretend and being foolish? Absolutely not. This is applying a fundamental principle of faith that is critical for your recovery. It requires you to become part of God's creative process, and it makes you a partner with God for your healing.

Along with speaking your health, you must ask God for His guidance. Is there something at the physical level that He wants you to do to participate in the healing process with Him? Pray and then be quiet so that you can hear God's voice clearly. You may be told to use herbs or you may be told to seek certain medical treatment or you may be told simply to receive your healing.

There are multitudes of options available, and God has a special path individually selected just for you so that your healing can be manifested. Go to your Heavenly Father. Ask believing that you have already received your healing. Let Him speak to you through the Holy Spirit and reveal your path to you.

Loving Father, sometimes I fall into the evil one's trap by continuing to voice my illness. Help me to stand on Your Holy Word and to see myself as You see me – whole and complete and healthy. Help me to speak Your truth. Guide me, Lord. Show me exactly what you want me to do so that I can manifest Your healing in my temple. In Jesus' name, I pray, Amen.

Day 84

One day as Jesus was standing by the Lake of Gennesaret, with the people crowding around him and listening to the word of God, he saw at the water's edge two boats, left there by the fishermen, who were washing their nets. He got into one of the boats, the one belonging to Simon, and asked him to put out a little from shore. . . . When he had finished speaking, he said to Simon, "Put out into deep water, and let down the nets for a catch." Simon answered, "Master, we've worked hard all night and haven't caught anything. But because you say so, I will let down the nets." When they had done so, they caught such a large number of fish that their nets began to break. So they signaled their partners in the other boat to come and help them, and they came and filled both boats so full that they began to sink. (Luke 5:1-7 NIV)

Because we do not understand the way things were done in Galilee, we miss the entire significance of this passage. Generally fish stayed around the rocks near shore, so fishing was done at night, near the shore, by using two boats which dragged a net between them. In this story Jesus tells Simon to do the exact opposite of the normal method – to go out in the daytime to deep water with one boat to catch fish. Look at the reply of Simon Peter to Jesus' suggestion. He tells Jesus that they have done it the way it was supposed to be done and they were still unsuccessful.

Nevertheless, Simon had three important characteristics. He had an open mind, he had faith in Jesus, and he had the willingness to follow the guidance he was given. Look at the results. So many fish were caught that they needed another boat and even then the catch was so huge that the boats began to sink under the weight of all the fish.

Are you willing to follow the example of this story with your life? Do you live in fear that you have to treat your illness according to "the way it is always done" or are you open and willing to hear the guidance of the Lord? God wants you to be well. Allow Him to speak to you and to reveal to you the way to your healing. It may be contrary to every method you have ever heard of – but, if it is God's path, be willing to act with the faith of Simon.

Wonderful Jehovah-rapha, too often I want to hold to the safety of old ways and old patterns. Open my ears so that I may hear Your voice clearly. Give me the courage to put my boat out into the deep water of faith and follow Your instructions for my healing. In Jesus' name, I pray, Amen.

Day 85

We remember the fish we ate in Egypt at no cost – also the cucumbers, melons, leeks, onion, and garlic. (Numbers 11:5 NIV)

Garlic is a marvelous food which has many powerful health benefits. A member of the onion family, garlic's pungent odor comes from its sulfur compounds, the most commonly known one being allicin.

Used in Biblical times as an antibiotic, garlic is still effective for that purpose today. It is a powerful stimulant to the immune system, and the various sulfur compounds that it contains are antagonistic to many types of microorganisms, including flu, colds, viruses, and bacteria. Its anti-viral, anti-bacterial, and anti-fungal action gives it several advantages over many antibiotics.

Throughout the world garlic has been used to combat intestinal infections, diarrhea, and diseases such as cholera and typhoid. When fighting an infection, people have learned to use small, frequently repeated amounts – either whole cloves of fresh garlic or hi-potency enteric-coated tablets. (Be careful not to select supplements which have had the allicin removed in order to be "odorless.")

Garlic has been used for centuries to lower high blood pressure. It improves cholesterol levels by raising HDL cholesterol and lowering LDL cholesterol. It has been used to help with cases of asthma and diabetes. In addition, it has been used to improve liver and gallbladder function. Garlic helps to remove mucus from the digestive and intestinal tract. It even has anti-cancer properties.

Studies are now showing that garlic can even help to improve your personality! People who eat garlic regularly have fewer mood swings and less anxiety, fatigue, and irritability.

Should you eat lots of garlic or take garlic preparations? Just because the list of benefits is long, don't assume that the answer is yes. Go in prayer and ask the Holy Spirit to reveal to you what you should do. And remember that the answer you receive is the answer for *today* and not the answer for the rest of your life.

Wonderful Jehovah-rapha, how grateful I am for the plants which You have provided in great abundance for my health and healing. Show me the best way that I can learn more about them and can use them wisely in the way You intended. Teach me, Lord. In Jesus' name, I pray, Amen.

And lest I should be exalted above measure through the abundance of the revelations, there was given to me a thorn in the flesh, the messenger of Satan to buffet me, lest I should be exalted above measure. (2 Corinthians 12:7 KJV)

Many people use these words of Paul as an argument that God not only does not always heal but that He also makes us sick. They believe Paul had eye trouble or some other ailment which God refused to heal.

The use of the word "thorn" as a figurative example of a problem occurs in the Bible in the Old Testament (i.e. in Numbers 33:55 and in Joshua 23:13). In this letter to the Corinthians, Paul uses it similarly, and he does not mean a literal physical illness or thing. Even today we refer to a problematic person as being a "thorn in our side."

Paul tells us exactly what the thorn is: it is a messenger of satan. It is a *personality* that is his problem, not a *thing* such as illness. The Greek word that Paul used is "angelos." In the Bible we find the word "angelos" 188 times. Seven times it is translated "messenger" and 181 times it is translated "angel." While some translations read that Paul asked God to take "it" (meaning the thorn) away from him, a translation by Weymouth says, " .. I besought the Lord to rid me of *him*." The thorn was one of satan's cohorts, coming at Paul again and again. The evil one does not want to leave the people of God alone. He will attack over and over. He seeks out the vulnerable places and tries to gain power. We have to put on the armor of the Lord and stand firm. Jesus rebuffed satan head on when satan came for Him.

The firmer you become in your faith and the more strongly you are willing to follow the Lord God Almighty, the more likely satan is to come after you. Even though he may send his messengers to harass you, they cannot succeed when you stand strong in the power of the Lord. Stand firm on God's Word which says, "My grace is sufficient for you, for my power is made perfect in weakness."

Almighty Heavenly Father, spread Your protective wings over me. I put on the Your armor and call upon Your name when the evil one tries to buffet me as he did Paul. Satan may try to come against me but I resist Him in Your name and in the name of Your Son Jesus Christ, who defeated Him fully for all of time. Your grace is sufficient for me and Your power is made perfect in my weakness. Thank You, Almighty Father, for strengthening me in Your service. In Jesus' name, I pray, Amen.

Day 87

This is the day which the Lord hath made; we will rejoice and be glad in it.
(Psalm 118:24 KJV)

Every day when you first open your eyes in the morning, say, "This is the day which the Lord has made. I will rejoice and be glad in it." Fill your soul with these words, and each cell in your body will receive the message, too.

Today is a gift. You can pick up the newspapers and read item after item from the front page to the back page about people for whom today did not come. Accept today as a precious treasure and say thank you.

What if you have felt sick for a long time? What if you are in discomfort or pain? What if the night has seemed very long and all the medical reports are grim and you really want an end to it all? When this is how you feel, "rejoicing and being glad in the day" seems beyond comprehension.

Your answers can be supplied only by God. Immerse yourself in the Holy Scriptures so that you can find faith to hold onto. "I have a plan for you and it is a plan for good." "I am the God who heals thee." "With God all things are possible."

Select the passages that speak to *you* and give you hope and purpose. Put them on a note card beside your bed and when you wake up in the morning, read each verse and then say, "God, I stand on your Word. I claim your healing and your purpose for my life. This is the day which You have made. I will rejoice and be glad in it." After you do this for a few days, you will be surprised at the difference you will begin to notice in yourself.

Spend time every day taking note of the things for which you can rejoice and be glad. No matter what your situation is, there are things worthy of thanksgiving. Focus on those. Rest in the Lord and praise His name.

Merciful God, there are times when I struggle and when I feel overwhelmed by my illness and by my situation. Give me courage, Lord, to see Your truth beyond the appearance that surrounds me. Fill me with Your strength and grace. Touch me with Your healing hand. Let me rise up every morning declaring, "This is the day the Lord God Almighty has made and I do rejoice in it." Thank You, God, for all Your many blessings in my life. In the name of Your Son, Jesus Christ, my Savior and my Redeemer, I pray, Amen.

Day 88

Look at the nations and watch – and be utterly amazed. For I am going to do something in your days that you would not believe, even if you were told. (Habakkuk 1:5 NIV)

What an astounding statement! Habakkuk has been complaining to God that everything around him looked really bad. There was violence and destruction, and there did not seem to be any justice. He calls out to God saying, "How long, O Lord, must I call for help, but You do not listen?"

When we are dealing with illness and disease, how often do we have the same feelings? Things within us don't seem to be looking good. There is a pain here and a pain there, a problem here, a problem there. One may seem to improve and two other problems pop up to take their place. The list goes on and on.

Like Habakkuk, we call out, "How long, O Lord, must I call for help? Are you there? Are you listening?" Deep inside, we are also saying, "I'm afraid. I'm so afraid."

Look at God's response. "Look and watch. And be utterly amazed. For I am going to do something in your days that you would not believe, even if you were told." Everything comes down to faith, trust, belief. God is willing to heal us. God wants us to be well. We have to absorb that belief into our innermost being so that God can work His mighty power and "utterly amaze us."

"You wouldn't believe it even if I told you," God told Habakkuk. But He did tell you! He sent His Son Jesus Christ not only to tell you but also to bear your sins and your infirmities on the Cross. God still has the same desire to save you and to "utterly amaze you" with His awesome healing hand. It has been done. You are redeemed. Accept the sacrificial act of Your Savior Christ Jesus and believe that "by His stripes You are healed."

O, Lord, how long must I call for help? There are times when I don't think You are listening. There are times when what is happening to my body seems so unfair. I know that these are times when the evil one is in control and is telling me lies. You are Jehovah-rapha. You have the power to utterly amaze me with Your mighty works. I believe, God; help my unbelief. Send Your Holy Spirit to guide me and to keep me on the path You would have me walk. In the name of Your Son Christ Jesus, my Redeemer, I pray, Amen.

Day 89 ✓

My son, attend to my words; incline thine ear unto my sayings. Let them not depart from thine eyes; keep them in the midst of thine heart. For they are life unto those that find them, and health to all their flesh. (Proverbs 4:20-22 KJV)

God's prescription for healing is this: if you want to be healed and to stay healed, listen to My Words and integrate them in the deepest part of your heart and soul. Then you will have health to all your flesh.

James warns us not to be "double-minded" by believing a little and doubting a lot. Here in Proverbs we are told essentially the same thing. God wants one hundred percent focus on Him. If we have our eyes on our symptoms most of the time, we are not looking at the Almighty. God's Word consistently guides us to life; our symptoms (which are manifestations of the handiwork of the evil one) lead us to death. We can't look at these two destinations at the same time.

Are there any exceptions listed? Are there any qualifications given? Does it say health to all their flesh – except, of course, for incurable diseases? Maybe not for brain cancer. Or multiple sclerosis. Or Alzheimer's disease. There are no exceptions listed or even suggested. God's Word plainly says, "health to *all* their flesh."

And look at the interesting choice of words about the connection between God's Word and life. *To those who find them,* God's Words are life. To those who *find* them. God always requires that we look for Him, that we choose Him. He is always available, never hiding.

God never forces us to believe in Him or to follow Him or to be obedient to Him. He simply says, "Here I am. I am the beginning and the end. All power is mine. With Me nothing is impossible."

So we must seek after the Lord. We are told to look for Him in the Holy Scriptures and to integrate His Word into our hearts and our total being so that we are filled with faith in Him. When that happens, there is no room for the seeds of the evil one to grow, there is no room for doubt, and there is no room for illness. Look on the Lord and you shall live.

Almighty God, there have been many times when I have allowed my focus to wander from Your Word, and I have allowed doubt to reside in the midst of my heart. I seek You now, God, fully and completely. You promise that those who look steadfastly on You will find health for all their flesh. Thank You, God, for healing me. In the name of Your Son, Jesus Christ, I pray, Amen.

As Jesus was on his way, the crowds almost crushed him. And a woman was there who had been subject to bleeding for twelve years, but no one could heal her. She came up behind him and touched the edge of his cloak, and immediately her bleeding stopped. "Who touched me?" Jesus asked. When they all denied it, Peter said, "Master, the people are crowding and pressing against you." But Jesus said, "Someone touched me; I know that power has gone out from me." (Luke 8:42-46 NIV)

This passage from God's Word compels us to take a look at the subject of energy. What is it? What place does it have in our being? And what place does it have in our healing? Sometimes people are afraid to discuss the subject of energy because they think that it is spooky or evil. Like everything else that is part of creation, it can be used for good or for evil – but it itself was born of God and was intended to be used for good.

Jesus was very aware of Divine energy. Even though Jesus was swarmed by mobs of people, He knew when a woman touched the hem of His garment with the belief that she would be healed. He felt His energy flow out to her. No one admitted at first to touching Him, and Peter even tried to convince Jesus that no one in particular had done anything but that He was just jostled by all the crowds. However, Jesus knew what He had felt.

Everything that God created has its own Divine energy. Find a tree and hug it. Allow yourself to feel the energy of the tree. It can be very healing to connect with God's creation in this way. Go to a natural area – beach, woods, meadow – and feel the energy in the air – how powerful and awesome. Reach down and pick up a stone or even some dirt. Hold it in the palm of your hand and feel its energy resonate in you.

Divine energy that God created is vital to your health. However, there is energy that satan has claimed, and it will mislead and destroy you. So make sure that you connect only to the energy that is God's. Call upon the Holy Spirit to fill you and guide you always. Ask for God's healing energy to transform you.

Almighty God, I awaken to experience Your Divine energy. Help me to be aware of Your Holy energy that flows within me and through every cell of my body. Help me connect to Your Divine energy which heals and restores me at every level of my being. Send Your Holy Spirit to fill me with this Godly energy. Help me to use it to Your glory. In the name of Your Son, Jesus Christ, I pray, Amen.

Day 91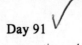

But the fruit of the Spirit is love, joy, peace, patience, kindness, goodness, faithfulness, gentleness and self-control. (Galatians 5:22-23 NIV)

While you need to be aware of your sins and of the ways you get out of alignment with God, it is more beneficial to keep your focus and attention on those things which bring you *into* alignment with God. These are the positive forces that make you strong spiritually, mentally, and physically and that fortify your shield of protection from the evil one.

Paul lists the fruit of the Spirit – love, joy, peace, patience, kindness, goodness, faithfulness, gentleness, and self-control. That is quite a list. When you feel sick, you need particularly to cultivate the fruits of positive qualities in your life and apply them not only to the people around you but also to yourself.

We often think it is selfish to be kind and gentle to ourselves. Yet Jesus plainly told us to love our neighbors *as ourselves.* Not more than or less than – but the same as. Frequently, one of the contributing causes to our illness has been our failure to treat ourselves lovingly and caringly. Applying the fruit of the Spirit is being self-*full*, not self-*ish.* It is part of fulfilling God's plan for us.

On this list of virtues one of the major elements needed in recovery is self-control. God requires that you be a partner in your healing. That means that you need to be willing to make changes where you have gone astray. Do you want to be healed enough to do your own part? Or are you wishing to be well so that you can keep doing what you have always been doing?

Doing what you did got you where you are. Be willing to make changes in your prayer and meditation time, in your diet, in your physical activity level, and in your thinking patterns. Wellness isn't just the absence of disease. It is a way of being. It is a way of living that allows God to work His will for you.

The fruits of the Spirit issue from a heart dedicated to the Lord. Turn every aspect of your life over to Him. Glorify Him in every action.

Wonderful Lord God Almighty, help me to stay focused on the fruits of the Spirit. Keep my eyes trained on You. Help me to fulfill Your will and Your purpose for me and to cultivate love, joy, peace, patience, kindness, goodness, faithfulness, gentleness and self-control. In the name of Your Son, Jesus Christ, my Savior and my Redeemer, I pray, Amen.

Day 92

You are my friends if you do what I command. I no longer call you servants, because a servant does not know his master's business. Instead, I have called you friends, for everything that I learned from my Father I have made known to you. You did not choose me, but I chose you and appointed you to go and bear fruit – fruit that will last. Then the Father will give you whatever you ask in my name. This is my command: Love each other. (John 15:14-17 NIV).

Repeatedly, Jesus exhorts us to do what He commands us to do. Notice that He uses the word "command." He does not tell us that He is making suggestions or offering ideas for us to consider. He tells us that what He is saying is part of the "musts" of life. You *must* do what I am telling you if you want the result I promise, He declares. You *have to* do it this way. There are definite strings to the gift that is offered.

What is the command? Love. We think we love others and we know we feel love for certain people. But love as a *feeling* is weak because love is *action*. It comes to life in what we *do*.

Take some time to make an accounting of the ways that you act your love. Set aside a few minutes at the end of the day to list five ways that you put your love in action during the day. Maybe you prepared dinner for your family with a song in your heart and love flowing into the food – instead of with complaints and pressure and unhappiness. Maybe you wrote a "thinking of you" card that you'd been putting off for days. Maybe you spent some extra time brushing your pet and giving him attention.

If we want to fulfill our purpose, we have to get in the love business. Remember the incident when at the age of 12 Jesus had gotten separated from His earthly parents in Jerusalem and was found teaching in the synagogue? He told Mary and Joseph that He had to be about His Father's business.

Here He tells us that we are now in the Father's business as well. Jesus has chosen us and He has told us everything we need to know. It is up to us to respond to the call.

Gracious Father, thank You for the love You shower on me every minute of every day. I want to be about Your business of spreading the Word of Your love and of being a living example of Your love to all who see me. Let me be a particular example for others as I walk the path of healing You have set before me. In the name of Your Son, Jesus Christ, Amen.

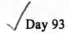

Day 93

There is no fear in love; but perfect love casteth out fear: because fear hath torment. He that feareth is not made perfect in love. (1 John 4:18 KJV)

There is no fear in love. When we absorb God's love into the depths of our being, we will be at peace. We all seem to strive for this, but few seem to attain it. Why is this so?

Fear is one of the primary tools of satan. He takes every opportunity to remind us of our fears and to keep us focused on them. We even learn to love our fears. And sometimes we become addicted to them. Being fearful allows us to seek reassurance from our family and friends over and over again.

This is especially true when the issues are health issues. Our symptoms can change every day or every week so there is always something new to be fearful about. Fear sucks us in and keeps us just where satan wants us. We are no longer focused on God's Word; we are no longer living in God's love; we are no longer trusting in God's will for our total redemption – soul and body.

To live in fear is a choice and to live in love is a choice. God allows us the free will to decide whether to choose love over fear. He extends His love to us every minute of every day and wants us to have it. His love is so boundless that He sent His Son for our salvation and healing.

Each time you feel fear about your health, stand firm on the Word of God. "I am the God who heals you." "By His stripes I am healed." "Himself took my infirmities and bore my sicknesses." "He healed them all." "If I have faith as a grain of mustard seed, I shall say to this mountain, 'move,' and it shall move. Nothing shall be impossible to me." "By faith in the name of Jesus, I am made strong." "He sent His Word and healed me."

Over and over again, speak the Word. Enforce it on every cell, tissue, gland, and organ of your body. Listen for guidance; trust; believe; and accept God's love with grateful thanks.

Dear Heavenly Father, surround me and enfold me in the perfect safety of Your love. Release me from the bondage of fear, and cleanse me of all patterns that keep me trapped in worry and anxiety. Deliver me from the evil one, Lord. I choose You, Your love, and Your healing. I choose to be well. I enforce Your Word on every cell in my body, and I ask that You fill every part of my temple with Your healing love. Stay by my side, Lord. Hold me in Your loving arms. In Jesus' name, I pray, Amen.

Day 94

Now for some time a man named Simon had practiced sorcery in the city and amazed all the people of Samaria. He boasted that he was someone great, and all the people, both high and low, gave him their attention and exclaimed, "This man is the divine power known as the Great Power." They followed him because he had amazed them for a long time with his magic. But when they believed Philip as he preached the good news of the kingdom of God and the name of Jesus Christ, they were baptized, both men and women. Simon himself believed and was baptized. And he followed Philip everywhere, astonished by the great signs and miracles he saw. When the apostles in Jerusalem heard that Samaria had accepted the word of God, they sent Peter and John to them. When they arrived, they prayed for them that they might receive the Holy Spirit, because the Holy Spirit had not yet come upon any of them; they had simply been baptized into the name of the Lord Jesus. Then Peter and John placed their hands on them, and they received the Holy Spirit. When Simon saw that the Spirit was given at the laying on of the apostles' hands, he offered them money and said, "Give me also this ability so that everyone on whom I lay my hands may receive the Holy Spirit." Peter answered: "May your money perish with you, because you thought you could buy the gift of God with money! You have no part or share in this ministry, because your heart is not right before God. Repent of this wickedness and pray to the Lord." (Acts 8:9-22 NIV)

The laying on of hands to heal the sick was taught to us by Jesus Christ. He specifically told us to do it, and in His last words before His ascension, He declared that it would be a sign of those who followed Him. It is real, it is important, and it is a gift from the Father.

Even though Simon was baptized and supposedly gave up sorcery, he hadn't gotten the message. He was a performer at heart and wanted to use the act of laying on of hands to dazzle others. Peter told him emphatically that such a display was from satan and not from God.

Today we still have some people who appear to use laying on of hands when, in fact, they are putting on a performance. Because such frauds exist, do not reject the laying on of hands as a valid means of healing. God sent the Holy Spirit as our Comforter. Stay grounded in God's truth, seek His counsel, and you will know whom to trust.

Wonderful Jehovah-rapha, thank You for sending the Holy Spirit. If You wish me to receive the laying on of hands, guide me to the right person. In the name of Your Son, Jesus Christ, my Savior and my Redeemer, Amen.

As you go, preach this message: "The kingdom of heaven is near." Heal the sick, raise the dead, cleanse those who have leprosy, drive out demons. Freely you have received, freely give. (Matthew 10:7-8 NIV)

In this passage of Holy Scripture Jesus gives detailed instructions to His disciples as He sends them out among the people.

What does He tell them to do? To preach the gospel and to heal the people. It is quite amazing to see how often and how consistently Jesus establishes a dual mission for His followers – to preach and to heal. There is never one without the other.

Jesus' disciples were ordinary people – several fishermen and even a tax collector. There were no doctors or people with medical training among them. Yet Jesus sent them out to do extraordinary things such as healing the sick, raising the dead, cleansing those who have leprosy, and driving out demons.

Jesus recognized that sickness came from the devil. He specifically instructed his followers to drive out demons. He wasn't talking just about people who were "out of their minds" or what we would today consider to be mentally ill. He was also referring to people who had been attacked by satan with illness in their bodies. The disciples were to throw the demons out and to make the people completely whole.

Imagine that you are in a village and see two men coming. They tell you, "The kingdom of heaven is near." They reach out, touch you, and heal you of your illness. And later you see Jesus walking up the same road. Run to Him, singing your song of praise, thanksgiving, and worship.

Jesus is Your Lord, Your Healer, Your Savior. It is His blood that has washed your soul clean and has healed every cell in your body.

Almighty God, I rejoice that You sent Your Son to save me and to heal me. Thank You for Your Holy Word. I need it so much, God. I need to see in passage after passage after passage that Your Son Jesus Christ sent ordinary people out with the mission to preach and to heal. I feel great strength in knowing that physical healing is important to You, that MY physical healing is important to You. O, God, thank You for healing me. Show me everything You want me to do to help this healing manifest fully in my body. In the name of Your Son Jesus Christ, my Savior and my Redeemer, I pray, Amen.

Day 96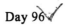

And whatever you do, whether in word or deed, do it all in the name of the Lord Jesus, giving thanks to God the Father through him. (Colossians 3:17 NIV)

Unless your recovery comes as an instantaneous healing from the Lord, there will be many actions you will probably take as your part in your partnership with God. There will be many temptations to stop following your program and to discontinue it.

The evil one wants to sabotage your healing and will throw up obstacle after obstacle to your recovery program. Life itself will get in the way. Friends and family will get in the way. How do you maintain the self-discipline to do what you need to do?

Dedicate every small action in following God's program for your healing to Him and to His Son Christ Jesus. "Whatever you do, do it all in the name of the Lord Jesus, giving thanks to God the Father through Him." That makes every step you take a prayer. Every herb you swallow for the healing of your liver is a prayer. Every step in a walk you take for the strengthening of your heart is a prayer. Every essential oil you apply for the healing of your joints is a prayer. Every weight you lift for the strengthening of your bones is a prayer. Every eyewash you use for the recovery of your sight is a prayer.

Even though the act itself is a prayer, pray while you are doing whatever you are doing. Thank God over and over again for your healing. Praise Him. Glorify Him. You may find that you begin to look forward to tasks that were once a chore. You sing and hum and pray while you are doing them, and they don't seem to take as long. You realize that you are bringing God's healing energy into your body and are vitalized by it.

A prayer is no longer just something you say; it is living praise to God as you carry out His will in your life.

Wonderful Jehovah-rapha, whatever I do, whether in word or deed, I do it all in the name of the Lord Jesus. I give thanks to You, Heavenly Father, and I am so grateful for Your constant love and guidance. I am awed by the sacrifice that was made for me on the Cross. My sins and all my infirmities were overcome there. I am saved. I am redeemed. I am healed. Show me my path for healing, Lord. I will do exactly as You instruct me, and I take every step in the name of Christ Jesus. Your will be done on earth as it is in heaven. I am Your instrument in Your service. In humble gratitude I pray in Jesus' name. Amen.

A cheerful look brings joy to the heart, and good news gives health to the bones. (Proverbs 15:30 NIV)

Laughter heals. Smiling heals. Joy heals. It is almost impossible to recover from illness if you spend all your time bemoaning your aches and pains and making every detail of the recovery process a chore and a burden. Yes, there is a time for serious attention to the steps you must take. But overall, you must learn to lighten up and to approach each day with cheerfulness and with joy in your heart.

We focus so much on the seriousness of Jesus, yet listen to these words: "I have told you this so that my joy may be in you and that your joy may be complete" (John 15:11). Jesus speaks of joy – His joy and our joy.

Just for a moment close your eyes and imagine Jesus standing before you. See Him step close and then see His eyes light up with delight. His mouth turns up into a big smile and then He breaks out into laughter. He speaks your name and says, "Share my joy. Laugh with me." And He laughs some more.

Smile. Laugh. Join Jesus in laughter. Throw your arms up into the air, and skip around like a little child for no reason other than the most glorious one of all – you are loved with an everlasting love by the Ever Faithful Father. Take your most troublesome problems and place them in a bubble. Release the bubble into the air and as it rises heavenward, laugh. Let your laughter grow and grow until the bubble pops.

How important it is to have a heart filled with joy! "This is the day the Lord has made. Let us rejoice and be glad in it" (Psalm 118:24). Sing your praise! Laugh your praise! Smile your praise! What better witness to others can you give than to show them your life filled with joy and gratitude for your loving God? There is no better testament.

When you know you are walking according to God's directions, you have not only peace in your soul but you also have laughter in your spirit and a smile on your face.

Wonderful Jehovah-rapha, it is Your joy that fills me, and it is Your good news that gives health to my bones. I have so many blessings to rejoice over. My cup truly runneth over. You are my mighty Protector and Healer. I sing and dance before You, and I seek to radiate to all who see me the joy of my faith and trust in You. Thank You, Father, for loving me, for saving me, and for healing me. In the name of Your Son, Jesus Christ, I pray, Amen.

He made him ride on the heights of the land and fed him with the fruit of the fields. He nourished him with honey from the rock, and with oil from the flinty crag, with curds and milk from herd and flock and with fattened lambs and goats, with choice rams of Bashan and the finest kernels of wheat. (Deuteronomy 32:13-14 NIV)

Also the food I provided for you – the fine flour, olive oil and honey I gave you to eat – you offered as fragrant incense before them. (Ezekiel 16:19 NIV)

For the Lord your God is bringing you into a good land – a land with streams and pools of water, with springs flowing in the valleys and hills; a land with wheat and barley, vines and fig trees, pomegranates, olive oil and honey; a land where bread will not be scarce and you will lack nothing. (Deuteronomy 8:7-9 NIV)

The references to olive oil as a good thing and as a gift of God appear over and over again in the Holy Scriptures. It is interesting that those people who consume rather large amounts of olive oil have low incidences of heart disease.

Since it is a versatile oil, it is useful both as a cooking oil and as a dressing on salads. It contains monounsaturated fats, which we now categorize as a "good" fat because it is used so beneficially in the human body. In addition to its helpful effect in preventing heart disease, it also contains substances such as steric and oleic acid, which may help to prevent breast cancer.

Olive oil can also be used to help in the recovery from particular ailments. Historically, some people have rubbed it nightly over their liver for detoxification. For centuries, people have flushed gallstones from their body by following a procedure involving the drinking of a mixture of olive oil and lemon juice.

The Holy Scriptures provide a wealth of information for guidelines for healthy living. Take the time to study them and to learn.

Wonderful Jehovah-rapha, I read Your Word but often I miss much of Your advice for healthy living. Today I am taking a new look at olive oil. Tell me clearly if You want me to incorporate it into my diet. If You do, I will spend some time deciding how I can best follow Your guidance. I understand that, if I make wiser choices in my foods, my health will improve. In the name of Your Son, Jesus Christ, I pray, Amen.

Day 99

When Jesus had finished saying all this in the hearing of the people, he entered Capernaum. There a centurion's servant, whom his master valued highly, was sick and about to die. The centurion heard of Jesus and sent some elders of the Jews to him, asking him to come and heal his servant. When they came to Jesus, they pleaded earnestly with him, "This man deserves to have you do this, because he loves our nation and has built our synagogue." So Jesus went with them. He was not far from the house when the centurion sent friends to say to him: "Lord, don't trouble yourself, for I do not deserve to have you come under my roof. That is why I did not even consider myself worthy to come to you. But say the word, and my servant will be healed. For I myself am a man under authority, with soldiers under me. I tell this one, 'Go,' and he goes; and that one, 'Come,' and he comes. I say to my servant, 'Do this,' and he does it." When Jesus heard this, he was amazed at him, and turning to the crowd following him, he said, "I tell you, I have not found such great faith even in Israel." Then the men who had been sent returned to the house and found the servant well. (Luke 7:1-10 NIV)

In the time of Jesus the Romans occupied Palestine, and the soldiers were generally brutal, causing much enmity between the Romans and the Jews. The Roman centurion in this story diplomatically contacts Jesus by sending Jewish elders with the message, "Just say the word that my servant be healed and I know it will be done. I believe your power has no limits, not even with regard to distance. So you don't even need to come. Just say the word."

Rarely do the Scriptures report that Jesus was surprised, but here we read that "Jesus was amazed." Why? Because the centurion's actions revealed two fundamental beliefs – first, that Jesus had the power to heal his servant, and, second, that Jesus' power was not limited in space. The centurion trusted that all that was necessary was for Jesus to speak the word of healing and it would be done.

Examine your own heart. Be careful where you place your trust. Do you have the centurion's kind of deep and total faith in the healing power of Jesus Christ? Stand on God's Word and the healing authority of Jesus. Make sure that the bedrock of your belief is Your Resurrected Lord.

Almighty God, strengthen me as I deepen my faith. I declare my belief in Your Son and I stand on Your Word. Thank you for healing me and for showing me the path to my recovery. In Jesus' name, I pray, Amen.

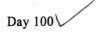

But [Satan is coming and] I do as the Father has commanded Me, so that the world may know (be convinced) that I love the Father and that I do only what the Father has instructed Me to do. [I act in full agreement with His orders.] (John 14:31 AMP)

Jesus tells us that every single thing that He does carries out an instruction of God. "I love the Father and . . . do *only* what the Father has instructed Me to do." The Amplified Bible explains that Jesus is "acting in full agreement with God's orders." Thus, the Holy Scriptures are clear that Jesus always manifested the perfect will of God.

Because Jesus walked with God and fulfilled His will, satan tried to influence Him and to separate Him from God. However, satan never succeeded with any of his attacks. It is interesting to note that Jesus suffered every trial and tribulation that we do except illness. There is no record of His ever being sick. Why? Because Jesus never allowed satan to enter the temple of His soul or of His body. Satan could attack from the *outside* but Jesus never allowed him to attack from *within*.

Be clear in your mind and heart that Jesus did *only* the will of God. Also be clear in your mind and heart that Jesus did *only* those things which He was commanded and instructed.

Consider the fact that Jesus healed *everyone* who received Him. The Scripture says it over and over and over again. He healed them *all*. He never told anyone that God wanted that person to remain sick. Now you must decide if you believe that Jesus' actions were only for the people of Galilee two thousand years ago – or if they apply to you right now in the twenty-first century.

Jesus knew His mission of salvation – healing the spirits and bodies of God's beloved children. God grieved when we lost the Garden so He sent His Son to redeem us. Through Jesus our sins are washed away and by His stripes we are healed. Open your heart to allow God's will for your healing to be manifested in your body.

Dear God, thank You for sending Your Son Jesus Christ to show me the way. I believe that everything that He did was according to Your will, Your commandment, and Your instruction. Your Son healed everyone who received Him. I receive Jesus Christ into my heart, my soul, and my body. I claim His healing now as Your will for me. Instruct me and guide me so that I may always act in accordance with Your Divine plan for my life. In the name of Jesus Christ, I pray, Amen.

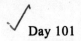

Day 101

"In those days, at that time," declares the Lord, "the people of Israel and the people of Judah together will go in tears to seek the Lord their God. They will ask the way to Zion and turn their faces toward it. They will come and bind themselves to the Lord in an everlasting covenant that will not be forgotten." (Jeremiah 50:4-5 NIV)

Sometimes we feel so overcome that we want to cry. A sense of despair fills us because we feel our fatigue and "unwellness" so deeply. When those times come, let the tears flow. Tears themselves can be healing if they are part of an honest outpouring of our sorrow. It is healthy to allow it to be expressed.

Notice, however, that this Scripture in Jeremiah focuses on a complete *process.* Many people stay stuck in their pain, tears, and sorrow and weep endlessly. But here we are shown the way to move through our valleys of despair.

In your tears, *seek the Lord,* as we are told in Jeremiah. No one knows your wounds better than God does. Offer your tears to God, and ask that they wash away emotions you have carried within your soul and within the very cells of your body.

Next *ask the way* and *turn your face* toward your goal. Keep your eyes on God and on His Son, Jesus Christ. Visualize Jesus as He heals all who receive Him, and visualize His healing *you*. Visualize the Divine light of God filling every cell in your body, and see each one living and functioning in a healthy manner.

Then *bind yourself to the Lord in an everlasting covenant.* God has declared His Word – "I am the God who heals you." Accept this covenant. Bind yourself to it. Let nothing separate you from God's love and God's will for you in your life.

Almighty God, today I weep. You know my heart, O God, and you know I am feeling hopeless and frightened. For a little while I have gotten lost and have strayed from Your path for me. I offer my tears to You, O God. Cleanse me. Cleanse my soul. Cleanse my body. I ask the way, O Lord God, and I turn my face toward the path You have laid out for me. I bind myself to You, Great Jehovah-rapha. Thank you for Your Son, Jesus Christ, who atoned for my sins and bore my sicknesses on the Cross. Wipe my tears, O Lord, and hold me in Your loving care. With grateful thanks I pray, in Jesus' name, Amen.

Day 102

Do not conform any longer to the pattern of this world, but be transformed by the renewing of your mind. (Romans 12:2 NIV)

You are healed through transformation of the spirit which changes the thoughts and attitudes of your mind. When you receive healing in your spirit and mind, then healing in your body will manifest itself.

The pattern of the world supports little true healing. We are flooded with advertisements for drugs which are, in fact, regulated poisons designed to eliminate symptoms rather than to heal the root cause of illness. We are encouraged to have body parts removed rather than to cleanse and nourish them so that they may recover their normal function. We are enticed with a myriad of "instant" remedies. All these patterns of the world seduce us into accepting the temporary appearance of healing instead of true healing.

God wants us to be healthy. Renew your mind by reading the Scriptures to see what God says about good health. Health is rarely supported by the patterns of the world, which looks for easy answers that do not require any change in your food, way of living, or your thoughts. God requires your complete attention and your complete commitment. When you renew your mind, you let go of your childish desire to do everything you used to do and still be healthy. That is what produced an environment in your body in which disease could live in the first place.

Through renewal, you accept responsibility for your part in creating an environment for illness to flourish – and you are transformed. Through renewal, you make the commitment to follow healthy living principles – and you are transformed. Through renewal, you change your thoughts to ones which support only recovery and health – and you are transformed. Through renewal, you praise God for healing you even if you do not see its manifestation in your body yet – and you are transformed.

Gracious, loving Lord, I confess that I have focused too long on the patterns of this world and my spirit, mind, and body have paid a heavy price for it. I no longer want satan to run my life, God, so I bind him as You have instructed me. I want You in control, Heavenly Father. Create in me a clean heart, a new heart. Transform me, God, into the person You want me to be. I am willing to give up blindly following the patterns of the world. Show me Your path for my healing and I will follow it. In the name of Your Son Jesus, I pray, Amen.

*I will take sickness away from the midst of thee. . . . the number of days I will fulfill.
(Exodus 23:25-26 KJV)*

God's promises are our strength. They are stars to guide us through the darkness of our confusion. They give us hope when we feel defeated and they give us strength when we feel weak. In this verse in Exodus God proclaims again that He is Jehovah-rapha, the God who heals you, when He says, "I will take sickness away from the midst of thee."

Make this promise of God a reality for yourself. To do that, first, visualize your illness. Take a moment to itemize your symptoms and all the difficulties that your illness causes you. Experience the emotional drain of the sickness and feel the fatigue within.

Now come before the Lord God Almighty. Hear Him say to you, "I will take sickness away from the midst of you." Repeat this verse of Holy Scripture aloud three times. Enforce the Word on your body and visualize every cell in your body functioning normally. Visualize every organ functioning according to God's design. Visualize yourself being whole, well, and healthy. Feel Divine energy fill you. Smile. Laugh. Allow joy to surround you and then penetrate deeply within.

Hold this vision of health and well-being. Think health. See health. Live health. Take the steps you need to take in the natural world to support your health, which will likely include using some of God's own remedies for your healing such as essential oils and herbs. Let God make that decision for you, and be bold enough to follow His direction. Allow God to work His healing wonders in your life.

God intends for you to fulfill the number of your days. He didn't want Adam to be robbed of the Garden by satan, and He doesn't want you to be robbed of a long life by actions of the evil one. Tell satan he can't have you because you have already been bought by the blood of Jesus Christ. Believe that God intends for you to live a long life as a glorious witness for Him.

Mighty Jehovah-rapha, You have proclaimed that You will take away sickness from my midst. You have promised that You will fulfill the number of my days. Thank You, God. There are times when I succumb to doubt. I put those doubts at Your feet, God. I know they didn't come from You, so I give them to You to cleanse and remove. You are The Great Physician, Lord, and nothing is beyond Your power. In Jesus' name, I pray, Amen.

Day 104

Bless the Lord, O my soul, O Lord my God, thou art very great; thou art clothed with honour and majesty. Who coverest thyself with light as with a garment: who stretchest out the heavens like a curtain. (Psalm 104:1-2 KJV)

The Psalms always lift us and reveal God's glory to us in the most beautiful way. Here we are given a vivid depiction of God, being clothed with honor and majesty, being covered with light as a garment, and stretching out the heavens like a curtain.

Isn't it a wonderful picture to visualize God being covered with light as a garment? The first thing that God created was light. Both physical earthly light and Divine spiritual light are crucial to our health. Jesus said, "I am the light of the world." We are told, "Let your light so shine . . . " When a person is filled with the light of Christ, their radiance is seen by everyone around them.

Close your eyes and visualize God's holy light streaming down from the heavens and coming into your head. See God's light flowing all the way down to your toes and penetrating into each cell of your body. Focus on the organs and areas in your body which are in the most need of healing. See God's light coming in a clear beam straight from heaven to those parts of your body.

Consciously relax and open up those cells to the Divine light. Some people like to visualize little hearts in the beam of light, symbolizing God's eternal love for them. Other people see little stars. As the light comes into you, visualize the little hearts or stars – or whatever you have selected – as remaining in each cell and continuing to emit God's holy love and healing you every minute of the day and night.

Doing this visualization every day accelerates your healing process because it intensifies your sense of partnership with Jehovah-rapha. Integrating healthy habits into your life focuses your intention and empowers the healing forces within you.

If you can do this meditative exercise while you are sitting, standing, or lying in the light of the sun, so much the better. Set aside some time every day for it, and rejoice in the healing that flows within your body.

Lord God Almighty, You are the God of the heavens and the earth. You are the God of light. Fill me with Your most Holy light, O Lord. Fill my soul with the light of Your love. Fill every cell of my body with the light of Your healing power. In the name of Your Son, Jesus Christ, my Savior and Redeemer, who is the Light of the world, I pray, Amen.

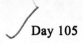

In righteousness you will be established: Tyranny will be far from you; you will have nothing to fear. Terror will be far removed; it will not come near you. If anyone does attack you, it will not be my doing; whoever attacks you will surrender to you. (Isaiah 54:14-15 NIV)

Be established in righteousness. Faith and acting on your faith will keep you from succumbing to terror and fear.

Isaiah makes it plain that attacks against you do not come from God. Attacks on your health do not come from God. Attacks on your health come from the father of lies, from satan. Satan may attack you outright or he may convince you to do foolish things that cause you to attack and destroy yourself.

What you must keep in your mind is that it is written, "If anyone does attack you, it will not be my doing." Don't point the finger of blame at God. If you get cancer, don't blame God. If you have a heart attack, don't blame God. It is not His doing. However, He is forever merciful, and, if you truly want recovery and are willing to do everything He tells you, He is the God who will heal you.

God sent His Son to liberate us from the evil one who attacks us. It is written, "God anointed Jesus of Nazareth with the Holy Spirit and power, and . . . he went around doing good and *healing all who were under the power of the devil,* because God was with him." Whoever attacks us must surrender to us since satan must leave in the presence of Jesus Christ.

God knows the emotions that you feel when you feel sick and have been injured. He knows the terror. He knows the fear. He knows the panic. He has provided the way out. Claim the authority of the Lord Jesus Christ. Do as He commanded.

Give thanks without ceasing that you are healed in the name of Jesus. Ask the Holy Spirit to give you revelation knowledge of any steps you are to take today for your recovery.

Merciful God, there are times when I am overwhelmed by the attack of the evil one. I know that this attack is not Your doing. Remove my fear, God. Help me to stand on Your Word and to follow the commands of Your Son Jesus Christ. When I take the time to pray and to allow the love of Christ to fill me, I feel great peace, comfort, and protection. I know then that satan must retreat. I give grateful thanks that You sent Your Son, Jesus Christ to bear my sins and my infirmities on the Cross. Thank You, Father. In Jesus' name, I pray, Amen.

Day 106

Elijah went before the people and said, "How long will you waver between two opinions? If the Lord is God, follow him; but if Baal is God, follow him." (1 Kings 18:21 NIV)

This is a fascinating question. "How long will you waver between two opinions?" Only one of them is from the true God, the One and Only Most High Lord God Almighty.

When you feel sick, you are given many opinions. Some come from family and friends, some come from natural health professionals, but most come from the medical profession. Even though these ideas are usually presented as facts, don't forget that they are really opinions. This is illustrated if you choose to see a second doctor – which is called seeking a second "opinion."

Why is this important to understand? Because the opinion that matters most is the opinion of God Almighty. For medical problems most people go to the doctor, get a medical opinion, follow it, and see what happens. For many the first time they call on God is just before they undergo treatment or surgery, asking for God's help. Yet they never asked God whether they should have had that treatment or surgery in the first place. Few go to God in prayer in every step along the way – from the first decision to the last. When God's opinion is not sought at *every* step, we are wide open for satan to slip in and begin working his destruction against us. Usually it is only after treatments fail to cure us, treatments create other health problems, or we are sent home to die that we turn fully to God.

It is God's will for you to be well. Medical treatment may be part of God's plan for your healing. But you will never know if you elevate medical authority to be equal with God's. Do not waver between two opinions. Go to God first and at every step along the way. Ask Him to speak to you. Ask the Holy Spirit to fill you clearly with God's truth so that you will know what actions to take at the physical level to complement God's own healing grace.

Great Jehovah-rapha, You are my ultimate authority. It is Your opinion which I seek. I know Your will for me, which is that I be well. I want every suggestion I follow to be in accordance with Your will and Your guidance. I vow to ask You at every step of the way from now on. I will not be divided any longer. Thank You, God for healing me. In Jesus' name, I pray, Amen.

Day 107

I will meditate on all your works and consider all your mighty deeds. (Psalm 77:12 NIV)

Praise the Lord, O my soul; all my inmost being, praise his holy name. Praise the Lord, O my soul, and forget not all his benefits – who forgives all your sins and heals all your diseases, who redeems your life from the pit and crowns you with love and compassion, who satisfies your desires with good things so that your youth is renewed like the eagle's. (Psalm 103:1-5 NIV)

What wise advice to meditate on all the mighty works of the Lord in your life! You are exhorted to "forget not all his benefits." Take a moment to assess your words and thoughts yesterday. Did you spend more time praising God for His mighty deeds in your behalf – or did you spend more time focusing on your problems and deficits and needs?

For the next week, make a commitment to yourself to keep a journal of all the mighty deeds of the Lord acting in your life. Remember that every positive event in your life is a "mighty" deed – so don't discount anything, no matter how "small" it might appear to you. For example, suppose you were able to slice a tomato without pain in your hands. Praise God and put it on your list. Or maybe you received a note from a friend. Or a little bird perched on a branch outside your window and sang a song to you. Maybe the sunset was especially beautiful. Or it rained. Or the sun shone brightly.

Take special note of every improvement in your physical condition. Big improvements will be easy to remember, but it is tempting to disregard the tiny ones. Keep your notebook handy so that you can jot down every blessing you notice.

At the end of each day, spend some time in prayer and meditation reviewing your list and giving grateful thanks for each item. Then close your eyes, and visualize the light of the Lord shining on you, penetrating deeply within your body, and healing every cell and every gland and every organ. Thank God for forgiving all your sins and healing all your diseases.

Wonderful Jehovah-rapha, I come to You with a grateful heart and I praise Your Holy name. I am awed by the mighty deeds that You are working in my life. My inmost being sings to You, O Heavenly Father, "Thank You, thank You, thank You.!" For thine is the kingdom and the power and the glory. In Jesus' name, I pray, Amen.

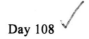

Day 108

See to it that no one takes you captive through hollow and deceptive philosophy, which depends on human tradition and the basic principles of this world rather than on Christ. (Colossians 2:8 NIV)

Do not be taken captive by beliefs that certain people have held for so long that they accept them as God's truth. One of the most prevalent and most devastating is that God does not want you to be well. Satan rejoices in the tradition of men that proclaims that it is not God's will to heal everyone. This is "a hollow and deceptive philosophy" and "depends on the basic principles of this world rather than on Christ."

When you feel tempted to believe this tradition, this "hollow philosophy," focus on the face of Jesus. Look at His life. When did He ever see someone who was hurting and fail to touch him with His healing hand? When did He ever see someone who was blind and fail to bring him sight? When did He ever pass a cripple and refuse to extend His hand and raise him to his feet?

Over and over and over again the Holy Scriptures tell us that the multitudes brought their sick and Jesus healed them *all*. Never once did Jesus refuse to heal someone because it was God's will that they be ill. Not one single time.

Furthermore, Jesus was very clear that He wanted all those who believed in Him to follow Him and do likewise. "I tell you the truth, anyone who has faith in me will do what I have been doing. He will do even greater things than these, because I am going to the Father" (John 14:12). He declared that those who believed in Him would "place their hands on sick people, and they will get well" (Mark 16:17-18).

Don't let satan deceive you. Follow the traditions of Jesus and not the traditions of men. "See to it that no one takes you captive through hollow and deceptive philosophy, which depends on human tradition and the basic principles of this world rather than on Christ."

Almighty God, keep me focused on Your Word and Your truth. Sometimes I get caught up in hollow and deceptive philosophies that depend on human tradition and the basic principles of this world, and I forget to stay grounded in Your Son Christ Jesus. Too often I look at my infirmities, let fear take hold, and become the captive of the evil one. I now bind satan and affirm that You have made clear Your will that I be well. Let Your will be done on earth in my body and in my life as it is in heaven. Thank You, God, for healing me. In the name of Your Son, Jesus Christ, my Savior and my Redeemer, I pray, Amen.

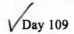

Day 109

When you fast, do not look somber as the hypocrites do, for they disfigure their faces to show men they are fasting. I tell you the truth, they have received their reward in full. But when you fast, put oil on your head and wash your face, so that it will not be obvious to men that you are fasting, but only to your Father, who is unseen; and your Father, who sees what is done in secret, will reward you. (Matthew 6:16-18 NIV)

Fasting was a common practice in the time of Jesus, a practice which He Himself observed. Few people fast today, which is regrettable since there are many health benefits that result. When you fast, you make a determination to refrain from eating either all foods or certain foods for a certain period of time. This allows the digestive tract to slow down and the energy of the body can be shifted to repairing organs and cells which need healing.

What is the difference between fasting and just skipping a meal because you are too busy to eat? The difference is intent. True fasting as practiced in the Bible is always accompanied by prayer.

The purpose of the fast is to allow both your mind and your body to become less busy so that you can focus on spiritual issues. As you bring your attention to your Creator, you bring your soul, mind, emotions, and body into harmony with the Divine will and purpose for your life.

Even though it is generally healthy to fast, do not assume that fasting is a wise choice for you. Ask the Holy Spirit first. Ask if you are to undertake a fast, and, if you receive a positive reply, ask what type of fast it should be and how long it should last.

If your body is very weak and you go on a three-day water fast without asking for guidance first, you may delay your recovery instead of accelerating it. Or if your pancreas is malfunctioning and you go on a three-day fruit fast without asking for guidance, you can create serious imbalances with your blood sugar levels. If you had asked for guidance, you might have been told to go on a vegetable broth fast for two days to give your digestive system a rest and yet provide plenty of nutrients for healing.

Always ask for guidance first whenever you have a decision to make regarding your health and recovery.

Wonderful Jehovah-rapha, today I come to You to ask if some type of fast would be helpful in my healing process. Reveal to me through the Holy Spirit if I should begin a fast. If so, tell me what kind of fast to do and what its length should be. In the name of Your Son, Jesus Christ, Amen.

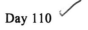

"As the rain and the snow come down from heaven, and do not return to it without watering the earth and making it bud and flourish, so that it yields seed for the sower and bread for the eater, so is my word that goes out from my mouth: It will not return to me empty, but will accomplish what I desire and achieve the purpose for which I sent it." (Isaiah 55:10-11 NIV)

Here in Isaiah we are told that God gave us His Word for a purpose. He means for it to accomplish something. Listen to Him speak, "So is my Word that goes out from my mouth: It will not return to me empty, but will accomplish what I desire and achieve the purpose for which I sent it."

The Holy Scriptures are God's Word. Jesus is God's Word. God wanted us to know what to do. He wanted His message of love for us to be clear, and He wanted His message of our redemption to be clear.

We are to receive the Word of God and to flourish and come to life under it. Isn't it a beautiful picture to see the rain and the snow coming down from heaven, watering the earth, and making the flowers and plants bud and spring to life? That is what God wants His Word to do for us.

God wants us not just to exist but to live fully according to His original plan for us. Look to the Garden of Eden and see the abundance of life there. Note the quality of life. Jesus told us, "I have come that you might have life and that you might have more abundantly" (John 10:10).

Allow God's Word to bloom in your heart. Set aside time every day to read His Word and to meditate on it. Hide it deep in your heart. Visualize all of God's healing words penetrating each cell of your body and remaining there.

God repeatedly tells us that His Word has power and authority. His Word is Divine truth. His Word can change your life if you will believe and have faith. It is written that Jehovah is the God who heals you. Trust Jehovah-rapha. Bloom and flourish according to His purpose.

Almighty God, thank You for Your Word, the Holy Scriptures. They instruct me, reprimand me, uplift me, comfort me. I am blessed to have Your positive words available to me at every moment of the day or night. No matter what my situation, Your Word is literally at my fingertips. All I have to do is to read it. Work Your purpose for my life in me, O Lord God. Let Your Word sow seeds in me that will bloom and flourish just as You intended. In the name of Your Son, Jesus Christ, I pray, Amen.

They did not understand that he was telling them about his Father. So Jesus said, "When you have lifted up the Son of Man, then you will know that I am the one I claim to be and that I do nothing on my own but speak just what the Father has taught me. The one who sent me is with me; he has not left me alone, for I always do what pleases him." Even as he spoke, many put their faith in him. (John 8:27-30 NIV)

Loneliness is one of the most painful feelings we experience. Everyone wants a sense of belonging. Everyone wants to feel loved. Within the circle of loving family and friends we feel secure and safe.

A surprising number of adults did not feel included in a circle of love when they were children. As a result, they still carry wounds of that loneliness and have various defensive mechanisms established to protect themselves from further hurts. These mechanisms may have been useful when they were children, but almost always they cause problems when the person has grown into an adult.

Have the courage to examine and release these old feelings. If you hold onto them, you will find that emotional turmoil often creates an inner chaos that eventually leads to physical illness.

Once you have released the old, painful feelings, you will be changed inside. Family members will make their own adjustments and you may still be close to them. Sometimes, however, you have to be apart from them in order to stop abuse and to establish a boundary of respect and kindness. In that case you may find that the feelings of loneliness continue, though in a different way.

Remember that these are just feelings and hold on to God's truth spoken by Jesus, "He has not left me alone." Through Jesus Christ, we are brought back into God's family. Look for others who share your love of God and will join in fellowship with you. Rejoice when you find them and treasure them. Jesus also tells us that our family is to be those who are doing the will of God. That points the way for us to identify them.

You are never alone. God loves you and will never forsake you.

Almighty God, there are times when I feel so alone. It is particularly hard when I feel bad physically, too. I want to cry and to hide. At those times I turn to Your Word and I am reminded that You have not left me alone. You are always with me. Help me to follow Your Son and do nothing on my own, but, instead, do everything according to Your plan and Your will. In the name of Your Son, Jesus Christ, my Redeemer, I pray, Amen.

Day 112

To keep me from becoming conceited because of these surpassingly great revelations, there was given me a thorn in my flesh, a messenger of Satan, to torment me. Three times I pleaded with the Lord to take it away from me. But he said to me, "My grace is sufficient for you, for my power is made perfect in weakness." Therefore I will boast all the more gladly about my weaknesses, so that Christ's power may rest on me. That is why, for Christ's sake, I delight in weaknesses, in insults, in hardships, in persecutions, in difficulties. For when I am weak, then I am strong. (2 Corinthians 12:7-10 NIV)

Paul was buffeted by a messenger of satan, one attack after another. It is very uncomfortable to be attacked by satan and his minions, to say the least, so Paul asked the Lord three times to do something to stop it. God's answer was that no matter what came at Paul, God's power would overcome it.

God does not mean for us to stay weak. Paul confirms that when he says, "For when I am weak, *then I am strong.*" It is the strength of the Lord which floods within him; it is the power of the Lord that lifts him up and carries him through whatever the evil one throws at him.

Paul knows that God makes wonderful lemonade from satan's lemons if we will only let Him. For that reason he is able to say, "That is why, for Christ's sake, I delight in weaknesses, in insults, in hardships, in persecutions, in difficulties."

Paul understands that, in a way, it is an honor to be buffeted by satan because it is the servants of the Lord whom the evil one wants most. Preferring your allegiance, he will settle for your fear. Paul had the right attitude and gave satan neither.

God is a God of freedom. He allows even satan the free will to exist and to act destructively. God never promises to stop satan from attacking us. He did not stop satan from attacking His own Son Jesus. But what He does promise is that He will give us the power to handle anything that satan dishes out. In our weakness, we are made strong, for nothing is too hard for God to handle. No power is mightier than His.

Almighty Lord, Your grace is always sufficient for me. Your power is made perfect in my weakness. Fill me with Your strength, O Lord, as I face my difficulties and problems. I will do my part to wear Your holy armor and to resist all attempts of satan to trap me. I rest in Your strength, Your power, and Your loving care. In the name of Your Son, Jesus Christ, I pray, Amen.

But the Lord said to Gideon, "There are still too many men. Take them down to the water, and I will sift them for you there." . . . There the Lord told him, "Separate those who lap the water with their tongues like a dog from those who kneel down to drink." . . . The Lord said to Gideon, "With the three hundred men that lapped I will save you and give the Midianites into your hands. Let all the other men go, each to his own place." . . . Gideon and the hundred men with him reached the edge of the camp. . . . The three companies blew the trumpets and smashed the jars. Grasping the torches in their left hands and holding in their right hands the trumpets they were to blow, they shouted, "A sword for the Lord and for Gideon!" While each man held his position around the camp, all the Midianites ran, crying out as they fled. (Judges 7:4-5, 7, 19-21 NIV)

Hundreds of thousands of men strong, the Midianite army swept into Israel. Hearing the Israelites crying to be saved, God selected Gideon to crush the enemy. Gideon gathered an army and prepared to fight. But the Lord God Almighty told him that some adjustments had to be made first "in order that Israel may not boast against me that her own strength has saved her" (v. 2). God required Gideon to reduce his army from over thirty-two thousand to only three hundred men.

Would you have had the courage of Gideon to follow God's orders? When we read this story, we may secretly be glad that we are not confronted with Gideon's situation. Yet if you have illness and disease in your body, you are under attack from the evil one. Your impulse may be to employ the most powerful arsenal of drugs, chemotherapy, radiation, and surgery than you can in order to win the battle. Before you embark on any such course, go in prayer to the Lord. Seek His advice and counsel with full faith and trust in your heart and with complete willingness to obey Him. What if He tells you to use juniper berries, uva ursi, and astragalus to heal a bladder infection instead of high-powered antibiotic? That may seem to you like pitting three hundred men against thousands upon thousands. Are you willing to do it if God asks it of you? Listen to His voice and obey.

Almighty God, my mind cannot conceive of the awesomeness of Your power. I get confused by the appearance of things and too often am afraid to follow guidance that doesn't seem reasonable to my human brain. Reveal to me Your truth, and give me courage to follow Your wisdom obediently and persistently. With Your help I bind the evil one, and I give grateful thanks for Your healing. In Jesus' name, I pray, Amen.

Day 114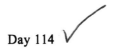

. . . the God who gives life to the dead and calls things that are not as though they were.
(Romans 4:17 NIV)

If you call things that are not as though they were, aren't you just wallow-ing in denial about your illness? The answer is no. Denial is pretending some-thing does not exist. Look carefully at Paul's words in Romans 4:17. You do not call something that *is* what is *not*. Instead, you call what is not as though it *were*.

For example, suppose you have had osteoporosis diagnosed. You do not say, "I don't have osteoporosis" and put your faith in that statement. At the moment your osteoporosis is real. It truly exists at the physical level. Acknowl-edge the diagnosis – but, having done so, do not dwell on it any longer or keep your attention focused there. Stop reinforcing your diagnosis by constantly voicing it.

Instead, ask yourself, "What is God's truth"? God is Jehovah-rapha, who is the God who heals you. God's will is that you be well and healthy. So speak in the way that God speaks. Call things that are not as though they were. Say, "I enforce God's Word on my osteoblast cells and command them to build new, strong, healthy bone cells in all the appropriate places. I declare my bones to be healthy according to God's design and purpose."

Put on the armor of Ephesians 6:10-18 and resist the devil. It is written that, if you resist him, he must flee. Command him to leave your body in the name of Christ Jesus. Bind him with God's Word. He has no authority over you and no place in any cell of your body. You have been redeemed by your Savior, who took not only your sins but also your illnesses to the Cross. It has already been done.

Stand on the Word. Speak it out loud several times each day. Enforce the Word on your body. Claim your health and speak it until it is manifested. Pay attention to guidance from the Holy Spirit, and walk the path to your healing that God wants you to walk. Be attentive, obedient, persistent, and faithful.

Wonderful Jehovah-rapha, nothing is too hard for You. Nothing is impossible for You. I get sidetracked by what I see and feel and touch. So often those things are not Your truth. Teach me to look beyond the appearance of things to Your reality. My body is the temple for Your Holy Spirit, and I want it to be whole and well so that I may use it fully and wisely in service to You. Bless me, Lord. I declare my faith and trust in Your path for my life and my recovery. In Jesus' name, I pray, Amen.

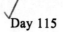
Day 115

Listen and understand. What goes into a man's mouth does not make him "unclean," but what comes out of his mouth, that is what makes him "unclean." . . . But the things that come out of the mouth come from the heart, and these make a man "unclean." For out of the heart come evil thoughts, murder, adultery, sexual immorality, theft, false testimony, slander. These are what make a man "unclean"; but eating with unwashed hands does not make him "unclean." (Matthew 15:10-11, 18-20 NIV)

It was important for Jesus to address the issue of clean and unclean foods in His ministry because what people ate was a major separating factor between Jews and non-Jews. According to Jewish law, people became *spiritually* unclean when they ate foods God had declared to be unclean.

Jesus makes it clear that the state of a person's soul has nothing to do with what foods they do or do not eat. Nor, He says, does eating with unwashed hands (also against Jewish law) make a person unclean spiritually. Have we committed a spiritual sin to eat the animals declared to be unclean? Jesus tells us that we have not, and He told His disciples to eat the food placed before them when they were visiting in someone's home.

Is Jesus saying that it is best to eat with dirty hands? Of course not. Jesus is not addressing a health or sanitation issue. He is addressing a moral and spiritual issue. Likewise, Jesus is not saying that food guidelines are useless and to be totally disregarded. Just as it is not healthy to eat with unwashed hands because the risk of contaminating our food is high, it is also not healthy to eat animals which carry an especially high level of toxins because the risk of contaminating our body with bacteria, viruses, and parasites is high.

God wants us to be well. Study God's Word. Learn what food recommendations were given to us. Then ask God how best to apply what you have learned to your life.

Almighty God, You have provided an abundance of food for me to eat. In studying Your Word I am learning about the foods that You have told us are unhealthy to eat. You know my heart, Lord, and You know how much I enjoy some of these foods. I know it is time for me to become a full partner with You in my healing process so I come to You now willing to make changes in my diet. Counsel me, advise me, and I will obey. In Jesus' name, I pray, Amen.

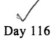

Day 116

Behold, the hour cometh, yea, is now come, that ye shall be scattered, every man to his own, and shall leave me alone: and yet I am not alone, because the Father is with me. These things I have spoken unto you that in me ye might have peace. In the world ye shall have tribulation: but be of good cheer; I have overcome the world. (John 16:32-33 KJV)

Jesus never promised that we would not have trials and tribulations. In fact, He told us that we would. Not only that, He told us that we would have many tribulations particularly because we were following Him. In this particular passage of Scripture, Jesus has just told His disciples that He is soon to be killed and that the disciples will run away and hide, each in his own home. In other words, satan was going to target Jesus, and satan was going to target the followers of Christ.

But that isn't the real message Jesus wants to leave with them. He says, I'm telling you this so you can understand not only what is happening but so that you can see beyond the appearance of things. I want you to have peace in your heart. I already forgive you for deserting me. And you must understand that I have overcome the world. I have overcome everything that satan has ever done or that satan can ever do. I have overcome it *all.*

It is interesting that the tribulations Jesus endured did not include illness. The arrest, trial, beating, torture by crucifixion, tyranny, rejection, and abuse that Jesus suffered were examples of the kinds of tribulations that the disciples and followers of Christ could expect later. Satan would throw at them every attack possible. Yes, that might even include sickness and disease. However, illness was not an adversity that Jesus wanted to hinder the mission of His followers, so the disciples were given power by Jesus and later by the Holy Spirit to heal all diseases in the name of Christ. They were taught by Jesus how to do this, and He expected them to follow His instructions and commands.

No matter what happens to you, be of good cheer! Jesus has overcome the world. Claim the peace of God not only to endure the tribulation but also to move through it. Keep your eyes focused on God, God's love, and God's promises. Don't let your gaze waver from Him.

Almighty God, sometimes I let fear born of the evil one distract me. Help me to keep my focus on You rather than on my current tribulations. Fill me with the peace of Your Son, who has overcome the world. Jesus reigns triumphant. He healed all who came to Him. I come, Father. Show me Your way to my healing. In Jesus' name, I pray, Amen.

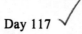

But the Lord said to Samuel, "Look not on his appearance or at the height of his stature, for I have rejected him. For the Lord sees not as man sees; for man looks on the outward appearance, but the Lord looks on the heart." (1 Samuel 16:7 AMP)

Samuel made a judgment about someone based on his appearance and God reprimanded him for doing so. God told Samuel that He looks beyond a person's appearance and sees into the person's heart and soul. In fact, God looks beyond the appearance of *all* things to see the heart of each matter. This is particularly important for us to remember with issues of health.

Sometimes we manifest serious diseases: cancer, osteoporosis, macular degeneration, lupus. The list goes on and on. All of them are "real." There are legitimate medical treatments for many of them based on information provided from our three-dimensional world. But how does God see these illnesses? Does He focus on the appearance? Or does He see beyond to the heart of the matter?

Satan loves to get us diverted by the appearance of our illness, by our symptoms, and by the logic of what we define as reality. This is a very effective method to separate us from God's will. By tempting us to focus on disease "facts," he makes us forget the fact that the members of the early church (who were ordinary people like us) healed people regularly in spite of the appearance of terrible diseases.

You must decide which reality to trust and which reality to live. God asks you to see His reality. God asks you to look beyond the appearance of your disease. Acknowledge your symptoms as appearance only. See yourself as God sees you – whole and healthy. Form a clear vision in your mind of every cell in your body functioning according to God's design and intent.

Repeat God's Word daily, hourly, or even minute by minute if necessary. Read God's Holy Word, believe, and trust.

O, God, I choose Your Divine will as my reality. Sometimes I look at my body and the appearance of disease looks overwhelming to me. Sometimes I feel so bad that I fail to see myself whole and well. In those times, Lord, help me to repeat over and over, "You are the God who heals me." Help me pray it until I fall asleep. Help me wake up saying it. Help me, God, to say it until I accept it deep in my heart as Your reality which You have proclaimed in Your Holy Word. Thank you, God, for loving me, for healing me and for guiding me. In Jesus' name, I pray, Amen.

Day 118

Love your neighbor as yourself. (Matthew 19:19 NIV)

Most Christians hear only the "love your neighbor" portion of these words of Jesus. They ignore the "as yourself" phrase because they are fearful of being accused of being selfish and self-centered. Consequently, Christians often have a great deal of trouble following this commandment.

The failure to do so is one reason that we frequently fall into ill health. We get caught up in taking care of others and fail to take care of ourselves with equal concern and diligence. Never forget that your body is your temple.

Helping others is a major way that we serve God, but if we do so without giving equal regard to our own temples, we violate God's will and plan for us. What priority do you give to living healthily and taking care of your own body?

Notice that Jesus did not say to love your neighbor either more or less than yourself – but equal to yourself. Jesus is telling you that you must be *self-full* rather than *self-ish*. What does it mean to be self-full? It means to be the best you that you can be. It means allowing God's love to fill you so that you take care of yourself lovingly, just as you take care of others.

Think about the little kindnesses you do for your family, friends, and neighbors. Think about the ways that you help them. Think of specific examples. Now, ask yourself when you applied those same kindnesses to yourself. Take a few minutes to reflect on how this has impacted your health. What do you need to do to make a change? What are some ways that you can get in partnership with God to facilitate your healing?

We live in a frantic world and our lives are filled to the brim with activities. We must refocus on what is God's plan for us. Jesus tells us that God wants us to serve Him by loving our neighbors and ourselves equally. Give Jesus any guilt you feel for taking care of yourself and then resolve to do as He instructs.

Almighty God, too often I don't follow this commandment that Your Son gave to me. I get caught up in my busy life, and I never seem to have enough time to do what I ought to be doing. Sometimes I feel guilty when I take time for myself. Help me, God, to learn to take the time to care for myself in a loving, nurturing way so that I can be Your partner in my healing. Thank you for the loving example of Your Son. In His name I pray, Amen.

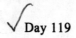

Day 119

He maketh me to lie down in green pastures. (Psalm 23:2 KJV)

Rest is essential for healing. In order to be restored, we must lie down and be physically still. When we are up and moving around, our bodies use large amounts of energy just to carry out the activities we are performing. While we are in a state of rest, the cells of our body can go about the task of repair and renewal.

We generally think of using energy to do vigorous activity and discount the effort it takes to perform simple, ordinary acts of living. When you are extremely ill, it is difficult simply to talk. You feel fatigue in every part of your body. Trying to form words with your mouth and summon the strength to push air from your diaphragm past your vocal cords seems a giant task. An action you did without effort thousands of times a day suddenly takes on new dimensions, and you realize how much energy is actually required to speak one tiny word.

Eating also requires a great deal of energy, so if you are seriously ill, you may find that you don't feel hungry. This is the body's natural response so that it can focus its energy in healing rather than in performing the task of digestion.

Adequate nutrition is vital, however, to provide the building blocks for recovery, so you may find that eating soup, vegetable juices, and nourishing broth provides the right balance between reducing the demands of digestion and providing the proper intake of nutrients.

Take time to ask God for guidance about the rest you need. Lie down (without feeling guilty) when your guidance tells you to do so. Make sure you are clear about your guidance. You know in your soul if you are using sleep and rest to retreat from the world, and, if this is the case, ask God for the steps you need to take to move out of your depression. Rest is not meant to be a hiding place. It is meant to be a healing time in the green pastures of restoration where the Lord, your shepherd, watches lovingly over you and returns you to health.

O, Lord, today I feel so tired and I feel so weary. I know there are times when I should be lying down to rest and instead I keep on pushing ahead. When I forget to listen to Your voice, make me to lie down, Lord, and watch over me as I rest. Thank You for being my shepherd, guarding me, protecting me, and healing me. In these green pastures, I rest in You, God, and in Your strength. In the name of Your Son, Jesus Christ, my Savior and my Redeemer, I pray, Amen.

Day 120

Then Jesus told his disciples a parable to show them that they should always pray and not give up. He said: "In a certain town there was a judge who neither feared God nor cared about men. And there was a widow in that town who kept coming to him with the plea, 'Grant me justice against my adversary.' For some time he refused. But finally he said to himself, 'Even though I don't fear God or care about men, yet because this widow keeps bothering me, I will see that she gets justice, so that she won't eventually wear me out with her coming!'" And the Lord said, "Listen to what the unjust judge says. And will not God bring about justice for his chosen ones, who cry out to him day and night? Will he keep putting them off? I tell you, he will see that they get justice, and quickly. However, when the Son of Man comes, will he find faith on the earth?" (Luke 18:1-8 NIV)

Have you ever noticed the first sentence in chapter 18 in the Book of Luke? "Then Jesus told his disciples a parable to show them that they should always pray and not give up." Always pray and not give up. There are people who pray for healing but who do not receive it because they give up too soon. They aren't persistent enough.

Praying persistently doesn't mean constantly begging God to heal you. Nor is it belligerent demanding. Notice the bottom line of the parable. The point of diligent prayer is that it exhibits faith.

So what is effective, persistent prayer? When you first notice a need, you say a prayer of request. You need not ask again because you know the Father has heard you. Now you must exhibit persistence and not give up. Now is the time to pray constant prayers of thanksgiving that you have been heard and that God will provide. Keep offering up your prayers of gratitude even when the appearance is that what you are praying for is not happening.

Pray asking for guidance from the Holy Spirit and being completely willing to *act* to follow the path of healing that God wants you to follow (even if it isn't the path *you* would choose). Stand firm, be persistent in your faith, and do not give up.

Wonderful Jehovah-rapha, I have prayed my prayer of request for my healing. Now give me diligence to stand strong on my faith and not give up. I know Your promise that You are the God who heals me. I let go of my own ideas for my healing and put myself totally in Your hands. Show me my part in my healing, Lord, and I will do it. Thank You, God, for healing me. Thank You, thank You. In Jesus' name, I pray, Amen.

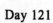

Day 121

For as he thinketh in his heart, so is he. (Proverbs 23:7 KJV)

Of all the sentences in the Holy Scriptures, this is one of the most profound ones. Our thoughts create our experience and our world. Although there are people who do not think that God exists, we, as Christians, have a relationship with God that is very real and very powerful. The thoughts of the atheist do not make God disappear, but they do change the way the atheist interprets everything in his life.

The same thing is true about illness. If we think that disease is defined solely by medical tests, then we cannot reach to the level where faith is the *substance* and *evidence* of things *unseen*. If we think that God made us sick, we are placed in a position of conflict to ask Him to heal us. If we think that we are being made ill in order for us to learn a lesson, we have an internal confusion over being well.

Most of us give medical reports great power. Occasionally, the conclusion of the report is that we have a condition for which there is no current medical cure. Sometimes there is a medical intervention, but it carries serious risks and causes severe side effects.

The problem comes when we limit our thinking to these possibilities and *only* these possibilities. We allow our thinking to be controlled by medical authorities instead of praying with our doctors and putting the final decision in the hands of The Great Physician. We are afraid to trust our ability to hear God's voice and to receive accurately the exact steps we are to take at the physical level to join in partnership with God for our healing.

As a man thinketh, so is he. If you think all healing must involve medical intervention, then so it is. If you think all medical opinions must be followed, then so it is.

On the other hand, if you think The Great Physician is both able and willing to tell you the exact actions to take to facilitate your healing, then so it is. If you think you can hear God speak to you clearly, then so it is. If you think God wants you to be well, then so it is. If you think God can make you well, then so it is. If you think God is healing you now, then so it is.

Dear God, I choose to change my thoughts. When the evil one plants thoughts of doubt, I choose to resist him. I bind him according to Your Holy Word. I choose to fill my mind with positive ideas and beliefs. I trust in Your will, Your guidance, and Your healing grace. In the name of Your Son, Jesus Christ, I pray, Amen.

For God hath not given us the spirit of fear; but of power, and of love, and of a sound mind. (2 Timothy 1:7 KJV)

God does not want us to be fearful. Repeatedly, He sends us angels who proclaim, "Fear not." Jesus' birth was heralded with the glorious announcement, "Fear not, for I bring tidings of great joy!" Paul delivers the same message to us again in 2 Timothy.

Fear is the tool of the evil one. It keeps us victimized by illness and by people's actions, and it makes us weak. Fear separates us from God and keeps us from accepting God's true gifts.

What does God give us? Power! Not power over people to control them, but power to transform ourselves. Power to fulfill God's purpose in our lives. Power to spread God's Word to others. Power to overcome obstacles in our path. Jesus told us He brought us power ("dynamis") over everything, including sickness and disease.

God also gives us love which is the core of our Heavenly Father's essence. Jesus kept telling us, "God loves you! As God loves you, love others. And as God loves you, love yourself. Love your neighbor *as yourself.*" When we connect to God's love and allow it to flow within our souls and our bodies, we are healed. Love is the most powerful force in existence. It is infinitely stronger than sickness.

Lastly, God gives us a sound mind, also translated as "self-control" or "self-discipline." These are our tools to do what we need to do. God always requires that we take action. We have to make the decisions to eat foods that are healthy for us, to get enough rest, to make time to play and laugh, and to walk, dance, or exercise.

All of this takes self-control and self-discipline. It is up to us to be willing to resist the temptations of the evil one and to align ourselves with God by following His guidelines for healthy living.

Wonderful Jehovah-rapha, thank You for giving me the spirit of power, of love, and of self-discipline, self-control, and a sound mind. I accept these gifts to help me fulfill Your purpose for my life. I accept these gifts to help me in my partnership with You for my healing. According to Your Holy Word, I command the evil one to leave my body. Give me the self-control to do those things which I know are healthy and to avoid those things which contribute to my illness. And keep on loving me, God, and holding me in Your protective arms. In the name of Your Son, Jesus Christ, I pray, Amen.

Day 123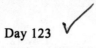

I am still confident of this: I will see the goodness of the Lord in the land of the living. Wait for the Lord; be strong and take heart and wait for the Lord. (Psalm 27:13-14 NIV)

How wonderful to be confident of seeing the goodness of the Lord in the land of the *living*. That is our goal while we are here on earth, to live fully and purposefully, carrying out God's will. A major key to our success is our willingness to wait for the Lord. It is easy to talk the talk of patience, but, oh, how difficult it is to walk that walk.

You must understand the role of patience in your healing. Miraculous healings occur in an instant and require only the patience of getting to that moment.

Many healings are not through instantaneous miracles, however, but are the result of a healing process. They are no less wondrous and no less God-given. They are just slower. We now live in a world that demands instant gratification. Waiting thirty seconds for a computer to respond irritates us. We speak of "hating" to wait in lines, at stoplights, etc.

Faith often requires waiting. God was not the author of your illness, but He can and will heal you if you ask Him and if you allow Him to work it out in His own way for your highest good. God can create something good from anything, no matter how horrible it began. God can always transform satan's handiwork.

You can sabotage your healing if you are not willing to wait for the Lord. If you constantly check your symptoms for improvement, you are operating on the basis of doubt and not of faith. When you see improvement, you believe. When you don't, you doubt. That is not faith. Living in such a way means that the evil one still has his hooks in you. You are not in alignment with God.

Wait for the Lord. Stand on His Word; enforce it on your body. Take the actions God tells you to take and then let Him work His mighty healing in you.

Almighty God, give me strength to wait for You to work Your healing power in Your own way and Your own time. I trust You, God. I will look beyond the appearance of my symptoms to Your truth – that nothing is too hard for You, that You love me, and that You are the God who heals me. In the name of Your Son, Jesus Christ, I pray, Amen.

Day 124

How much better to get wisdom than gold, to choose understanding rather than silver.
(Proverbs 16:16 NIV)

Being well is not an accident that happens to you or a gift that comes no matter what you do. It involves a partnership between you and God. Satan seeks to undermine that relationship and will do so at every opportunity.

This proverb exhorts you to cultivate wisdom and understanding. How do you do this in relationship to your health?

First, give God the unquestioned authority to make all your health decisions, and you will be wise indeed. To do otherwise leaves you in the position of being a victim to the opinions of others who, no matter how much technical knowledge they may have, are limited by their own biases and by their human capacity.

You must be willing to take responsibility for your own health and for your part in creating either illness or wellness. Without this attitude, God doesn't have a lot to work with. It is rather like your asking a friend for money, and as quickly as he gives it to you, you burn it or put it in a shredder and then ask for more. If you do not know how to care for your body properly and *do it*, then you will not be healthy no matter how often God heals you.

Second, learn about your body. The more you know, the more in awe you will be at God's magnificent creation – including not only your body, but the plants and herbs that meet your body's needs. Do not be foolish by focusing on your symptoms and medicating them into silence. Since the underlying problem is still there and nothing will have been done to change it, satan has deceived you into looking for an easy way out. You are in deeper trouble than you realize. The problem is simply driven deeper into the body and the consequences are often disastrous.

Instead, follow the path of wisdom. Learn what is really happening in your body and make your corrections at the core.

Almighty God, I seek Your wisdom. You know my heart and my soul and my body, and I know that You want me to be well. I choose to rely only on You. You are the One who created my body. Help me to learn about my temple, Lord. Help me to find the books and teachers I need. I appreciate the opinions of others, including my doctors, but, Lord, I want You to tell me which advice to follow and which path to walk. I will elevate no person above You, God. You are my Creator, my deliverer, and my healer. In Jesus' name, I pray, Amen.

Day 125

Then the king ordered Ashpenaz, chief of his court officials, to bring in some of the Israelites from the royal family and the nobility – young men without any physical defect, handsome, showing aptitude for every kind of learning, well informed, quick to understand, and qualified to serve in the king's palace. . . . The king assigned them a daily amount of food and wine from the king's table. . . . But Daniel resolved not to defile himself with the royal food and wine, and he asked the chief official for permission not to defile himself this way. Now God had caused the official to show favor and sympathy to Daniel, but the official told Daniel, "I am afraid of my lord the king, who has assigned your food and drink. Why should he see you looking worse than the other young men your age? The king would then have my head because of you." Daniel then said to the guard whom the chief official had appointed over Daniel, Hananiah, Mishael and Azariah, "Please test your servants for ten days: Give us nothing but vegetables to eat and water to drink. Then compare our appearance with that of the young men who eat the royal food, and treat your servants in accordance with what you see." So he agreed to this and tested them for ten days. At the end of the ten days they looked healthier and better nourished than any of the young men who ate the royal food. So the guard took away their choice food and the wine they were to drink and gave them vegetables instead. (Daniel 1:3-5, 8-16 NIV)

As this story of Daniel illustrates, "choice food" often makes us sick. The food at the king's table was filled with delicacies and rich, tasty preparations, but it was heavy, hard to digest, and unhealthy. Daniel asked for only vegetables to eat and water to drink. This was a diet high in complex carbohydrates and loaded with minerals and vitamins. At the end of ten days he and his friends were healthier and better nourished than the young men who ate the rich, "royal" food.

Often following the example of Daniel by eating only vegetables and fruits for ten days helps a sick person to recover. Do not assume that you should do so, however, without first going to God in prayer and asking what path you should follow. Ask if Daniel's diet is appropriate for your recovery at the present time. If you receive an affirmative response, then ask for information on the length of the diet and exact recommendations for specific foods. Follow all guidance that you are given.

Almighty God, I am grateful for this story of Daniel in Your Holy Word. Reveal to me Your guidance on the diet that You want me to follow, and I will be obedient to Your instructions. In Jesus' name, I pray, Amen.

Day 126

Do to others as you would have them do to you. (Luke 6:31 NIV)

How do you treat other people? What you sow, that you also will reap. If you want to be healed, you have to take a look at the actions you are taking in your life. Careless, thoughtless, hurtful acts will eventually come full circle and attack you in ways you never anticipated.

Treating others as you want them to treat you is easy when all is going well in your life and in your relationships. The hard part comes when we feel hurt or unjustly treated. We feel innocent, and we are wounded by rejection, carelessness, or perhaps willful acts of maliciousness. Whatever the reason, we end up feeling resentful, angry, and sad.

All too often these words of Jesus are interpreted to excuse people from being held accountable for their actions under the guise of returning good for evil. But stop to think about this for a minute. What is best for *you* – to be held accountable for your actions or not? We can grow and mature only when we accept responsibility for ourselves and for the choices we make.

Therefore, when you feel hurt by someone, it is your responsibility to tell him in a way that does not attack him but stays focused on your own experience of the events and on your own feelings. If the person hears you and shares his own feelings, then you can continue the relationship. If you are not received, then it is up to you to determine what you need in order to continue the relationship. For example, you may say that you need to be respected and to be treated with kindness.

Once you have said what you need, "shake the dust off your feet" as Jesus directed, and let the other person have time to decide what he wants to do. He may choose to honor your request and rebuild the relationship, or he may choose to go his separate way. You have to be willing to allow him to make a free choice and to send your blessing no matter which decision he makes.

Ask God to help remove from you all the hurt, sadness, and anger. If these emotions remain in your heart, they also fester in your body and create illness. Let God cleanse you, renew you, and make you whole.

Gracious God, help me to treat others with the respect that I want for myself and truly to do unto others as I would have them do unto me. Give me the courage to be honest in my relationships and to accept with peace the decisions of others. Thank You for bringing supportive, loving people into my life. In Jesus' name, I pray, Amen.

Day 127

Why do you look at the speck of sawdust in your brother's eye and pay no attention to the plank in your own eye? How can you say to your brother, "Brother, let me take the speck out of your eye," when you yourself fail to see the plank in your own eye? You hypocrite, first take the plank out of your eye, and then you will see clearly to remove the speck from your brother's eye. (Luke 6:41-42 NIV)

If you focus on the faults of others, you are creating an unfavorable environment in your soul, your mind, your body, and the world around you. Being critical and negative is not only a major hindrance to healing, but many times it is at the root of illness and disease. A constant fault-finding attitude often characterizes a person who is unforgiving. Creating more than spiritual and emotional wounds, resentment also leads to physical imbalances within the body.

Negativity actually upsets your immune system by depleting your energy and draining vitality from your cells. It was no accident that Jesus, the Master Healer, consistently taught the importance of forgiveness and of approaching life with a positive, loving heart.

As an experiment, carry a little notebook around for a few days. Each time you make a remark that is critical of some person, event, or thing, jot it down, along with the time. At the end of the day, take a look at your list. Is there any pattern that is apparent? Are there particular times of day when you were more negative? For example, were you more negative when you were involved in certain activities, such as driving or doing certain chores or being with particular people?

Decide whether you want to end these habits of negative criticism. If so, turn to God in prayer to ask for His assistance in releasing you from your resentments and for His healing of all emotional wounds that contribute to your staying stuck in negative thought patterns.

Each time that you find yourself becoming stressed and critical, take a deep breath, say a prayer to release your irritation, and allow God's love and joy to fill your mind, your soul, and every cell in your body. Say "thank you" to God for transforming, changing, and redeeming you.

Almighty God, help me to release my negative thought patterns and flood me with your positive love, joy, and energy. Help me to stop being critical of others and to look instead with eyes of compassion and wonder at the world around me. This is the day that You have made. Let me rejoice and be glad in it. Thank You, Lord. In Jesus' name, I pray, Amen.

Day 128

Is any one of you in trouble? He should pray. Is anyone happy? Let him sing songs of praise. Is any one of you sick? He should call the elders of the church to pray over him and anoint him with oil in the name of the Lord. And the prayer offered in faith will make the sick person well; the Lord will raise him up. If he has sinned, he will be forgiven. Therefore confess your sins to each other and pray for each other so that you may be healed. The prayer of a righteous man is powerful and effective. (James 5:13-16 NIV)

James speaks of a specific ordinance for healing. We are told to call the elders of the church to pray over us and to anoint us with oil in the name of the Lord. The power of this anointing is particularly strong because we are in the midst of those who not only believe in Jesus Christ but who also believe in God's will and ability to heal us. We are anointed by those in the church who are strong in their faith and whose prayers are not weakened by doubt.

While those few churches today which observe this anointing ordinance use olive oil or something similar, the disciples and the followers of the early church were taught to use true essential oils. These oils had therapeutic, healing qualities that aided in the person's recovery, making the anointing more than a symbolic act.

Anointing also brings our intention into focus. Intention is a key factor in everything we do – and this is especially so in our prayer requests. In a manner of speaking, the oil has been bathed in the fervent intention of the faithful of the church that the sick be healed.

The anointing is done *in the name of the Lord*. It is done as though Jesus were standing there Himself. Intercessory prayers are offered up just as Jesus would have done if He were still living in the body on earth. And what is the result we can expect? To be healed in our body. And to know that our sins are forgiven.

Essential oils are available to us today. Find them, learn about them, and utilize them in your healing. Find a church which honors the practice of anointing with oil, and experience the blessing of healing through this powerful ordinance.

Dear God, help me to find a church where the faithful will anoint me with oil and pray in Jesus' name for my healing. I need the help of a community that believes there is a path for my healing. I need help in keeping my intention clear and my faith strong. Guide me, Lord, and I will follow. In the name of Your Son, Jesus Christ, I pray, Amen.

Day 129

And whosoever shall not receive you, nor hear your words, when ye depart out of that house or city, shake off the dust of your feet. (Matthew 10:14 KJV)

Jesus made this statement to his disciples when He sent them out to preach the gospel and to heal the people. He knew that not everyone would welcome His followers; He Himself had not been received in His own hometown of Nazareth. Since no one is ever forced to believe, Jesus instructs His followers to leave places where they are not accepted and to move on where they are wanted and understood.

You, too, need to be on guard as you walk the path of your healing. You often receive many suggestions and opinions about what you should do. Many of these opinions come from family members whom you love; other opinions come from authority figures in the medical profession. Some conclusions that they draw are not only persuasive but frightening – foretelling dire circumstances (and even death) if you do not follow a particular treatment method.

Go to a quiet place, place your concerns before God, and let Him tell you what to do. Ask the Holy Spirit to reveal Divine truth to you. It is written, "Ask and you shall receive." Once you have God's truth and God's instructions, you know the path you are to walk.

If your advisors – whether friends, family, or health care professionals – encourage you to ignore the instructions you have been given by the Holy Spirit, see if they will join you in going to the Lord in prayer. If not, do as the disciples were taught and shake the dust off your feet and move on.

It is vital that those around you be able to listen to your words. They do not have to agree but they must accept your decision to follow God's path as it has been revealed to you. When Peter, out of his love for Jesus, tried to persuade Jesus not to follow the path that would lead to His crucifixion, Jesus said to him, "Get behind me, satan." Peter's concerns touched Jesus at a vulnerable point, but Our Lord remained firm in following God's will. Follow His example and do likewise, walking God's path to your abundant health.

Almighty God, I have prayed for instructions about what I should do at the physical level to join with You on my path to healing, and I have received Your Holy guidance. Now give me the strength to follow that guidance faithfully and to shake from my feet the dust of those who cannot hear me and support me in following You. In Jesus' name, Amen.

Day 130

"For I know the plans I have for you," declares the Lord, "plans to prosper you and not to harm you, plans to give you hope and a future. Then you will call upon me and come and pray to me, and I will listen to you. You will seek me and find me when you seek me with all your heart. I will be found by you," declares the Lord, "and will bring you back from captivity." (Jeremiah 29:11-14 NIV)

Here in Jeremiah God tells us again that He has plans for us. For every single person alive He has a special plan. He says very clearly that He will not harm us. His plan, instead, is one to prosper us and to fill us with hope and a future. Surely, sickness and disease do not fit that definition of the plan as God describes it.

God even tells us why He has this particular plan. It is to help re-establish the relationship that He had with us in the Garden when Adam was a companion to Him. They walked together and communed together – and God wants that again.

Our Heavenly Father wants us to talk with Him. "Pray to me," He says, "and I will listen." God wants open communication with each one of His precious, beloved children.

God tells us He is fully and completely accessible to us. "Seek me and you will find me," He says. Seek how? With our whole heart. We can't hold part of ourselves back. We can't hold onto our doubts and misconceptions and expect to have the kind of relationship that is described in Jeremiah.

One more time God tells us clearly that He wants us to be free. God does not want us shackled by the lies of the evil one. He never wanted us to know evil in the first place, but He has allowed us the freedom to make that choice. Never forcing us to come to Him, God always beckons and offers us the option to accept Him. He sent His Son to pay the full price for our redemption and to set us totally free.

Call upon the Lord. Seek Him with all your heart. Learn the plans He has that will give you hope and a future.

Gracious God, thank You for setting me at liberty. It is comforting to know that You are always there, listening to me, and answering my call. I want the future You describe and in the name of Your Son Jesus I claim it. Every day I seek to walk the path of Your plan for me. I know that it is a plan for my good. Grant me the wisdom to listen to You and to make wise choices for my health. In the name of Your Son, Jesus Christ, my Savior and my Redeemer, I pray, Amen.

Day 131

Then the angel of God, who had been traveling in front of Israel's army, withdrew and went behind them. The pillar of cloud also moved from in front and stood behind them, coming between the armies of Egypt and Israel. Throughout the night the cloud brought darkness to the one side and light to the other side; so neither went near the other all night long. (Exodus 14:19-20 NIV)

As you travel on your road to recovery and healing, imagine mighty forces of the Lord traveling with you just as the angel of God and the Lord God Himself went with the Israelites on their journey from Egypt. You, too, are being led out of your imprisonment.

You have been held in bondage by your illness or physical infirmities, but you do not have to remain a captive. Jehovah-rapha has declared Himself the God who heals you and the God who frees you.

Jehovah-rapha is more powerful than any disease which may inhabit your body at the present time. Re-read this powerful story of protection in Exodus when the Lord Himself leads His people to safety against impossible odds. See The Lord God Almighty walking before you by day and by night. See Him and His mighty angels standing between you and the evil one.

When you feel overwhelmed and when you feel discouraged, stop the mental chatter in your head that may be flooding your being with negative messages of despair and hopelessness. First, take three deep breaths. Remember Genesis 2:7 in which God breathed in Adam the breath of life. As you inhale deeply, say to yourself, "I breathe in the breath of life from Jehovah-rapha."

Next, close your eyes and visualize in your mind the angel of God standing between you and your health problem. *Feel* the power of the Lord God Almighty fill every organ and every cell in your body with His healing presence.

Trust that God loves you every moment, protects you every moment, and heals you every moment. Relax in the power, protection, and healing of Jehovah-rapha.

Wonderful Jehovah-rapha, be my pillar of cloud by day and my pillar of light by night. Send Your mighty angel to stand between my illness and me. Lead me out of bondage, Lord. Bring me safely into the Promised Land where I can serve you in health and in joy. In the name of Your Son, Jesus Christ, my Savior and my Redeemer, I pray, Amen.

Day 132

Freely you have received, freely give. (Matthew 10:8 NIV)

Pass it on! Pass it on!

These are Jesus' words with an important message. We are to pass on what we have received.

And what is it that we have received? The answer is in the sentence just before this one: "As you go, preach this message: 'The kingdom of heaven is near.' Heal the sick, raise the dead, cleanse those who have leprosy, drive out demons."

Incredible! Jesus is saying that He has given us the message of our spiritual salvation and our physical healing. We are to receive both, and we are to pass them on.

What an awesome message! Jesus gives to us freely. And He Himself is doing just as He is telling us here in Matthew to do. Jesus Himself freely received from the Father, and He freely passes it on to others as the Father wishes Him to do. Yesterday, today, and forever.

God is a personal God. He desires a personal relationship with each one of us. From the beginning He created a Garden where He could walk personally with each of His children. He has always wanted this and He has never changed. When we made the disastrous choice to know evil and to walk with evil, God found a way to redeem us.

This redemptive message of salvation is a glorious one. It is a message of our complete restoration, soul and body. God needs us to spread this message. Each person who receives healing must pass it on to someone else.

We have to let people know that God wants them to be well. We have to form a chain of love with each person passing on what he or she has received. One by one we stand linked together, and each one of us then becomes stronger than we could ever be on our own. Our healing magnifies as we stand together linked to our Lord.

Almighty God, thank You for Your abundant mercies. Thank You for my healing. Help me to be a witness to others of Your grace, Your love, and Your healing power. Many people are hurting today, God, and they don't know that You want them to be well. Use me according to Your plan for me and for others. I am willing to follow the directions of Your Son who said, "Freely you have received, freely give." Guide me always. In Jesus' name, I pray, Amen.

Day 133

Then they brought him a demon-possessed man who was blind and mute, and Jesus healed him, so that he could both talk and see. (Matthew 12:22 NIV)

It is interesting to note that the Scriptures often refer to people who are ill as being demon-possessed. Today it is certainly politically incorrect to refer to people in such a manner. Was the gospel wrong or out-dated? Or were people simply lacking in modern scientific terminology?

Sometimes the description of the demon-possessed seems to indicate to us a person who was either mentally ill or epileptic. But here in this passage in Matthew the man is described as blind and mute – and demon-possessed. Undoubtedly, the scientific community today would have an explanation of the exact cause of the blindness and muteness and would be able to prove the man's condition was entirely due to certain physical malfunctions.

Nevertheless, in the Holy Scriptures we repeatedly see Jesus driving demons out of people. In His commands to His followers in His last moments on earth before ascending into heaven, we find Him telling them that a sign of those who believe in Him will be that they will also drive demons out "in His name." Was Jesus deluded?

Of course not. Jesus had no doubts and no questions about the will of God. He knew that God's will was not for people to be ill. He knew that God's will for people in the Garden of Eden and in heaven was for people to be well. He knew that He had been sent to tell people that God loved them and that they must repent their sins. He knew that He had been sent to heal all who came to Him. He knew that it was satan who was the source of illness and disease. Therefore, people who are ill have been attacked by the father of lies in one way or another.

Jesus has told us how to be healed. *"In my name,"* Jesus says, rebuke satan. All power and authority has been given to Christ. Call on that power and enforce it on the evil one. Demand liberty for your body. Stand on God's Word. Claim the healing of Jehovah-rapha.

Almighty God, I call to You in the name of Jesus Christ, and I command all forces of satan which may be any place in my body, soul, or mind to leave me now. I am washed in the blood of my Savior and I am made whole. I joyfully proclaim that "by His stripes I am healed." Thank You, Lord, for delivering me and bringing my salvation. In the name of Jesus Christ, my Savior and my Redeemer, I pray, Amen.

Day 134

But for you who revere my name, the sun of righteousness will rise with healing in its wings. (Malachi 4:2 NIV)

Here in Malachi is another prophecy of the coming of the Christ and another expression of His mission – to heal us in soul, mind, emotions, and body. Joy of joys, the Redeemer did come! He came bright and clear as the sun with the light of healing.

Let your soul and your heart and your body soak up more passages from Holy Scripture of the healing power of Your Lord and Savior Jesus Christ. Notice the appearance of the word "all." Notice Jesus' response to those who came. Put yourself in the midst of the crowd and accept His healing.

When the apostles returned, they reported to Jesus what they had done. The he took them with him and they withdrew by themselves to a town called Bethsaida, but the crowds learned about it and followed him. He welcomed them and spoke to them about the kingdom of God, and healed those who needed healing. (Luke 9:10-11 NIV)

As soon as they got out of the boat, people recognized Jesus. They ran throughout that whole region and carried the sick on mats to wherever they heard he was. And wherever he went – into villages, towns or countryside – they placed the sick in the marketplaces. They begged him to let them touch even the edge of his cloak, and all who touched him were healed. (Mark 6:54-56 NIV)

Jesus left the synagogue and went to the home of Simon. Now Simon's mother-in-law was suffering from a high fever, and they asked Jesus to help her. So he bent over her and rebuked the fever, and it left her. She got up at once and began to wait on them. (Luke 4:38-39 NIV)

Wonderful Jehovah-rapha, thank You for sending Your Son Jesus Christ – the sun of righteousness with healing in His wings. I am awed by His example and graced by His compassion and love. Thank You, Lord, for Your many blessings my life. In Jesus' name, I pray, Amen.

Day 135

And Jesus went forth and saw a great multitude and was moved with compassion toward them and he healed their sick. (Matthew 14:14 KJV)

Think for a moment about compassion, which is an awareness of the distress of others along with a desire to lessen or remove it. Here in Matthew we read that Jesus was filled with sympathetic understanding, and from that compassion He reached out and healed the multitude. As the Son of God, He showed us who God is and what God is doing for us.

God is conscious of our distress and our suffering, and He wants to alleviate it. In the beginning He put us in the Garden where everything was good, but we changed the plan by deciding to know evil.

In order to restore us, God had to resort to drastic measures. Evil had to be defeated at the level that it was lost – on earth, by someone at the physical level. God sent His Son in a physical body to live with us as we live. God wanted us to see His compassion in action through the work and example of His Son. Jesus repeatedly told us that He saw our suffering, and He repeatedly brought healing for both our body and our spirit.

God is filled with mercy and compassion for us, and He proclaims that He is the God who heals us. Likewise, Jesus is filled with compassion. He went forth and He healed. Jesus is the same yesterday, today, and forever. He is still filled with compassion as He sits at the right hand of the Father. He still heals.

Accept God's will for your healing and His mercy towards you. Close your eyes, breathe deeply, and imagine God enfolding you in His loving arms. Feel His healing power fill every cell in your body. Allow His compassion to penetrate deeply within you like the warm rays of the sun. See your Risen Lord Jesus Christ smile at you with Divine grace and reach out and touch you with His healing hand.

O, Gracious Heavenly Father, thank You for Your compassion for me. I have struggled a long time and I need Your healing peace. Embrace me with Your compassion; enfold me in Your desire to alleviate my suffering. Thank You for sending Your Son, Jesus, who lived on earth to show me the way. Lift me up; cleanse me at every level of my being; touch me. I thank You for Your great compassion for me and for Your healing. I stand firm on Your Holy Word and enforce it on every cell in my body. With gratitude and praise, I pray in Jesus' name, Amen.

Day 136

You have let go of the commands of God and are holding on to the traditions of men. . . . Thus you nullify the word of God by your tradition that you have handed down. And you do many things like that. (Mark 7:8, 13 NIV)

Jesus makes some very profound statements here as He is talking to the Pharisees and teachers of the law. These are the people in authority, the people who are supposed to have answers, the people who are supposed to know what is the "right" way to do things. These learned men have criticized Jesus and His disciples for failing to adhere to the "right" way to behave. Specifically, the disciples were seen eating some food without washing their hands first. Jesus tells them that they are nullifying the Word of God by holding onto the traditions of men.

Remember this when you feel sick. Family, friends, and health care professionals are quick to try to enforce on you the traditions of men. That is the path that they know and that is the path that they are comfortable walking upon. Stand firm on the words of Jesus and seek the "commands of God." Go in prayer both with your health advisors and also by yourself to determine what *God's* path to your healing is. It might be to follow men's traditions. On the other hand it might be some other path that seems foolish or risky to others.

Remember the time that God led the Israelites to a position between the sea and the pursuing Egyptians. Remember the time God told Noah to build a boat when there was no rain. Remember the time God told Joshua that great walls would tumble down at his shout. The path to your healing may be extremely unconventional. God will show you the way, and He will not fail you.

Almighty God, help me to honor Your commands, especially during the times when I feel pressured to follow the traditions of men. I am told that terrible things will happen if I do not follow certain medical procedures, and I am afraid of making the wrong decision. I want to live, Lord, but I don't know what to do. If I follow others and they are wrong, I can say I did my best and it wasn't my fault. If I don't follow them and something goes wrong, then I will feel foolish and stupid, and it may be too late to try what they suggest. Lord, I struggle for clarity in knowing what the exact path is that You want me to follow. Make Your will known to me, God, so clearly that I am absolutely sure. I will obey You and Your command. I trust You to heal me. In the name of Christ Jesus, my Savior and my Redeemer, I pray, Amen.

Day 137

I am the Lord who heals you. (Exodus 15:26 AMP)

When Moses asked God who He was, God replied, "I AM who I AM" which is translated Yahweh or Jehovah. Later in the Holy Scriptures, God reveals Himself and His Divine essence by using seven expansions of His name:

Jehovah-Rapha – the Lord who heals us

Jehovah-Shammah – the Lord who is always there

Jehovah-Shalom – the Lord our Peace

Jehovah-Ra-ah – the Lord our Shepherd

Jehovah-Jireh – the Lord who provides

Jehovah-Nissi – the Lord our Banner, Victor, and Captain

Jehovah-Tsidkenu – the Lord our Righteousness.

How wonderful it is that one of the most important things that God wanted us to know about Him was that He is a Healer. He created Adam and Eve without sickness, and it was only after they came to know evil through their choice of disobedience that they were subject to illness and disease.

Since God's plan was made perfect in the Garden, we know that sickness was not part of God's plan for man. It was part of satan's plan to separate man from God. But God is more powerful than satan. Hallelujah! God is perfectly faithful to us, His beloved creation, His beloved children. And He knows how devastating illness can be. So He covenants with us that He has the power to make His plan prevail.

God sent His Son and we were fully redeemed – spirit and body. Jesus carried not only our sins to Calvary's Cross but also our illnesses. No matter what sickness or infirmity may befall us, Jehovah-rapha is there, to heal us and restore us if only we will ask for help, obey the guidance we are given, and receive our healing.

Almighty God, I give you grateful thanks for revealing Yourself as the great Jehovah-rapha, the mighty God who heals me. I give grateful thanks that you are above all sickness and disease. I fix my eye on the Garden, your perfect plan for me. I focus on Your healing power. Touch every malfunctioning cell, tissue, gland, and organ with Your healing hand and restore them all to wholeness according to Your design and plan. I trust you, Lord. You are the God who calls what is not as though it were, so I declare my faith as You bring my health into being. Show me what actions You want me to take to work in partnership with You. In the name of Jesus Christ, my Savior and my Redeemer, I pray, Amen.

Day 138

He will love you and bless you and increase your numbers. He will bless the fruit of your womb, the crops of your land – your grain, new wine and oil – the calves of your herds and the lambs of your flocks in the land that he swore to your forefathers to give you. (Deuteronomy 7:13 NIV)

Ziba answered, "The donkeys are for the king's household to ride on, the bread and fruit are for the men to eat, and the wine is to refresh those who become exhausted in the desert." (2 Samuel 16:2 NIV)

The first miracle that Jesus did was to change water into wine (John 2:7-11) and in the ordinance of the Last Supper He offered wine to His disciples as a symbol of the blood He was soon to shed for us. We find numerous references in the Holy Scripture to the wise and moderate consumption of wine.

Today there is much new research being done about a component of red wine, called resveratrol, which appears to inhibit certain cancerous tumors. Various studies have shown effectiveness in dealing with colon, liver, and breast cancer. Thusfar, it appears that resveratrol helps the cells to maintain healthy DNA and prevents cells from mutating into cancerous forms. In addition, studies show that cholesterol is lowered with the consumption of resveratrol.

Red wine and grapes are high in antioxidants – particularly biologically active flavonoids. Flavonoids are effective in lowering LDL cholesterol, preventing arteriosclerosis, and preventing blood clots.

The Holy Scriptures are quite clear that the key to the consumption of any alcoholic beverage is that it be done in moderation. Isaiah warns, "Woe to those who rise early in the morning to run after their drinks, who stay up late at night till they are inflamed with wine" (Isaiah 5:11).

For those who would like the benefits of the grape and of red wine without the hazards and problems of alcohol, there is now an alcohol-free wine which is available. Also the addition of a few grapes to the diet adds to good nutrition.

Almighty God, today I give grateful thanks for the grape – and the many substances You placed in it for my nutrition, well being, and healing. Help me to use this fruit wisely in a positive, healthful way. I seek always to join with you in partnership for my recovery and healing. Keep showing me my path and I will walk it. In the name of Your Son, Jesus Christ, my Savior and my Redeemer, I pray, Amen.

Day 139

O give thanks unto the Lord; call upon his name: make known his deeds among the people. . . . He brought them forth also with silver and gold: and there was not one feeble person among their tribes. . . . And he brought forth his people with joy, and his chosen with gladness. (Psalm 105:1, 37, 43 KJV)

In Psalm 105 the psalmist is recounting the promises that God made to Abraham and the events that occurred as God kept His promises.

He tells of the captivity of the Israelites in Egypt and of the way that God delivered His people. In this amazing account, the psalmist declares "and there was not one feeble person among their tribes." After years and years of captivity often under harsh conditions there was not one feeble person among all the tribes that made the exodus from Egypt. What an astounding fact!

Not one feeble person. God brought them out with joy and gladness – and with health in their bodies. God's healing power is awesome. He has revealed it over and over and over again. We have only to believe. In verse 7 of Psalm 105 we read, "He hath remembered his covenant for ever, the Word which he commanded to a thousand generations." God never forgets His covenant; He never forgets His promises to us.

God's story is one of redemption for His children. He wants us to be redeemed, saved, and brought back to Him. Our redemption is not just for our souls but for our entire selves. That includes for our bodies, too. When Jesus came, he repeatedly healed the sick, and He said, "Your faith has made you well" (Luke 17:19 NIV).

Your redemption has been won. Your sins and infirmities were taken to the Cross two thousand years ago by Jesus Christ. It is done. God wants you to go forth with joy and gladness. He wants you to be well. Thank Him for your healing and let His healing love fill you with joy.

O Gracious Lord, I rejoice that I can trust Your covenant with me. As You led the Israelites, lead me, God, and I will follow. Help me to remember these stories of long ago and to draw strength from them. I stand on Your Word and claim Your healing grace. I glory in Your Holy name and sing to You my songs of praise and thanks. Give me strength to follow Your path for me in my healing. In the name of Christ Jesus, my Savior and my Redeemer, I pray, Amen.

Day 140

This, then, is how you should pray: Our Father in heaven, hallowed be your name, your kingdom come, your will be done on earth as it is in heaven. Give us today our daily bread. Forgive us our debts, as we also have forgiven our debtors. And lead us not into temptation, but deliver us from the evil one. (Matthew 6:9-13 NIV)

Every Christian has repeated this prayer thousands of times. In fact, we often say it mechanically without even hearing the words or absorbing their meaning.

What is this prayer about? Is it a prayer Jesus Himself would pray? No, because it includes a request for forgiveness for sins, and He was without sin. It was a prayer for us. I will teach you how to pray, He said. This is the way to do it.

Think of the number of times you have said, "Your will be done on earth as it is in heaven." Stop for a moment to consider what God's will *is* in fact like in heaven. There is no sickness and disease in heaven. It stands to reason that there are no physical illnesses since people have left their earthly bodily temples behind. However, there are other types of illnesses – both mental and spiritual – and we all believe that none of those illnesses exist in heaven either. Heaven is a totally spiritual "place" where God's will is expressed perfectly.

God created the Garden of Eden to reflect the spiritual qualities of heaven and also to embody the physical realm. It was Adam and Eve's desire to know evil that created the problems – when humans desired to place their own will above God's.

In the Lord's Prayer, Jesus tells us to ask God to manifest His will on earth as He does in heaven. Everything Jesus did was to do just that. He healed every single person who came to Him and who needed healing. He did that not just to convince people who He was but He did it to fulfill His purpose of seeing that the Father's will was done on earth as it was in heaven.

Jesus told us that He followed the Father's will always, without ever deviating from it. Trust Jesus' words. Trust Jesus' actions. Pray the Lord's Prayer with feeling and with intent for your healing.

My Father in heaven, hallowed be Your name, Your kingdom come, Your will be done on earth as it is in heaven. Give me today my daily bread. Forgive me my debts, as I also have forgiven my debtors. And lead me not into temptation, but deliver me from the evil one. In the name of Your Son, Christ Jesus, my Savior and my Redeemer, I pray, Amen.

Day 141

One of the teachers of the law came and heard them debating. Noticing that Jesus had given them a good answer, he asked him, "Of all the commandments, which is the most important?" "The most important one," answered Jesus, "is this: 'Hear, O Israel, the Lord our God, the Lord is one. Love the Lord your God with all your heart and with all your soul and with all your mind and with all your strength.' The second is this: 'Love your neighbor as yourself.' There is no commandment greater than these." (Mark 12:28-31 NIV)

Love is the ultimate healing force. Why? Because God *is* love. It is because God loved us that He made us. It is because God loved us that He gave us the wonderful Garden of Eden. It is because God loved us that He sent His Son Jesus Christ to redeem us when we made the fatal decision to know evil and to suffer all the consequences of evil. It is because God loved us that He sent His Son Jesus Christ to heal every single person who came to Him, without one exception.

Notice what Jesus told us about love. We are to love God, first and foremost. We are to love our neighbors. And we are to love *ourselves*. The last one is often the hardest. When we feel sick, we often beat ourselves up with guilt or shame. We think that, if we were better people, we wouldn't be sick. When we stay in that emotional place, we are not loving ourselves, and it is highly unlikely that we will heal. Such negative thoughts only add to our health problems and exacerbate them.

Visualize the love of God streaming down from heaven and up from the earth, covering you and warming you. Feel yourself in a cocoon of perfect love. Feel that love penetrate through your skin and deep inside of you. Feel it pass into every cell in your body. Concentrate it in those areas which are the most wounded and the most damaged by illness or injury. Feel yourself relax and feel your fears lifting and floating away.

Remain bathed in this love as you resume your activities for the day. Repeat this exercise often, and allow God's love to bring you His peace and His healing.

Gracious God, I seek always to love You and honor You as the One True Jehovah-rapha. Help me to love my neighbors and to forgive those who trespass against me. And help me, God, to love myself. Sometimes I don't know how You can love me because I keep doing so many things that I know You don't want me to do. Help me to see myself through Your eyes of compassion, and help me to love and honor myself as Your child. In the name of Christ Jesus, my Savior and my Redeemer, I pray, Amen.

Day 142

Commit your way to the Lord; trust in him and he will do this: He will make your righteousness shine like the dawn, the justice of your cause like the noonday sun. (Psalm 37:5-6 NIV)

This is love for God: to obey his commands. And his commands are not burdensome, for everyone born of God overcomes the world. This is the victory that has overcome the world, even our faith. Who is it that overcomes the world? Only he who believes that Jesus is the Son of God. (1 John 5:3-5 NIV)

God does not promise healing without any conditions. In order to receive it, we must make a commitment to Him. We have to give Him our full faith and allegiance. We have to trust Him first and foremost in our lives. And we have to obey His commands.

To some people those requirements sound heavy and depressing. Yet listen to the Apostle John, who says, "His commands are not burdensome." And why is that so? Because "everyone born of God overcomes the world."

No matter what problems may come to you from the world, God and His Son Christ Jesus are victorious over it. The world is the place where satan "prowls around like a roaring lion looking for someone to devour." He seeks to destroy us and one of his tools is disease.

However, we are not to remain subject to the devil because our Lord and Savior Jesus Christ has overcome the world. It is written that on the third day Christ Jesus rose from the dead, effectively defeating satan forever. Therefore, by confession of faith in Jesus Christ we overcome any weapon that the devil may use to attack us.

Commit yourself to God's Word. Commit yourself to living victoriously according to your confession of faith in Christ Jesus. Enforce the Word upon every cell in your body, and believe without doubt that God is healing you.

Almighty God, I commit my life to You – body, mind, and soul. I trust You to defend and save me, to raise me victorious above the attacks of the evil one. I commit myself to obey Your commands. I give glorious thanks that I am born again into Your salvation and that through Jesus Christ I overcome the world. I believe in Your Son Jesus Christ, who bore my sins and my infirmities on Calvary's Cross. In Jesus' name, I pray, Amen.

Day 143

On the seventh day, they got up at daybreak and marched around the city seven times in the same manner, except that on that day they circled the city seven times. The seventh time around, when the priests sounded the trumpet blast, Joshua commanded the people, "Shout! For the Lord has given you the city!" . . . When the trumpets sounded, the people shouted, and at the sound of the trumpet, when the people gave a loud shout, the wall collapsed; so every man charged straight in, and they took the city. (Joshua 6:15-16, 20 NIV)

Do you have the faith of Joshua? It's important to notice how often the stories in the Holy Scriptures reveal God's asking His people to take actions that were completely unconventional – and often seemingly ridiculous.

Here we see Joshua at war. God tells him to march around Jericho and on the seventh day on the seventh lap to blow the trumpets and to shout. What an absurd requirement! It is as ridiculous as building a boat when there is no rain in sight. Or putting blood on your door so the angel of death will pass over. Or putting mud on your eyes in order to recover your sight.

It is written in the Old Testament that God often referred to His people as "stiff-necked" and "stubborn" and "disobedient." In many ways we are far worse now because we insist on holding everything up to the standard of "science" and "reality."

Generally, science is defined as being separated from God and all things spiritual. It reveals the "truth" through "impartial" tests and the application of scientific "facts." Of course, we conveniently ignore our history of changing these "facts" as our understanding changes. For example, where once the scientific community was positive the world was flat, we now believe it is round.

All "facts" are based on the understanding of the mind of man. God gave us intelligence to use. He gave us curiosity to seek and to discover and to invent. Yet He constantly reminds us that He exceeds anything we can possibly imagine and that His power is never bound by any rules, theories, or "facts" that we may proclaim.

Wonderful Jehovah-rapha, I want to be well. I put aside my assumptions, Lord, that my treatment and recovery has to be a certain way. Help me to be like Joshua, to listen for Your voice, and then to follow Your instructions exactly as You give them. I am willing to take action, God. I am willing to be bold and to stand firm. In Jesus' name, I pray, Amen.

Day 144

For in the time of trouble he shall hide me in his pavilion: in the secret of his tabernacle shall he hide me; he shall set me up upon a rock. And now shall mine head be lifted up above mine enemies round about me: therefore will I offer in his tabernacle sacrifices of joy; I will sing, yea, I will sing praises unto the Lord. (Psalm 27:5-6 KJV)

In the midst of our difficulties we can sing praises of joy to the Lord. Why? Because those songs come from our faith. We know that no matter what our situation is we are set upon the rock of the Lord. No matter what.

When times get tough, the tough get going. Tough times never last, but tough people do. Whatever enemies surround you, the Lord God Almighty will lift your head up above them. The battle is the Lord's, and you cannot be defeated because the battle has already been won. Jesus Christ has already atoned for your transgressions; he has taken your sins and your infirmities to the Cross.

You are now blessed with the opportunity to look beyond the appearance of things and to keep your eyes focused on God's truth as He reveals it to you through meditation and through the Holy Scriptures. This does not mean that you ignore the appearance around you, such as symptoms of your illness. You must ask for guidance for the best way for you to handle them. They exist and you must deal with them.

Nevertheless, do not define yourself by them or see them as God's truth for you. Look beyond them, and ask for your healing, believing that you have already received it, according to God's Holy Word.

Becoming grounded in God's love creates a spring of gladness and thanksgiving within. You know you are loved. You know you are protected. You know the evil one cannot have dominion over you. So the music of your soul pours out naturally to your Creator. And the more you sing and the more you give thanks, the more your body will respond.

God implanted multitudes of healing mechanisms within each cell, and each song of joy and gratitude activates those mechanisms. Offer your songs to the Lord. Sing, sing, sing.

Almighty God, in this time of trouble, hide me in Your tabernacle. Set me on a high rock. Lift my head above the struggles and challenges around me. Thank You, God, for delivering me. I offer my songs of joy and songs of praise to You, Lord. Thank You for Your mercies and Your blessings. In the name of Your Son, Jesus Christ, I pray, Amen.

Day 145

Now to each one the manifestation of the Spirit is given for the common good. To one there is given through the Spirit the message of wisdom, to another the message of knowledge by means of the same Spirit, to another faith by the same Spirit, to another gifts of healing by that one Spirit, to another miraculous powers, to another prophecy, to another distinguishing between spirits, to another speaking in different kinds of tongues, and to still another the interpretation of tongues. (1 Corinthians 12:7-10 NIV)

Paul lists a number of gifts of the Holy Spirit and tells the people of Corinth that some members of the church are gifted in one area more than others. Does this mean that the Holy Spirit confers only one such gift per person? Are only some people supposed to be wise? Are only some people to have faith? No. That wouldn't make sense. He means that some people are given "extra doses," so to speak. You have all the gifts of the Holy Spirit, although you may be stronger in one area than in others.

Let us focus on one particular gift of the Spirit: the message of knowledge. The King James Version calls this "the word of knowledge," referring to knowing something you "couldn't" know from any of the facts you have ever learned.

Jesus acknowledged that Peter had received a word of knowledge when Peter answered that Jesus was the Christ, the Son of the living God. Jesus said to him, "Blessed are you . . . for this was not revealed to you by man, but by my Father in heaven" (Matthew 16:17 NIV).

The word of knowledge can be a great blessing to you when you feel ill. Through your connection to the Father, Son, and Holy Spirit, you can receive this revelation knowledge to point you in the right direction in your path to healing. You "know" things that it is not possible for you to know otherwise. One of the signs that you have received revelation knowledge is that you will feel a great internal confidence and peace about this information even though it may seem ridiculous to others. Ask the Holy Spirit for revelation knowledge as often as you wish, but ask only if you are willing to act on the word of knowledge that you receive. Ask and you shall receive. Reach out for God and walk with Him.

Almighty God, thank You for the many gifts of the Holy Spirit. Help me to use them with awe and wonder, with reverence and humility. Today I give special thanks for revelation knowledge which guides me on the path You wish me to follow for my healing. In Jesus' name, I pray, Amen.

Day 146

Jesus said to them, "If God were your Father, you would love me, for I came from God and now am here. I have not come on my own; but he sent me. Why is my language not clear to you? Because you are unable to hear what I say. You belong to your father, the devil, and you want to carry out your father's desire. He was a murderer from the beginning, not holding to the truth, for there is no truth in him. When he lies, he speaks his native language, for he is a liar and the father of lies. Yet because I tell the truth, you do not believe me! Can any of you prove me guilty of sin? If I am telling the truth, why don't you believe me? He who belongs to God hears what God says. The reason you do not hear is that you do not belong to God." (John 8:42-47 NIV)

Jesus is very clear about the existence of satan. And He is also very clear that the mission of satan is to deflect us from God's path for our lives. One of the primary ways that satan does that is to interfere with our ability to hear God speak to us.

Jesus describes this situation vividly in this account as written by John. "Why is my language not clear to you? Because you are unable to hear what I say." It ought to be the easiest thing in the world to hear God speak to us especially since every child is born with a strong connection to his Creator. Children speak to God with innocent clarity, and they often see and speak with angels. Somehow we lose that closeness and connection as we grow older.

Hearing God means listening to the still, small voice inside. Satan whispers to you also as he tries to confuse and trick you. So how do you know which voice is which? Identify which voice is connected with fear. If you hear that you should have a certain treatment and you feel afraid that something bad will happen if you do not, then it is likely that this is the whisper of the evil one.

God does not motivate you through fear. When you are centered in God, fears diminish rather than increase.

Do not doubt your faith. Doubt your doubts. The father of lies wants to deceive you. Stand firm in God's truth and be counted as one who belongs to God wholeheartedly.

Almighty God, help me to hear Your voice and Your voice alone. I resist the evil one and declare that he must flee. I am Yours, God. I call on the name of Jesus Christ the Resurrected One and stand washed in His blood. Speak to me, Lord. Show me Your truth and give me the courage to follow it. In the name of Your Son, Jesus Christ, I pray, Amen.

Day 147

Then shall thy light break forth as the morning and thine health shall spring forth speedily: and thy righteousness shall go before thee; the glory of the Lord shall be thy reward. (Isaiah 58:8 KJV)

Isn't this a wonderful picture of recovery that Isaiah gives us? Say this Scripture out loud. "Then shall thy light break forth as the morning and thine health shall spring forth speedily: and thy righteousness shall go before thee; the glory of the Lord shall be thy reward." Repeat it again. And once again for the third time.

Visualize your body shrouded by shadow. Slowly God's light breaks forth as the morning and begins to illuminate you. Feel the warmth of this light on your face, your arms, and your legs. Feel this light penetrate deep within your body until it permeates every single cell. Feel God's light transforming each cell and bringing it into Divine alignment. Feel yourself radiating this light as your own.

Now visualize your health springing forth speedily. Imagine your cells and your organs functioning normally. Speak to your cells, and command them in the name of Jehovah-rapha and the name of Christ Jesus to work according to God's Divine plan. Enforce the Word on every part of your body.

Ask God for forgiveness of your sins. See His Holy light washing you clean inside your heart and your soul. Come before God with your whole self – soul, mind, emotions, and body. Offer all of you to Him.

Allow the glory of God to fill you and let your life be an example to others of the majesty and magnificence of Jehovah-rapha. There are many people who are hurting, and they don't believe that there is a way out and a way through. Reach out to them, and show them how they, too, can receive the glory of God as their reward.

Almighty and most merciful God, I love this passage from Your Holy Scripture. Sometimes I feel stuck in the shadow and I feel afraid. I know that fear does not come from You. It is You who are my ever-present source of Divine light – having it burst on me like the sunrise. I particularly like the words "thine health shall spring forth speedily." I must admit that is what I want, God. A really speedy recovery. But help me to be willing to wait on You, Lord, and to follow Your path, whatever it is, trusting that it is perfect for me. In the name of Your Son, Christ Jesus, I pray, Amen.

Day 148

Do you not know? Have you not heard? The Lord is the everlasting God, the Creator of the ends of the earth. He will not grow tired or weary, and his understanding no one can fathom. He gives strength to the weary and increases the power of the weak. (Isaiah 40:28-29 NIV)

Do you not know? Have you not heard? Our Creator is the everlasting God! How glorious! Nothing – absolutely nothing – is beyond the power of God.

Often when we are ill, we feel tired, tired, tired. The weariness seeps through us down to our very bones. Every chore looms like a giant hurdle and every task seems like a heavy burden. Sometimes our eyes fill with tears, yet we don't even have the strength to cry.

At these moments turn your face to the Almighty God, your Creator. Let yourself feel His awesome power. Let yourself feel His mighty strength. He does not grow tired or weary. Not ever. And He is willing to pour His strength and power upon you in an everlasting flow of Divine energy and love. Our Lord Jesus Christ told us, "Ask and you shall receive." So ask for God's strength. Claim it. Feel it surrounding you and filling you. And say thank you.

Now give God your cares, your worries, and your fears. Name them, wrap them in a bundle, and lay them at the feet of the Lord God Almighty. Only after you do this are you ready to rest unencumbered by burdens that hinder the healing of your soul and your body.

Often it helps to envision the loving arms of God gathering you up just as a tender parent embraces a hurt and weary child. Sink into God's lap. Snuggle against His strong shoulder. Feel the Divine healing power of God on your skin as you lean fully on Him. Now feel that warmth, love, and grace penetrate deep within you and flow into every cell in your body. Smile and rest in the Lord.

Almighty God, You are the everlasting God. You are my Creator and the Creator of the ends of the earth. I feel weary; give me strength. I feel weak; increase my power. O, Lord, I claim Your Word in this Scripture. I need hope today. I need healing today. Be with me. Comfort me. Enfold Your loving arms around me and hold me close to you. Let me rest in Your strength, O God. Renew my soul. Renew, restore, and transform every cell in my body. Help me to fulfill Your mission and Your purpose for me. With grateful thanks I pray in the name of Your Son, Jesus Christ, my Savior and my Redeemer, Amen.

Day 149

By him therefore let us offer the sacrifice of praise to God continually, that is, the fruit of our lips giving thanks to his name. (Hebrews 13:15 KJV)

Like a child who flings his arms around the neck of a loving parent with an exuberant hug, we run to God with prayers of gratitude, saying, "Thank You, thank You, thank You!"

The writer of Hebrews reminds us to say "thank You" *continually, which means to keep on doing something without stopping. Amazing. We are to say* "thank You" without interrupting our songs of praise. Why? Because every good gift comes from God and the least we can do is to be grateful.

An attitude of gratitude is vital for those who feel ill because the easier path is often to be critical and hard to please. It is easy to give in to depression, listlessness, and crankiness. The more you allow yourself to spin in negative thoughts, however, the deeper your illness penetrates into your body and your soul.

Post little notecards in the rooms of your home. All they have to say is "Say thank you." Be sure to put two or three in your kitchen. Put one on your refrigerator and one on your kitchen cabinet where you keep your dishes.

Why is the kitchen important? Because nutrition provides the building blocks at the physical level for you to heal. Saturating your food in generous amounts of gratitude will have a positive effect in the way you digest your meals and in the way you assimilate the nutrients.

What a difference gratitude makes. Saying thank you, thank you, thank you a hundred times a day brings the healing power of love into your body. Gratitude can actually create a change in your body chemistry as positive energy flows through you.

As you reach up to God with thanksgiving, He smiles down on you with His healing grace. The "You're welcome" of God and the Holy Spirit is a shower of healing water that purifies you and washes you clean.

Wonderful Jehovah-rapha, thank You, thank You, thank You. Every minute of the day is a gift from You. I joyfully sing my praises of thanksgiving and I declare my gratitude for the many blessings You shower upon me. I choose to be positive. I choose to focus on Your goodness and mercy. I choose to maintain an attitude of gratitude. And I choose to look up and reach for the stars. In the name of Your Son, Jesus Christ, my Savior and my Redeemer, I pray, Amen.

Day 150

O Lord, how manifold are thy works! In wisdom hast thou made them all: the earth is full of thy riches. (Psalm 104:24 KJV)

God made everything that is in the natural world *in wisdom*. That means that everything has a place in creation and a purpose in creation (even if most of us are still trying to figure out the necessity for the mosquito). Think about the implication of this for a moment. It means that God made what we call "germs." God made bacteria and viruses – and interestingly, He made them in great abundance.

In the past hundred or so years, the scientific community has developed two predominant theories of health in relation to these germs. One viewpoint is the germ theory expounded by Pasteur, which is based on the belief that germs are the cause of disease. The other viewpoint is the "law of the terrain," which is based on the belief that imbalances in the body are the cause of disease because they create an environment favorable to the survival and growth of germs. It is interesting that Pasteur at the end of his life came to recant his belief in the germ theory and to state that "the germ is nothing, but the terrain is everything."

Today most of us are caught up in the fight to kill all viruses and bacteria we deem as harmful. This external focus on an invading "bug" allows us to keep on doing just exactly what we want to do in our personal lifestyles – and we find that the germs simply mutate and become more and more resistant to our drugs. We need to stop playing victim to germs and to turn to God for instruction on building a strong terrain within our bodies. We have to accept responsibility for our health and for our daily decisions that affect our well-being. Just as satan cannot live in a soul that is working in harmony with God, neither can disease live in a body that is functioning in harmony with itself and with the Lord.

God made bacteria and viruses just as He made us. He established rules for our good health and knew that, if we are obedient, good health will follow. Turn to the Lord. Ask the Holy Spirit to reveal to you what you need to change in your life so that you can create an environment within that promotes health.

Almighty Lord, I take responsibility for having made mistakes in taking care of my body. You made the universe, you made germs, and you made me. Show me what You want me to do, and I will do it so that my temple will be well and strong to glorify Your name. Thank You, Jehovah-rapha, for healing me. In Jesus' name, I pray, Amen.

Day 151

David said to the Philistine, "You come against me with sword and spear and javelin, but I come against you in the name of the Lord Almighty. . . . All those gathered here will know that it is not by sword or spear that the Lord saves; for the battle is the Lord's and he will give all of you into our hands." (1 Samuel 17:45, 47 NIV)

When illness looms above us, it can seem as big and as mighty as Goliath looked to the Israelites. Read the entire story of David and Goliath in 1 Samuel 17. A nine-foot-tall giant stomps up and down, hurling insults and challenges to the Israelites. "Come on, I dare you. Send over your best man to try to kill me. If you win, we Philistines will be your subjects. If you lose, then you must be our subjects."

What was the response of the Israelites? Fear. Then young David comes in from tending his father's sheep and says, "Hey, what's this guy doing? Somebody needs to stop him." His brother calls him conceited and tries to make David be quiet. However, David goes to Saul and offers to fight Goliath. After trying on some heavy armor, he takes it off and picks up five smooth stones. He goes before Goliath, tells him that "the battle is the Lord's," and then he kills the giant.

This story offers a model for dealing with disease which comes to us as Goliath. The evil one wants to claim us and he uses disease as his mighty giant. However, God does not want us to be subject to illness. We may feel as scrawny as young David, but the battle is not ours – the battle is God's.

What is our weapon? It is the power of the Lord. When we look for earthly weapons to fight disease, think about the example shown to us by David. He took a look at the man-made weaponry, but what was he led to use? One of God's natural substances – which happened to be a smooth stone. Be open to allow God to work through you with His natural substances. He has provided them for us for a reason and a purpose. Goliath, satan, and disease must fall when confronted with the face of Jehovah.

Mighty Lord, thank You for the example of David. I face my own Goliath – this health condition that wants dominance over me. The battle is Yours, God. As I ask Your Divine guidance for the pathway to my healing, I choose among my weapons Your natural remedies. Disease has no power in my life. Disease has no authority over me. You alone are Lord. You alone are Jehovah-rapha. With grateful thanks, I pray in the name of Your Son, Jesus Christ, my Savior and Redeemer, Amen.

Day 152

Be not overmuch wicked, neither be thou foolish: why shouldest thou die before thy time?
(Ecclesiastes 7:17 KJV)

Why die before your time? God wants you to fulfill all your days. He wants you to fulfill His purpose for your life. Here in Ecclesiastes it is put clearly before us that it is usually up to us whether we die before our time. Notice what the major sources of dying before our time are according to Ecclesiastes – either being too wicked or being too foolish. Aren't these interesting reasons?

The health consequences of being foolish are myriad – and obvious. If we live on hamburgers and French fries, we are likely to develop heart disease. If we gorge ourselves on candy and sweets, we are likely to develop diabetes. If we breathe in smoke, we are likely to develop emphysema.

Many diseases are a result of our own foolishness and stubbornness. They are not the result of God's will but of *our* own will and our determination to do just exactly what we want when we want to do it. There is a price to pay, but often that accounting does not occur until years and even decades of abuse. We lie to ourselves and think that we are getting away with our actions. Led further and further astray by the father of lies, we end up trapped and ill.

The health consequences of being sinful are less obvious. When we have anger and bitterness in our hearts, our bodies are affected. When we are filled with desire for revenge, our bodies are affected. When we gloat over taking advantage of others, our bodies are affected.

None of these negative emotions are of God; they are tools of the evil one and they set up an internal environment for illness. The more quickly we recognize that we are out of step with God, the more quickly we can ask forgiveness and make our correction to get back into alignment.

Don't choose to die before your time. Ask for forgiveness, and make the changes you need to make in your life so that you may fulfill your days.

Almighty God, forgive my sins. Deliver me from the traps of the evil one, and cleanse me of the negative emotions that are harmful to both my body and my soul. Warn me when I am being foolish and help me to walk with You in joy and obedience. Keep me on track, God, so that I may follow Your will for me. In the name of Christ Jesus, my Savior and my Redeemer, I pray, Amen.

Day 153

Know also that wisdom is sweet to your soul; if you find it, there is a future hope for you, and your hope will not be cut off. (Proverbs 24:14 NIV)

Wisdom is sweet to your soul – and to your mind, your emotions, and your body. *If you find it,* there is a future hope for you. We get so caught up in the daily whirlwind of our jobs, school, errands, chores, clubs, and activities that we take little time to seek wisdom.

Jesus told us that, if we would seek, we would find. We have both the Holy Scriptures and the Holy Spirit as voices of wisdom and guidance for us. God's health laws are among the wisdom we have to be willing to seek. If we find them, there is a future for us, and our lives will not be cut off prematurely by our own foolishness and disobedience.

How do we know what foods are wise choices and which are unwise? Turn to God's Holy Scripture. First, look for things that God specifically tells us are to be food for us. Read Genesis 1:29 (seeds, nuts, fruits, and vegetables) and Genesis 3:18 (plants of the field), for example. Also read Leviticus 11:2-23 (animals that are not scavengers).

Second, look for items that God tells us not to eat. Read Leviticus 7:23 (cover fat of cattle, sheep, or goats) and Deuteronomy 12:16 (blood of animals).

Third, look for edible things that God gives as gifts. Read Ezekiel 16:19 (whole grain flour, olive oil, and honey) and Exodus 16:13-15 (quail and manna).

Fourth, look for food that Jesus ate or gave to others to eat. Read Matthew 15:36 (whole grain bread and fish) and Isaiah 7:15 (curds and honey).

Fifth, look for food that Jesus used in His stories and parables. Read Matthew 7:9-11 (fish and whole grain bread) and Luke 11:11-13 (fish and eggs).

God blessed our bodies with thousands of internal healing mechanisms. In order for them to function properly we have to provide our bodies with appropriate food and nutrition. We must seek the wisdom that will provide us with a healthy future according to God's plan.

Almighty God, sometimes I want my future the easy way, my way. I seek your wisdom, knowing that it is healing to my soul and to my mind and to my body. Only in Your wisdom is there a future hope for me which will not be cut off. I am seeking, Lord. Teach me. In Jesus' name, Amen.

Day 154

Then he said to them, "Suppose one of you has a friend, and he goes to him at midnight and says, 'Friend, lend me three loaves of bread, because a friend of mine on a journey has come to me, and I have nothing to set before him.' Then the one inside answers, 'Don't bother me. The door is already locked, and my children are with me in bed. I can't get up and give you anything.' I tell you, though he will not get up and give him the bread because he is his friend, yet because of the man's boldness he will get up and give him as much as he needs. So I say to you: Ask and it will be given to you; seek and you will find; knock and the door will be opened to you. For everyone who asks receives; he who seeks finds; and to him who knocks, the door will be opened." (Luke 11:5-10 NIV)

Keep praying, Jesus tells us. Ask once for what you want and then pray prayers of thanksgiving over and over again. Boldness and persistence are valuable and important traits, and they are extremely useful tools in your healing.

Does this mean that God can be manipulated into healing us and that all we have to do is to browbeat God into making us well? Of course not. God does not "perform on command." Seeing directly into our hearts, He *knows* our innermost thoughts and feelings. It is only earnest faith-filled prayers which are heard.

Notice that Jesus tells us to ask and to seek. At first glance, they might seem to be the same thing, but they are not. Our asking for God's help comes when we pray.

But what about the seeking? Our seeking comes when we are quiet and listen for God's guidance. It is only then that we will find our answers, and frequently they are unexpected ones. For example, we may have asked for guidance about using a particular herb for an intestinal problem, yet in the stillness we are told, "Forgive your brother."

Be bold in going to Jehovah-rapha for your healing. Be willing to hear His instructions. Be joyful in giving thanks for His many blessings in your life.

Almighty God, I come to You as Your Son Jesus Christ told me to do – boldly and persistently. I ask Your help and Your healing, God, and I know that it will be given to me. I seek Your guidance and I know that I will find it. I knock at Your door, Jehovah-rapha, and I know that it will be opened to me. All these things are written in Your Holy Word and I claim them as my truth. Guide me, God, and I will obey. In the name of Your Son, Jesus Christ, my Savior and my Redeemer, I pray, Amen.

Day 155

As Jesus went on from there, two blind men followed him, calling out, "Have mercy on us, Son of David!" When he had gone indoors, the blind men came to him, and he asked them, "Do you believe that I am able to do this?" "Yes, Lord," they replied. Then he touched their eyes and said, "According to your faith will it be done to you"; and their sight was restored. (Matthew 9:27-30 NIV)

Here is a short, simple story of Jesus as He healed two blind men. We don't know from this Scripture what had caused each of the men's blindness. What scientific explanations would we use today? Glaucoma? Macular degeneration? Diabetes? Injury? Blindness is as frightening a diagnosis today as it was in Jesus' time. Think about going to a doctor who has vast knowledge about eyes and hearing him say, "I'm sorry. You are going blind. There is no known cure. Maybe we can try some new procedures or drugs." What do you do now?

You have to put aside your emotional feelings of fear and despair. You even have to put aside your logic (remember Noah). What you must do now is to go to God in prayer, meditation, and silence. Be open to God's voice and *only* God's voice so that you can hear clearly what God has to say. Satan loves to deceive us. He especially loves to get us to equate scientific fact based on the knowledge and mind of man with Divine fact based on the wisdom and mind of God. He loves to get us to believe only in the tangible "facts" that we can see and hear and touch. He wants us to believe all test results are conclusive.

When the blind men came to him, Jesus asked, "Do you believe I can do this?" What is your answer today? Do you believe in the power of your illness or do you believe in the power of God? Do you believe that science defines reality for you? Your healing depends on what you believe and what you trust.

"Your faith has made you whole," Jesus said. Go to God in faith and in quietness. Go to God believing that He wants you to be well. Go to God believing that He can heal you. Go to God believing that He is healing you. Ask for His guidance and He will tell you what to do.

Dear Heavenly Father, You have declared Yourself as Jehovah-rapha – the God who heals me. Sometimes man's reality and man's truth seem overwhelming to me. Help me to see myself with Your eyes. Reveal to me exactly what You want me to do for the manifestation of my healing. Help me to follow Your guidance even if it seems foolish to me and those around me. Thank You for healing me. In Jesus' name, I pray, Amen.

Day 156

O Lord my God, I called to you for help and you healed me. O Lord, you brought me up from the grave; you spared me from going down into the pit. (Psalm 30:2-3 NIV)

When Jesus had finished saying these things, he left Galilee and went into the region of Judea to the other side of the Jordan. Large crowds followed him, and he healed them there. (Matthew 19:1-2 NIV)

God's Word is filled with acts of healing. From the Psalmist in the Old Testament who declares "You healed me" to the healing ministry of Jesus in the New Testament, we are given account after account of God's healing power.

Take heart that God wants you to be well. Where His will is worked perfectly – in the Garden of Eden, in heaven, and in the life and ministry of His Son Jesus Christ – there is no illness. Accept that into your consciousness at every level and dimension of your being. Eliminate phrases in your prayers such as "if it be Your will, please heal me." Stand on God's Word and pray instead, "I claim Your healing, Jehovah-rapha; let Your will be done on earth and in my life and in my body as it is in heaven."

Understand what is going on in your body so that you know what the imbalances are within your organs and cells. Then speak to these imbalances and command them to come into alignment with the Lord God Almighty. Command your cells to function as God intended them to function. For example, in the name of Jesus command the cells of your pancreas to secrete proper amounts of insulin or command the cells of your skeletal system to build healthy, strong bones. Enforce the Word of God on the organs and cells of your body.

Listen for God's instruction about the ways that you are to participate in your healing – whether it be to undergo certain treatment or to use certain healing methods. Always be obedient to God's voice.

Wonderful Jehovah-rapha, I call to You for help and You heal me. O Lord, You sent Your Son to carry my sins to the Cross and to bear all my infirmities. I need Your healing touch in my life. O, God, I want to be Your full partner in my healing process. I joyfully proclaim my healing, and I rest in Your power and grace. Thank You, God, for all Your mercies to me. Help me to live in full service to You. In the name of Your Son, Jesus Christ, my Savior and my Redeemer, I pray, Amen.

Day 157

I can do all things through Christ which strengtheneth me. (Philippians 4:13 KJV)

Paul had been imprisoned, beaten, stoned, shipwrecked, robbed, hungry, and cold. Certainly, he had endured far more tribulations than most people ever encounter in one lifetime. Despite all these hardships here he is proclaiming that "I can do all things through Christ which strengtheneth me." He knew that there was no attack powerful enough to separate him from the love of God and Jesus Christ. As long as Paul kept his eyes focused steadfastly on his Risen Lord, he would emerge victorious.

The source of illness is the evil one. When you are attacked in your body, look to Christ Jesus for your strength and for your healing. You can do all things with the help of the Lord if you are willing to do your part. You must be willing to see how you have allowed yourself to become vulnerable to satan's attack and look for the ways that you contributed to your situation. What things could you have done differently to keep your body and immune system strong and more resistant to infection and disease? Ask the Holy Spirit to reveal to you anything you may have overlooked.

Then go in prayer asking how to handle your illness or infirmity. Pray with complete trust. Pray with expectation of results. Pray believing that your request, which is in accordance with God's will that His children be well, is already being answered. Hold fast to your faith. Listen for the instructions of the Holy Spirit for your healing and follow them exactly.

While you are in the process of recovery, do not focus on all the negative aspects of your situation. Paul said that he had "learned to be content whatever the circumstances" (Philippians 4:11). He knew that you can't proclaim faith and belief and simultaneously be negative, critical, and worried. Maintaining a positive frame of mind is an integral expression of faith. No matter what challenges you face today, rejoice. Your life is a glorious witness to the awesome power of the Lord to overcome it all.

Wonderful Jehovah-rapha, I can do all things through Your Son Jesus Christ who strengthens me. I am determined to stop saying words of despair and defeat and to stop looking at my world with negative eyes. I claim the positive vision and power of Christ Jesus who carried my infirmities to the Cross. In Jesus' name, I pray, Amen.

Day 158

He will die for lack of discipline, led astray by his own great folly. (Proverbs 5:23 NIV)

Self-discipline is a major issue in healing and recovery from illness. There are many things that we know we should do, and we struggle to find the time to do them. Then on the other hand, there are many things that we know we should *not* do, and yet time after time we find ourselves doing them. The worst part is that we judge ourselves by our failures and then use our failing as an excuse to give up.

If you are having these problems, take a deep breath and welcome yourself to the human race. Lighten up. Smile. And begin again. This time focus on just one part of your healing program. For example, suppose you are working on your eyes and your guidance is to use an herbal eyewash. You know you should do it, and you managed to do it for about a week, but then your schedule got crowded, your energy was low, and you felt too irritable to do it.

Go in prayer to God. Tell Him about your struggles and your difficulties. Check with Him to make sure that you are still to continue the eyewash, and make sure that you are clear about the particular herbs to use. Once you are certain about God's guidance, ask for help in making this part of your healing a priority in your life.

Spend some time in meditation to see if there are any emotional blocks to your being healed. In this example, is there anything in your life – past, present, or future – that you don't want to see? Ask God to reveal to you what you need to know in order to allow healing to flow freely to you.

Then ask God to help you to integrate the details of your healing program into your life. Make a commitment to God to exercise self-discipline. Don't allow the evil one to sabotage your healing and lead you down the road of folly.

Claim God's mighty power and offer each step in your program to God. Do it in His name and for His glory.

Wonderful Jehovah-rapha, I don't want to die for lack of discipline, led astray by the evil one and my own great folly. Help me to be disciplined, Lord. I offer every part of my healing program to You. I perform each act in Your name and for Your glory. I am determined to walk the path to my healing that You want me to follow. Thank You, God, for leading me every step of the way. In the name of Your Son, Jesus Christ, I pray, Amen.

Day 159

In the same way, count yourselves dead to sin but alive to God in Christ Jesus. Therefore do not let sin reign in your mortal body so that you obey its evil desires. Do not offer the parts of your body to sin, as instruments of wickedness, but rather offer yourselves to God, as those who have been brought from death to life; and offer the parts of your body to him as instruments of righteousness. For sin shall not be your master, because you are not under law, but under grace. (Romans 6:11-14 NIV)

Health is a decision you make. Health is the result of your taking responsibility for the condition of your body, spirit, emotion, and mind. Satan wants your soul and he seeks control over your body as a way to get power over you. If he cannot get you to worship him and follow him spiritually, he will settle for getting you to live in a state of fear – whether it is fear of people around you, fear of your environment, or fear of your illness.

Paul warns you not to let sin reign in your mortal body nor to offer parts of your body to sin. Remember that your body was created by the Lord God Almighty. Your body is the temple of the Holy Spirit. It is to be reverenced and treated with respect. Your body should be an instrument of God, and through it you are to be a witness of your faith and your belief.

Satan will tempt you, however, to make your body become an instrument of sin and self-destruction instead. You may be tempted to eat foods that God did not intend for food, and consequently your body is invaded and destroyed by parasites, bacteria, and viruses. You may be tempted to collapse on the sofa after a day of sitting behind a desk instead of walking or dancing or moving your body.

You may be tempted to use mood-altering alcohol or drugs in an attempt to suppress the pain from emotional wounds you do not have the courage to face. You may be tempted to use your body in promiscuous or immoral sexual acts.

God first breathed the breath of life in you and He has brought you from death to life once again. Offer every part of your body to Him as an instrument of righteousness.

Wonderful Jehovah-rapha, I offer my body to You as the temple of Your Holy Spirit. You have brought me from death to life, and I offer all of me as an instrument of righteousness. God, I am under Your grace totally and completely. In the name of Your Son, Jesus Christ, I pray, Amen.

Day 160

And a woman was there who had been subject to bleeding for twelve years, but no one could heal her. She came up behind him and touched the edge of his cloak, and immediately her bleeding stopped. "Who touched me?" Jesus asked. (Luke 8:43-45 NIV)

Jesus was very aware of the Divine energy that was within Him. When God created each one of us, He breathed in us the breath of life, *His* breath of life, which carried with it His Divine energy. It is a glorious gift which we must treat with awe and respect.

As you increase your awareness of energy, you will begin to observe that those things which were made by the Creator have His Divine energy inside and those things made by man do not. Go outside and pick a flower, a leaf, or some growing plant. Place it between the palms of your hands, and ask the Holy Spirit to help you to feel the Divine energy of the plant. Eventually you will feel the life force of God's creation. As a contrast, hold a piece of plastic or synthetic fabric, and you will discover it has no Divine energy at all. Instead, it has a reversed, "jangly" kind of energy.

Learning to sense energy as Jesus did is an important tool for you in your healing. Suppose you have been guided by the Holy Spirit to use herbs for your healing. Pick up a bottle of herbs, hold it in your right hand, and place it against your body just above your navel. Ask the Holy Spirit to fill you and to help you to feel the Divine energy of the herbs. Then listen and feel. High quality herbs have a strong Divine life energy; poor quality herbs do not.

Try holding a bottle of herbs and then holding processed cane sugar. Practice using different substances. Do so with reverence and intention. You aren't learning a trick to show off to others. You are learning to become attuned to God's Divine energy as Jesus was. This technique can be a useful tool to assist you in making wise choices about appropriate food, herbs, supplements, and medicine.

Be sure to ask the Holy Spirit to guide you so that you will not be misled by the evil one. Use this Divine energy to facilitate your healing by increasing your awareness of it. Give grateful thanks for the gift of God's Holy energy.

Almighty Lord, thank You for putting Your Divine energy in me and all Your creation. As You help me to attune myself to it, send the Holy Spirit to guide me and to help me to use it wisely for my healing. In the name of Your Son, Jesus Christ, my Savior and Redeemer, I pray, Amen.

Day 161

Submit yourselves, then, to God. Resist the devil, and he will flee from you. Come near to God and he will come near to you. (James 4:7-8 NIV)

The words sound rather simple, "Submit yourselves to God. Resist the devil and he will flee from you." The reality can be quite difficult. All godly people will be attacked by the devil because those are the ones he especially wants to control. And he will use any tool he can to accomplish his goal.

If we feel sick, we know that the evil one has found a vulnerable spot and has been successful in getting through to us. Ultimately, he cannot win if we resist him. But it can be much harder to resist him than we think if we do not get clear about the ways that he attacks us.

Your physical illness is often entangled with your emotional issues. At the core are often the pain of loneliness and a fear of not being loved. Those two factors drive us to do everything for everyone, to take abuse repeatedly, and to ignore our own needs in the process.

The evil one convinces us to deceive ourselves that we are going the second mile when in fact we are not loving ourselves as we love others. The result is that we deplete our physical energy, we deplete our financial resources, and we deplete our emotional stamina. Finally, many of us break down, either physically or emotionally or both.

Who has won? Whose purpose has been served? And what will the people do who just could not get along without you? Unless they decide to change, they will keep on doing what they were doing. They will make whatever adjustments they are forced to make and they will go on.

To resist the devil means to be willing to make the changes we need to make in our lives. Yes, we need to pray, but we have to act as well. We must identify what is causing us pain and then release those destructive emotions. We must embrace the truth that we are loved with the everlasting love of Jehovah-rapha. God will always help us. As we come near to God, He will come near to us.

Almighty God, help me to identify those places in my life where I make myself vulnerable to the evil one. I choose to resist the devil, Lord. I am willing to let go of the emotional pain that is hurting me and am willing to make changes in my life. I am willing, God; I am. I come to You freely, asking that You cleanse me and make me whole. Thank You, Heavenly Father, for staying near to me and for healing me. In Jesus' name, I pray, Amen.

Day 162

When the sun was setting, the people brought to Jesus all who had various kinds of sickness, and laying his hands on each one, he healed them. Moreover, demons came out of many people, shouting, "You are the Son of God!" (Luke 4:40-41 NIV)

Jesus healed them all. The question you must decide in your own mind is whether he is available to heal *you*, today, now, two thousand years later. Many people believe that the healings of Jesus were part of the signs and wonders to "prove" he was the Son of God. Therefore, it was a display only for the time that He was to be on earth. But, if that were true, He wouldn't have had to heal *everybody*. For example, Elijah raised a boy from the dead and Isaiah healed Hezekiah with a fig poultice. God's power was demonstrated quite well in each case by one spectacular healing. The same thing could have happened with Jesus. But it didn't. He healed them *all*.

Scripture repeatedly tells us why. Jesus tells us he came to do the will of the Father and to set at liberty all who are oppressed of the devil. He came to bear our infirmities as well as our sins. We do not question that He took the sins of *all* people to the Cross. We know He didn't die for the sins of just the people living two thousand years ago but that He also died for our sins as well. And He died for the sins of every person yet to be born who will believe in Him. Jesus redeemed all God's children for all time to come.

Pay attention that it is written that "demons came out of many people" as they were healed. Notice the words, "many people." Not all of those who were ill had demons within, but many did. Today some people are not healed because they are not willing to consider the possibility that they, too, may have a demon inside. There is some vulnerability where the evil one has seized control.

Don't assume that the language about demons is a figure of speech based only on people's ignorance. Jesus was not naïve or stupid or lacking in knowledge. He knew exactly what He was doing and why He was doing it. Go to Jesus in prayer, and ask Him to rebuke any demons that may be within you so that you may be healed.

Wonderful Jehovah-rapha, the glorious news is that Your Son came and He healed every single person who came to Him and who needed healing. I know that the evil one is the author of disease. Cleanse me physically, emotionally, and spiritually. Cast out any demons that may be within me. Thank You, Father, for healing me. In Jesus' name, I pray, Amen.

Day 163

A man with leprosy came to him and begged him on his knees, "If you are willing, you can make me clean." Filled with compassion, Jesus reached out his hand and touched the man. "I am willing," he said. "Be clean!" Immediately the leprosy left him and he was cured. (Mark 1:40-42 NIV)

It is interesting to note that there are only a couple of places recorded in the Holy Scriptures where someone comes to Jesus for healing and does not assume that Jesus will heal him. Here we see the man with leprosy saying, "if you are willing, heal me."

Notice the response of Jesus. He was filled with compassion for the man, and He immediately reached out to touch him, saying, "I am willing." Since Jesus was the perfect expression of God's will, every act and every statement reflected the will of Jehovah. With regard to healing, Jesus left no one sick for any reason. Therefore, when the leper came questioning Jesus' will to heal him, Jesus wanted to make sure that that issue was settled immediately. "I am willing. Be clean."

Using the phrase "if it be thy will" with regard to a request for healing does not stand on God's Word since such a statement relies on hope rather than faith. It is an expression that says, "Maybe God will heal me and maybe He won't." Questioning God's intent undermines your faith and, therefore, diminishes the likelihood of your healing.

"If it be thy will" is a completely appropriate prayer when you are trying to determine if you should move to a certain city, marry a certain person, or choose a certain career. These answers depend on a revelation from the Spirit and are not found in the Holy Scripture.

But God's healing will *is* declared in the Holy Scripture, and the actions of Christ Jesus fulfilled God's Word perfectly by healing *everyone* who came to be made well.

Thank Your Heavenly Father for declaring that He is the God who heals you. Thank God for sending His Son Christ Jesus to carry your infirmities to the Cross. Thank the Lord God Almighty for revealing to you the path to your healing.

Wonderful Jehovah-rapha, I stand on Your Holy Scriptures. You are the God who heals me. The question is not "if" but "how." I know that You have a special pathway for my healing. Reveal it to me and I will obey all Your instructions. Thank You, God, for healing me and making me whole. In the name of Your Son, Jesus Christ, my Savior and my Redeemer, I pray, Amen.

Day 164

Show me your ways, O Lord, teach me your paths; guide me in your truth and teach me, for you are God my Savior and my hope is in you all day long. (Psalm 25:4-5 NIV)

How easy it is to get off God's path. This is especially true when we are making decisions about our health. Even when we are clear about God's guidance, temptations abound to keep us from making healthy choices for our lives. We must remember "my hope is in you all day long." That means every moment of every day. No matter what.

As hard as it is to do what we need to do for our health when we know what the right thing is, it is harder still to find God's path when we are in doubt. Most health problems can be handled in several different ways. How do we know which is the path God wants us to take? Which is the particular way that God wants for us?

Often we are given very firm medical opinions that demand a certain path for treatment. To consider doing something different may be very frightening. Usually, too, our family and friends have definite opinions about what we should do – and to fail to comply with their wishes is also unsettling. Remember, the voice of fear drowns out the voice of God so we must hand our fears to God as often as it is necessary.

Retreat into the heart of this psalm. "Show me YOUR ways, O Lord. Teach me YOUR paths." The opinions of others are important and it is right to give them prayerful consideration. However, your ultimate, final authority is the Almighty God. Quieten your mind. Go within. Ask God to reveal clearly to you what He desires you to do. Take deep breaths and put aside your fears. Tell your intellectual self to relax and be still and to put aside all assumptions.

Reach beyond yourself and rest in the heart of God. Listen for guidance. If you don't "hear" anything, then tell God you need help hearing Him. Ask Him to "speak up" and to make His pathway clearly known to you.

Almighty God, I need Your help. I hand my fears over to You. I see my symptoms, and I feel in my body how my lack of health affects me. Everyone around me seems to know what I should do, God. And most of them seem so sure of themselves. I come to You, O God, because You are The Great Physician. I stand on Your Holy Word and I look beyond the appearance to Your truth. Let me hear Your voice clearly. Teach me to relax so that I can listen well. Send me Your guidance in the form I can hear it best. In Jesus' name, I pray, Amen.

Day 165

Therefore, I urge you, brothers, in view of God's mercy, to offer your bodies as living sacrifices, holy and pleasing to God – this is your spiritual act of worship. (Romans 12:1 NIV)

Paul exhorts you to offer your body to God as a living sacrifice and as a spiritual act of worship. Would it make a difference in your choices if you thought of every movement of your body and every act you do *for* it and *to* it as an act of worship to the Lord God Almighty?

Most of the things we do are accomplished without much conscious thought at all. Our nose itches and we scratch it. Our muscle feels cramped and we stretch it. Our stomach growls and we eat. Our bodies feel ill and we reach for a drug. Rarely do we think of any of these things as an act of worship.

Whether you feel sick or whether you feel well, offer your body to God as a living sacrifice, holy and pleasing to Him. God is your Creator. He made you, and, therefore, your body is pleasing to Him as a reflection of His majesty and creative power. Your body was designed as a temple, the temple of the Holy Spirit. It is a magnificent instrument for God's purpose.

There is no human being who understands how an egg and a sperm can unite and ultimately form a being of trillions of cells, each one filled with life, each one having a specific function, and each one fulfilling its purpose in harmony with the others. No one ever will. We may dangerously experiment with cloning life that already exists, but it is the breath of God and God alone that creates life.

Because your body is God's Holy creation, you should look to God for instruction on its care. Let God's Holy Word show you the proper nourishment and food for it. Let God guide you to the use of His own remedies through essential oils or herbs or to treatment by spirit-led medical personnel. Let God be your sole authority, and let everything you use regarding your health function as an instrument for working God's will. God has breathed in you the breath of life and He wants you well. He wants you to glorify and worship Him with your body.

Wonderful Jehovah-rapha, I offer my body to You as a living sacrifice. May it be holy and pleasing to You, God, as Your awesome creation. I honor and respect my body and treat it lovingly and with care. I enforce Your Word upon it and claim healing for it in the name of Your Son Christ Jesus. Thank You, Jehovah-rapha, for healing me. In Jesus' name I pray, Amen.

Day 166

Philip said to Him, "Lord, show us the Father [cause us to see the Father – that is all we ask]; then we shall be satisfied." Jesus replied, "Have I been with all of you for so long a time, and do you not recognize and know Me yet, Philip? Anyone who has seen Me has seen the Father. How can you say then, 'Show us the Father?' Do you not believe that I am in the Father, and that the Father is in Me? What I am telling you I do not say on My own authority and of My own accord; but the Father Who lives continually in Me does the (His) works (His own miracles, deeds of power). Believe Me that I am in the Father and the Father in Me; or else believe Me for the sake of the [very] works themselves. [If you cannot trust Me, at least let these works that I do in My Father's name convince you.]" (John 14:8-11 AMP)

Jesus tells Philip that everything He is doing is of the Father. He is very clear about that. And Jesus says that it is the Father who does the healing, who performs the miracles.

Jesus says something else that is very interesting. He tells Philip to believe Him because He is telling him the truth – but that, if his words are hard to accept, then to believe Him *for the sake of the works themselves*. What were the works of Jesus? He taught people about God's love for them. He taught people about the kingdom of heaven. He healed the leper. He gave sight to the blind. He made the cripple to stand up and walk. And He raised the dead.

Look at what I am doing, Jesus says. Look at all the things I am doing in my Father's name. I am working my Father's will. When I tell you to love one another, I am doing that because God wants you to love one another. When I heal you, I do that because God wants you well.

Let the works of Jesus convince you that God wants you to be well. Jesus Himself pleads with you to do this. Listen to Him. Believe Him. Give thanks that He has already paid the price for you – soul and body. It is written. Command the evil one to leave your body and enforce the words of Jesus on it. Declare your concentrated, focused faith and belief in your healing.

Dear Heavenly Father, I accept the message of Your Son Jesus Christ, who asks me to let His works convince me that He is the Son of God and that He does only Your will. I accept the Gospels into my heart. I do believe, Father. I seek ever to follow Your Son and to obey You, Lord. Thank You for teaching me; thank You for saving me; thank You for healing me. In Jesus' name, I pray, Amen.

Day 167

He sendeth the springs into the valleys, which run among the hills. They give drink to every beast of the field: the wild asses quench their thirst. By them shall the fowls of the heaven have their habitation, which sing among the branches. He watereth the hills from his chambers. (Psalm 104:10-13 KJV)

Water is essential for life. God has provided it in great abundance both outside our bodies (the earth is about 70 percent water) and inside our bodies (we are about 65 percent water). Without sufficient water we can survive only a few days because the cells of the body cannot function properly without it. For example, water is critical in our eliminative process and in the regulation of our body temperature. Many illnesses come upon us after many years of partial dehydration of our bodies.

Thank about the water described in this lovely Psalm and then consider what we do to water. We routinely dump waste materials into our water supply and then add more chemicals to attempt to clean it up enough to drink. We add fluoride, which is a potent poison, on the erroneous assumption that it prevents cavities in teeth. In our folly, we end up with bones filled with brittle fluoride (having replaced calcium) and with bone fracture rates 2-3 times as high as those who drink unfluoridated water.

We also add chlorine to kill bacteria, which it does very effectively. Unfortunately, however, studies as old as the 1930s show that chlorine is also linked to various types of heart disease – now the leading cause of death in our country. Are these health problems God's will? Of course not. He plainly told us that He gave us dominion over the earth (Genesis 1:28). We are listening to the lies of the evil one, killing ourselves, and then blaming God for it.

In order for you to be healthy, it is vital to drink large amounts of pure, wholesome water. You must find the healthiest supply you can – whether it be distilled water with added minerals or truly healthy spring water. God will not be mocked. To be well you must return to the basics and water is one of the most essential.

Almighty God, Maker of heaven and earth, I seek to return to Your plan for life by consuming healthy water. I have taken water for granted and haven't made the effort to see that I drink and bathe in water that promotes my good health. I understand now, God, how I have contributed to my health problems and I return to Your plan for pure water. In Jesus' name, I pray, Amen.

Day 168

"Go back and tell Hezekiah, the leader of my people, 'This is what the Lord, the God of your father David, says: I have heard your prayer and seen your tears; I will heal you. On the third day from now you will go up to the temple of the Lord. I will add fifteen years to your life. And I will deliver you and this city from the hand of the king of Assyria. I will defend this city for my sake and for the sake of my servant David.' " Then Isaiah said, "Prepare a poultice of figs." They did so and applied it to the boil, and he recovered. (2 Kings 20:5-7 NIV)

Living in the time before Jesus has come to atone for all, Hezekiah, king of Judah, is still under the curse of Adam. He becomes gravely ill, and the prophet Isaiah goes to him, tells him to prepare for death, and then leaves. Hezekiah immediately turns to the Lord and cries out to Him. "Remember, O Lord, how I have walked before you faithfully and with wholehearted devotion and have done what is good in your eyes."

God responds to Hezekiah by intercepting Isaiah before he can even get out of the courtyard. "I have heard thy prayer. I have seen thy tears," God says as He extends his mercy on Hezekiah and promises to heal him. In only three days the healing will be accomplished.

God chooses different healing methods for different people. With some He simply speaks His Word and they are healed. With others, there is a process of healing requiring actions at the physical level. In Hezekiah's case, the Lord reveals to Isaiah to prepare a poultice of figs. We usually think of figs as a fruit to eat; however, it is little known fact that they are one of the most alkaline of all foods and have a powerful anti-acid effect. Therefore, they have historically been used for ulcers (of both the mouth and the stomach), heartburn, boils on the gums, and also to help remove bad odors from cancers. Holy Scripture tells us that figs were applied to Hezekiah's boil according to God's instruction and he recovered.

Let Jehovah-rapha show you His plan for your path to healing. Perhaps, like Hezekiah, it will involve the use of some of His abundant herbs, essential oils, or plants. Be open to whatever guidance you are given and follow it with gratitude.

Wonderful Jehovah-rapha, like Hezekiah I cry to You for my healing. Send revelation knowledge to me and my advisors to show me the exact remedies You want me to use at the physical level for my recovery. I will follow Your guidance without question or hesitation. In Jesus' name, I pray, Amen.

Day 169

Blessed is he who has regard for the weak; the Lord delivers him in times of trouble. The Lord will protect him and preserve his life; he will bless him in the land and not surrender him to the desire of his foes. The Lord will sustain him on his sickbed and restore him from his bed of illness. I said, "O Lord, have mercy on me; heal me, for I have sinned against you." . . . All my enemies whisper together against me; they imagine the worst for me, saying, "A vile disease has beset him; he will never get up from the place where he lies." Even my close friend, whom I trusted, he who shared my bread, has lifted up his heel against me. But you, O Lord, have mercy on me; raise me up, that I may repay them. I know that you are pleased with me, for my enemy does not triumph over me. In my integrity you uphold me and set me in your presence forever. Praise be to the Lord, the God of Israel, from everlasting to everlasting. Amen and Amen. (Psalm 41:1-4, 7-13 NIV)

This is a fascinating psalm of David, who has become sick and who is praying to God for help and healing. Notice that he assumes that God will heal him. He very firmly declares, "The Lord will sustain him on his sickbed and restore him from his bed of illness." He doesn't doubt either God's power or God's desire to heal him.

He makes a very interesting confession. "Heal me," he says, *"for I have sinned against you."* He admits that he has violated some of God's laws – whether they be physical laws of good health or whether they be spiritual ones that make a person vulnerable to attacks of the evil one – and that he is now suffering the consequences of his actions. Illness has overcome him and he needs healing.

David raises another vital issue in healing concerning the opinions of others. He says his enemies are "imagining the worst." And even his closest friend is not giving him his support. You, too, may find that your friends and family are focused on the worst and are filled with thoughts of fear about you. Refuse to accept their negative view of your situation; instead, choose to be like David and focus on the healing power of Jehovah-rapha. Remain firm in your belief that He will raise you up.

Dear Heavenly Father, I relate well to the psalm of David. I, too, have sinned against you, and I ask your forgiveness and Your healing touch. Don't let me listen to negative voices imagining the worst about my illness. Instead, let me hear only the voice of the Holy Spirit telling me each step in the path to my healing. In Jesus' name, I pray, Amen.

Day 170

All the days of the oppressed are wretched, but the cheerful heart has a continual feast.
(Proverbs 15:15 NIV)

Joy in your body brings health; sadness, despair, and depression do not. It can be hard to be cheerful when you feel sick, but the paradox is that the more you focus on gladness, the more you create an internal environment for healing.

This concept was popularized most spectacularly by Norman Cousins who became very ill with a collagen disease in the mid-1960s. Even though he was in constant pain and felt like crying all the time, he embarked on an experiment using laughter to stimulate his healing. He found movies, jokes, and stories that were funny, hilarious, and just plain silly. The more he laughed, the less pain he felt. He used joy to activate his immune system and endocrine system into proper functioning.

When he had succumbed to the oppression of the disease, Cousins felt wretched. When he developed a cheerful heart, he found he had a continual feast of gradually improving recovery. Ten minutes of belly laughter produced two hours of sleep without pain. Hours of laughter each day produced more and more healing in his body which was confirmed by consistent laboratory tests.

This was not a case of Dr. Cousins' willing himself to be a Pollyanna. This was a situation of immersing himself fully in joy and allowing his soul, mind, emotions, and body to unite in harmony in the positive experience of cheerfulness.

How much do you laugh during the day? Do you take your life and your illness or injury so seriously that there is no room for joy to fill you? Every cell in your body can feel the vibrations of God's joy. Make a list of the things that make you laugh the deep-down, roll-on-the-floor belly laugh – humor that is so funny to you that you laugh until tears roll down your cheeks. That is the laughter of healing.

Create your own "Laugh for Health" collection. Ask your friends and family members to send you clippings or jokes – anything to add to your collection and to give you fresh material. Make a commitment to spend time every day immersed in humor and in laughter. Make a joyful noise to the Lord. Come before Him with gladness.

Thank You, God, for the healing power of a cheerful heart. Thank You for the pure joy of laughing and laughing and laughing. In the name of Jesus Christ, my Savior and my Redeemer, I pray, Amen.

Day 171

How beautiful on the mountains are the feet of those who bring good news, who proclaim peace, who bring good tidings, who proclaim salvation, who say to Zion, "Your God reigns!" (Isaiah 52:7 NIV)

Be willing to share with others the good news you have learned about healing. The sad fact is that most people haven't heard this message. Each day by the thousands, people are dying before they have fulfilled their days because they do not know that Jehovah-rapha is the God who heals them.

Each day by the thousands, people are dying before they have fulfilled their days because they do not include the counsel of the Holy Spirit in their medical decision-making process. And each day by the thousands, people are dying before they have fulfilled their days because they do not know anything about God's own remedies and God's own health laws.

Jesus told us in Matthew 7:13-14, "For wide is the gate and broad is the road that leads to destruction, and many enter through it. But small is the gate and narrow the road that leads to life, and only a few find it."

This truth is as valid for our physical selves as it is for our spiritual souls. More would find the road to vital, healthy life if only they had someone to guide them to it. It is easy to be swept along with what everyone else seems to be doing. The road seems wide and there appears to be safety in numbers.

When you feel strong in your own understanding and faith, tell your story to those who will listen. Don't try to convince anyone. Those who are ready to hear you will hear and those who are not ready will not. You have to bless those who cannot hear you and move on. Be careful not to allow others to confuse you and weaken your faith. Hold fast to your beliefs and do not succumb to arguments.

God calls you to be a beautiful witness for Him. Answer His call. Carry the good news to someone today.

Wonderful Jehovah-rapha, help me to share Your glorious healing news with others. Help me to proclaim Your peace, Your good news, Your good tidings of healing, Your message of salvation to all who will listen. You have declared You are the God who heals us. You sent Your Son to us to give us life abundant here on earth and then life everlasting in heaven, when our days are fulfilled. Keep my faith strong, Lord, and my intent clear. In Jesus' name, I pray, Amen.

Day 172

For you have heard of my previous way of life in Judaism, how intensely I persecuted the church of God and tried to destroy it. I was advancing in Judaism beyond many Jews of my own age and was extremely zealous for the traditions of my fathers. But when God, who set me apart from birth, and called me by his grace, was pleased to reveal his Son in me so that I might preach him among the Gentiles, I did not consult any man, nor did I go up to Jerusalem to see those who were apostles before I was, but I went immediately into Arabia and later returned to Damascus. (Galatians 1:13-17 NIV)

Tradition says that God wants certain people to be sick and that He is glorified by their illness. If that is true, then Jesus was constantly interfering with God's glory because He healed every sick person who came to Him. In fact, of one blind man, He said that God was to be glorified by His recovery of sight, not by His blindness.

Think about the number of hospitals, doctors, nurses, and medical treatment facilities we have in this country. If we truly believe that it is God's will for people to be ill and that some Divine purpose is worked in their lives by their being sick, then all these facilities and all these people are working contrary to the will of the Lord God Almighty. It is a strange but common phenomenon of human beings that we go to church on Sunday and pray that we can accept God's will to accept and bear our illness bravely and then turn around on Monday and race to the doctor to be made well.

Jesus was very clear that every act He did was according to the will of God. And He was also very clear that every sick person who came to Him would be healed if he wanted it. One tradition says that these acts of Jesus were miracles only for the people who lived two thousand years ago. But in His last words to us as written in Mark 16:17-18, Jesus said, "and these signs will accompany those who believe: . . . they will place their hands on sick people, and they will get well." Do you believe Him?

Paul warns of the hazards of zealously following the traditions of men. Pray with your family, friends, and health care advisors. Place your ultimate trust in your Creator. Listen to His advice and follow His path for your healing.

Wonderful Jehovah-rapha, teach me to follow Your way only and to put Your advice before any other. I stand on Your Word. I trust and believe You, God. Use my life for Your glory and Your service. Thank You for leading me to my healing. In Jesus' name, I pray, Amen.

Day 173

"This is why I speak to them in parables: 'Though seeing, they do not see; though hearing, they do not hear or understand.' In them is fulfilled the prophecy of Isaiah: 'You will be ever hearing but never understanding; you will be ever seeing but never perceiving. For this people's heart has become callused; they hardly hear with their ears and they have closed their eyes. Otherwise they might see with their eyes, hear with their ears, understand with their hearts and turn, and I would heal them.' " (Matthew 13:13-17 NIV)

Jesus presents an important lesson in these few words. He pleads with us to listen to the voice of God. As He often does, He returns to the written Word of God. Here He quotes the prophet Isaiah and speaks of people who have eyes that do not see and ears that do not hear. He is not talking about the senses of vision and auditory reception. He is talking about receiving the Word and voice of God.

Divine truth has only one source and that is God. We must learn to quieten ourselves within, to connect to the Holy Spirit, and to listen. God will speak to us about every aspect of our lives – and that includes our health.

Jesus, quoting the prophecy of Isaiah, says God is telling us that if we would see and hear and understand, He will heal us. Heal how? At every level of our being. Heal our souls, our minds, and our bodies.

We can't know God's path for us if we don't listen. God's Word makes it clear that He intends for us to be well. But there are many avenues to healing. How do we know which ones to take? By asking God for direction and then by listening.

After we hear and understand clearly, then we must have the courage to act on the revelations we have received. As long as we are clear about God's instructions, we must let no one dissuade us from following the path to healing that we have been shown.

Almighty God, show me clearly Your path for my healing. I need Your guidance. Sometimes I hear so many voices that I get confused. I know my family, friends, and health advisors want what is best for me. But only You know everything about me. Only You are the Great Physician. Only You, Lord. I affirm my faith in You. I come to You with reverence and with an open heart and soul. I am listening. And I will act according to Your instruction. In Your Holy name, I pray, Amen.

Day 174

For this purpose the Son of God was manifested, that he might destroy the works of the devil. (1 John 3:8 KJV)

Just exactly what were the works of the devil that Jesus destroyed? Look at His life and His ministry. What did He do? Acts 10:38 tells that "He went around doing good and healing all who were under the power of the devil."

Jesus set people free again and again and again. If the devil had attacked them with illness in their bodies, he healed them. If the devil had led them into prostitution, He told them to go and sin no more. If the devil had made them mentally ill, He healed their minds. If the devil had convinced them to steal from others, He healed their spirit and led them to repentance and atonement.

Have no doubt that the source of illness is the devil. If you feel sick, satan has a foothold in your body. If you want him to leave, then enforce the Word of God on him and on the illness that is present. Follow the example of the Lord God Almighty and of Jesus Christ and *speak* God's truth into being.

Speak with authority to your illness. Command it to leave in the name of the Almighty and the blood of Christ Jesus which conquered the devil and defeated him. Talk to the cells that are malfunctioning, and tell them to resume normal activity. Talk to the organs of your body, and tell them to stabilize and perform their functions according to the Divine plan of the Almighty.

Name each system of your body – immune, digestive, intestinal, nervous, glandular, endocrine, urinary, skeletal, reproductive, respiratory, sensory, and circulatory – and command each one to be made whole in the name of Jesus Christ and to be filled with the Divine energy of Jehovah-rapha. Command each body system to function normally according to its Divine purpose.

Then "whatever you ask for in prayer, believe that you have received it, and it will be yours" (Mark 11:24 NIV).

Almighty God, in the name of Your Son Christ Jesus, I command satan to leave my body. I enforce Your Word on every cell in my body and I command illness to leave me. In the name of Jesus, I command every cell, every gland, every organ, and every system to function normally. I claim Your healing. I vow to follow all instructions You give me as I join with You in partnership for my recovery. Thank You, Jehovah-rapha, for healing me. In Jesus' name, I pray, Amen.

Day 175

God be merciful unto us and bless us; and cause his face to shine upon us; that thy way may be known upon earth, thy saving health among all nations. Let the people praise thee, O God; let all the people praise thee. (Psalm 67:1-3 KJV)

Great is the Lord, and most worthy of praise, in the city of our God, his holy mountain. It is beautiful in its loftiness, the joy of the whole earth. (Psalm 48:1-2 NIV)

But as for me, I will always have hope; I will praise you more and more. My mouth will tell of your righteousness, of your salvation all day long, though I know not its measure. I will come and proclaim your mighty acts, O Sovereign Lord; I will proclaim your righteousness, yours alone. Since my youth, O God, you have taught me, and to this day I declare your marvelous deeds. Even when I am old and gray, do not forsake me, O God, till I declare your power to the next generation, your might to all who are to come. (Psalm 71:14-18 NIV)

Sing to the Lord a new song; sing to the Lord, all the earth. Sing to the Lord, praise his name; proclaim his salvation day after day. Declare his glory among the nations, his marvelous deeds among all peoples. (Psalm 96:1-3 NIV)

The Holy Scriptures are filled with praise for the Lord God Almighty. How many times during the day do you praise the Lord? When something good happens, say, "Praise the Lord" and "Thank You!" When something upsetting happens, praise the Lord for sending you a solution, whether you are clear what it is or not. Turn the problem over, thank God for the answer that is on the way, and be receptive to the voice of the Holy Spirit telling you what you need to do.

Be creative in incorporating praise into your daily life. Music offers a joyful way to express your praise, and it provides healing vibrations to all the cells in your body at the same time. Play it while you do your housework and other chores. Sing as often as you can, offering your voice in gratitude and thanksgiving.

Almighty Lord, I praise You and glorify You. I delight in sharing with others the story of my healing, and I praise You for showing me the way to my recovery. I sing my praises every day and I am grateful for Your many blessings. In the name of Your Son, Jesus Christ, I pray, Amen.

Day 176

But when he saw the multitudes, he was moved with compassion on them, because they fainted, and were scattered abroad, as sheep having no shepherd. (Matthew 9:36 KJV)

Jesus had been traveling around the countryside, visiting many cities and villages, teaching in their synagogues, proclaiming the good news (the Gospel) of the kingdom, and curing all kinds of disease and every weakness and infirmity. He was in action, fulfilling His dual mission of preaching and healing. Healing what? *All* kinds of disease. *Every* weakness and infirmity.

What is the situation described in Matthew 9:36? The Amplified Bible uses these words: "When He saw the throngs, He was moved with pity and sympathy for them, because they were bewildered (harassed and distressed and dejected and helpless), like sheep without a shepherd." What a vivid description!

We think that modern society is unique in its stresses, yet look at this account of people two thousand years ago. Can you relate to feeling bewildered and harassed? To feeling distressed and dejected? To feeling helpless? Many in the crowd felt ill and their illness magnified their anxiety. Sickness can certainly make you feel trapped and stranded, like a lost sheep who has gone astray.

Jesus' message was that God cares for the lost sheep. God is moved with compassion, pity, and sympathy for you, and He has sent Jesus as The Good Shepherd to find you and bring you back to safety. The Good Shepherd does only the will of the Father and He heals all who come to Him.

Sometimes you may feel faint and scattered inside, overwhelmed by business schedules, housework, financial concerns, meetings, and daily activities. Illness adds more than you can bear. Give it all to Jesus, your Shepherd. He calls you gently to Him and enfolds you in His loving, healing arms.

Merciful Lord, look on me with compassion. There are times when I feel bewildered and harassed, distressed and dejected. Modern life seems overwhelming and there are many demands on my time and my energy. I feel lost. Find me, Lord. I feel wounded and hurt. Heal me, Lord. You are my Shepherd. In You I find my refuge, my safety, and my healing. With a grateful heart, in Jesus' name, I pray, Amen.

Day 177

While Jesus was still talking to the crowd, his mother and brothers stood outside, wanting to speak to him. Someone told him, "Your mother and brothers are standing outside, wanting to speak to you." He replied to him, "Who is my mother, and who are my brothers?" Pointing to his disciples, he said, "Here are my mother and my brothers. For whoever does the will of my Father in heaven is my brother and sister and mother." (Matthew 12:46-50 NIV)

Sometimes you have to create a new family – or perhaps an extra family – in your walk of recovery. Many people find that their family and relatives are the most resistant to the God-directed healing path. You may find that the same is true for you.

Your revelation knowledge may lead you to the use of natural substances for your healing and away from synthetic pharmaceuticals. Or your revelation knowledge may lead you to say no to standard medical treatments that destroy the immune system. It is frightening to those who love you to see you reject what they accept as the only sensible way to deal with illness. You will find it is futile to try to change them. Pray for them to have peace concerning your choices, and pray that God will reveal to them your understanding in His time.

Remember that your focus is to do the will of God. That and only that. Find people who are able to support you in this. Bring them into your life as your family.

Jesus did not reject his mother and his brothers nor did He imply that they *were not* following the will of God. Jesus knew that sometimes people live in pain and anguish, wanting love and support that their blood family cannot give them. Instead of letting go, they try to make their family act the way they believe they should. Jesus points out that relationships based on a common love of God and true joy in being together are far more important and are what constitute a real family.

Family is a matter of the heart and soul, rather than blood. Hold fast to those who support you in following God's will and direction to the best of your ability. Embrace them, love them, and tell them how grateful you are to have them as your true family of the heart.

Gracious God, keep me strong in my resolve to follow Your path even though some of my family and friends do not understand what I am doing. Thank You for sending people to me who can support and help me in my healing. I am grateful for them in this journey and I welcome them as my new family. In the name of Your Son, Jesus Christ, I pray, Amen.

Day 178

In his heart a man plans his course, but the Lord determines his steps. (Proverbs 16:9 NIV)

To whom do you give control of your life? Is it God? Or is it yourself? What course do you follow when you feel sick? God's? Or your own?

We need to get clear that the Lord God Almighty is to order our steps because we can become deceived very easily. Sometimes what looks like illness is, in fact, really the cure.

A good example is the common cold. With this ailment our immune system has become weakened (which is the real problem) and a virus has taken hold inside our body. We start sneezing; our eyes water; our nose fills with mucus and becomes clogged; we cough. We feel awful.

God has created the body to take all these actions to rid itself of the virus. Since the body has gone into appropriate action to remove the germ, the cold symptoms aren't the disease; they are the cure.

But what do most people do? They follow their own (erroneous) understanding and take every medicine they can to suppress the symptoms that are annoying and unpleasant. By focusing on the symptoms and trying to eliminate them, they are not dealing effectively with meeting the needs of their body according to the steps that God has determined.

Instead, what is the proper solution? Let God determine your steps so that you can strengthen your immune system as quickly as possible and, thus, allow your body to restore its proper function.

Go to God in prayer and ask the Holy Spirit to reveal to you the proper course to take. It is quite likely that you will hear to use God's own herbal remedies and essential oils. Or you may hear to use homeopathics. Or a combination of these and other options. There are many ways to assist your body in moving through the healing process quickly.

Give God total control in your life. Do not make assumptions for your healing. Allow God to determine your steps, knowing that He wants only good for you.

Almighty God, there are times when I become willful and stubborn. I pretend that I am in control and I charge ahead without asking You for direction first. Slow me down, Lord. I trust You to guide me along the path to my recovery that is for my highest good. In the name of Your Son, Jesus Christ, my Savior and my Redeemer, I pray, Amen.

Day 179

The Lord said to Moses, "Say to the Israelites: 'Do not eat any of the fat of cattle, sheep or goats. The fat of an animal found dead or torn by wild animals may be used for any other purpose, but you must not eat it." (Leviticus 7:22-24 NIV)

The controversy continues to rage over fat – how much to eat, what kind to eat, etc. Man-made food rules seem to change weekly. Turn to God's Word. The instructions in Leviticus are clear – do not eat the fat of cattle, sheep, or goats. The fat being referred to is the cover fat of the animal, rather than the fat that is marbled in the muscle tissue.

What makes the cover fat a problem for us? It contains higher amounts of toxins and contaminants than other tissue. Many people think that all toxins are eliminated by the body, but this is not the case. The various systems of an animal's body do attempt to remove toxic substances through eliminative channels; however, many toxins are simply stored. One of the major depositories is cover fat, which also happens to be high in saturated fats.

Notice that the Holy Scripture does not advocate a no-fat or extremely low-fat diet. In fact, God's Word makes frequent reference to the consumption of olive oil and nuts – which are foods with high essential fatty acid content. Olive oil is high in monounsaturated fat, and those people in the Mediterranean areas who eat large amounts of it (sometimes consuming 35% of their diet in these fats) have a very low rate of heart disease.

"Good" fats are critical to our good health. Dr. Nathan Pritikin, who advocated an extremely low-fat diet in order to protect himself from heart disease, died instead of leukemia. We now know that extremely low fat consumption often leads to death from leukemia.

God calls us to balance, to moderation, to obedience, and to wise choices. In general, it is healthy to eat moderate amounts of fats found in the plant kingdom (such as nuts, seeds, grains, and natural oils) and small amounts of fat from the flesh of animals approved by God for food. Make no assumptions for your own particular situation, however. Ask the Holy Spirit to guide you in what is healthy for your body at this time.

Almighty God, I want to be aware of developing dietary information, but help me to overcome the temptation to act on it without first asking for Your guidance. Help me to choose healthy fats and healthy foods for the nourishment and healing of my body. In Jesus' name, I pray, Amen.

Day 180

Come unto me, all ye that labour and are heavy laden, and I will give you rest. Take my yoke upon you, and learn of me; for I am meek and lowly in heart: and ye shall find rest unto your souls. For my yoke is easy, and my burden is light. (Matthew 11:28-30 KJV)

Stress kills. One of the most difficult lessons for many people is to learn to rest in the Lord. We proclaim faith with our lips and yet worry ourselves into stress, illness, and sometimes even death. We profess the Lord as our Savior and yet live frantic lives, racing from one "to-do" list to the next, never stepping back to ask the Lord to guide our path and set our priorities.

Jesus knows very well that high stress levels make people sick, and, if relief is not found, those illnesses often become fatal ones. Negative stress causes physiological changes throughout the body and especially taxes the nervous system. It also causes constriction of blood vessels, threatening the health of the heart, brain, eyes, organs, and glands.

"Handling" stress is really not the solution. You need a method of living that acknowledges stressful situations and events but then *transforms* them into positive growth experiences. It is Jesus Christ who can perform the transformation for you. He tells you clearly that He will exchange all the burdens you have for His own yoke – which He says is light and easy.

Jesus doesn't say you will have no yoke at all, but what He does promise is that He will take the one that is overwhelming to you and will give you one instead that is light enough for you to carry it easily.

Are you feeling overwhelmed by the situations in your life? Do you have health problems? Or financial problems? Or relationship problems? Or career problems? Or all of them? Is there too much to do and too little time? Do you dare to trust that Jesus means what He says when He tells you to give your problems to Him?

First, get clear about what your stress is really about. Write all the things that are having a negative impact on you at the present time. Now, sit in a comfortable chair, close your eyes, quieten your soul, hold your list in your hand, and offer it to Christ Jesus. Ask for guidance in your life and then be bold to follow it.

Heavenly Father, I feel stressed and overwhelmed. Your Son told me to give Him my burdens so I offer them up now. Show me clearly what I am to do and restore peace to my soul and confidence to my spirit. Lift me up, Lord, and teach me Your way. In Jesus' name, I pray, Amen.

Day 181

Thou art snared with the words of thy mouth; thou art taken with the words of thy mouth.
(Proverbs 6:2 KJV)

Words are potent – both those spoken and unspoken. What you think and what you say reveal who you really are. These words provide the spiritual environment in which you exist. If your thoughts and words are positive, healing ones, you are bathing your soul and your body in a soothing stream. If your thoughts and words are negative, doubt-filled ones, you are floundering in a pot of boiling water.

Do you spend a lot of time expressing your doubt that you will be healed? Do you itemize your ailments over and over, emphasizing any increase in symptoms and describing them as further indications of your deterioration? Do you sigh and *wish* you had faith and then sigh some more?

We build our own prisons with our words. Satan is standing by ready to help us and encourage us, for he seeks always to trap and bind us. Satan loves to convince us that we are "just being honest." He wants to confuse us and keep us off balance. He knows that we will sink – or rise – to the level of our words and our thoughts. Every statement or thought that "I'll never be well" or "I'm not getting any better" or "This is as good as I'll ever be" insures that that will indeed be our situation because we are declaring it as our truth.

Abraham had to "face the fact" that he and his wife could not possibly have a child – yet he also had to learn to look beyond the appearance and speak words of belief and faith in the promise of God. Face your own "facts." Faith isn't playing pretend. Don't ignore symptoms, "hoping" they will go away. Acknowledge the appearance of your health situation. Then take every element of it to God in prayer. Make no assumptions about what you should or should not do.

Let God be in total control. Let Him decide what path you should take – whether it be through His own instantaneous healing power, through prayers of the elders, through natural healing methods, or through medical intervention. Follow God's guidance for the perfect solution for you. Voice your belief in God's goodness and speak powerful words of faith and trust.

Almighty God, help me to watch the thoughts that I think and the words that come out of my mouth. Let them be words of trust, belief, and faith in Your goodness, Your healing grace, and Your power. In Jesus' name, I pray, Amen.

Day 182

My people are destroyed for lack of knowledge. (Hosea 4:6 KJV)

Information has never before been so voluminous. We are inundated by studies, reports, and new discoveries. There is no one who is not overwhelmed by it all. It would certainly seem that we have too much knowledge, rather than any lack of it. So is Hosea outdated? Unfortunately, not. This Scripture is still relevant today – especially in the area of recovering our health.

We can look around us and see hundreds and hundreds of herbs and natural substances that are beneficial for our health. Are these just serendipitous results of evolution? No, they are intentional gifts from God, and He expects us to use them. Ironically, while the majority of the people of the world values these God-given plants, most Americans know almost nothing about them. We have convinced ourselves that our inventions are better than the creations of the Almighty. Surely God must weep for us.

Many of us expressed outrage when God was purged from the educational system, and we see evidence that we are reaping what we have sown. Yet no one seems even to notice that God is also purged from our medical system. One system nourishes minds and the other nourishes bodies. Both need the presence and participation of the Almighty.

There is much to change. Pray that people will learn about God's remedies and will turn to them first when they become ill. Pray that scientists will act in partnership with God, insuring that all experiments and discoveries will be made according to revelation knowledge and in harmony with God's purpose for His people. Pray that doctors will pray with and for their patients so that treatments will not be automatic knee-jerk responses to test results but will be given only on the specific instruction of The Great Physician. Pray that both those seeking to be healed and those gifted with healing abilities will look to the Great Physician for guidance and direction.

Dear Heavenly Father, we have strayed from Your path. And we are dying as a result of it. Help me to do my part to bring You back into our health care system. Guide me to teachers and courses that will show me how to use Your essential oils and herbs for my healing and recovery. I pray now for all doctors, medical personnel, and support people. Help them to make You a part of their work. In the name of Your Son, Jesus Christ, I pray, Amen.

Day 183

We do not want you to become lazy, but to imitate those who through faith and patience inherit what has been promised. (Hebrews 6:12 NIV)

Sometimes God's path for our healing takes only an instant. But at other times it is a slower process.

We have to hold to our faith, to remain patient, and also to be diligent in our efforts so that we will inherit what has been promised. We have already been redeemed – body and soul – by Jesus Christ on the Cross. The promise is that the healing that has already been accomplished through Jesus Christ can be made manifest in our own body and life.

The writer of Hebrews tells us to have patience. That means to allow God to work in His own way. Refrain from judging your recovery by signs of change in your symptoms. Don't judge your healing by the appearance of things – whether your vision is still blurred or your hands still shake or your rash is still red.

To base your belief according to the appearance of your symptoms undermines your faith because your inner voice is really saying, "If my vision is still cloudy, then I'm not healed." That is the voice of doubt. The father of lies wants to keep you focused on anything that can make you doubt Jesus' redemption of your soul and body. He loves to keep you checking and double-checking for signs of improvement.

Yes, it is hard to be patient. And there are certainly times when it seems that the devil throws up every obstacle he can find to hinder your progress. At these times keep your eyes on the Cross. When you look at your body, see the Cross there. See the Cross in your eyes, on your hands, on the rash. Then ask for guidance for the specific step you need to take for that day to be a partner in your healing.

Once you receive your instruction, you must be diligent in carrying it out. It is easy to be lazy and say, "Tomorrow . . ." That is again the father of lies speaking to you.

Trust in God. Thank Him for healing you. And so it is.

Dear God, teach me to be patient and to stay focused on Your guidance for my life and my healing. Help me not to be lazy; give me the strength to do what I need to do as a partner with You in my recovery. Stay by my side. Let me be an example to others of a faithful follower of Your Son Jesus Christ so that I may manifest in my body, mind, and soul the promise of His redemption. Thank You, O God, for Your many mercies upon me. In the name of Your Son Jesus Christ, I pray, Amen.

Day 184

Shout for joy, O heavens; rejoice, O earth; burst into song, O mountains! For the Lord comforts his people and will have compassion on his afflicted ones. (Isaiah 49:13 NIV)

Over and over again we are taught the connection between expressions of joy and our healing. Here in Isaiah we have a beautiful poetic verse: "Shout for joy, O heavens; rejoice, O earth; burst into song, O mountains! For the Lord comforts his people and will have compassion on his afflicted ones."

How can you put this part of God's Word into effect in your life? How often have you ever shouted for joy? Think of three things for which you are grateful. Now do something that may feel really silly. Say out loud the first item on your list and then shout, "Yay, God! Thank you!" Then repeat the process for the remaining two items. Do you feel joy bubbling up and maybe a chuckle or two?

Now find some exuberant music filled with praise and worship for the Lord. Sing along with all your heart and your soul. Dance to it if you are able. Let the music fill you, lift you, and energize you. Your blood flows better and your breathing increases. More healing oxygen and nutrients get to your cells.

Now it's time to make a different selection of music. Find songs that are filled with tranquil worship – songs that tell the story of God's love and compassion, of His strength and His power, of His amazing grace. Let the music and the words cradle your soul and heal your body.

As you listen, see yourself as a little child, hurt and afraid, climbing up into the lap of your heavenly Father. See yourself being enfolded in the arms of God. Feel the enormous compassion and love that flows from Him into you. Feel how soothing and gentle His touch is. Allow His comforting presence to abide with you.

O merciful Lord, joyful, joyful, I do adore thee. I join with the heavens and shout for joy. I join with the earth and rejoice in Your great goodness. I burst into song with the mountains. You shower on me so many blessings, Lord. Too often I forget that truth when I focus on my ailments. You are filled with compassion for my afflictions and You have sent the Comforter to be with me always. You sent Your precious Son Jesus Christ to carry my sins and my infirmities to the Cross. Thank You, gracious Father. Thank You. In the name of Your Son, Jesus Christ, I pray, Amen.

Day 185

"I will make you a wall to this people, a fortified wall of bronze; they will fight against you but will not overcome you, for I am with you to rescue and save you," declares the Lord. "I will save you from the hands of the wicked and redeem you from the grasp of the cruel."
(Jeremiah 15:20-21 NIV)

Do you have times in your life when you feel overwhelmed with problems and difficulties? You may have small children who need a great deal of attention, an elderly parent who needs special help, a teenager who is troubled, or a spouse with whom you are having problems communicating. You may have an adult child who is dependent on you financially, or you may be a part-time or full-time caretaker for your grandchildren. You may be unhappy with your career or you may be in financial difficulties. The list goes on.

No matter what situation occurs, the Lord can protect you if you will let Him. God does not promise that these difficulties will not come, but He does promise that He will help us to get through them. "I am with you to rescue you," God tells us. "I am with you."

What is required of us? We must go in prayer and see what our part is in all our problems. How are we contributing to the situation? Many people feel afraid of letting someone else down. So they go and go until they have depleted themselves.

What they have done is to let *themselves* down instead and to violate Jesus' command to love your neighbor as yourself. Satan has the upper hand when he can get you to ignore your own needs and to place everyone else's needs above your own. Don't fool yourself. When you don't stand up for yourself and for your needs, satan is in control of your life and not God.

Your health cannot improve if God is not in control of your life. So what are the solutions? You must first set the boundaries of what you can and cannot do. Then God will fortify them and help you stick to them. God has a purpose for your life. All Him to strengthen you so that you can do His work.

Almighty God, I cry out for your help. I feel overwhelmed. Give me the courage to set my boundaries. Fortify the walls of my life, Lord, and protect me. Strengthen me so that I may fulfill Your purpose for my life. In the name of Your Son, Jesus Christ, I pray, Amen.

Day 186

Now when John in prison heard about the activities of Christ, he sent a message by his disciples and asked Him, "Are you the One Who was to come, or should we keep on expecting a different one?" And Jesus replied to them, "Go and report to John what you hear and see: The blind receive their sight and the lame walk, lepers are cleansed (by healing) and the deaf hear, the dead are raised up and the poor have good news (the Gospel) preached to them. And blessed (happy, fortunate, and to be envied) is he who takes no offense at Me and finds no cause for stumbling in or through Me and is not hindered from seeing the Truth." (Matthew 11:2-6 AMP)

When you find yourself filled with doubt and yet you are castigating yourself for feeling that way, remember this story about John the Baptist. Here was a man who had baptized Jesus himself. After Jesus' baptism and He had come up out of the water, John had seen the Spirit of God descending like a dove and lighting on Jesus. And he had heard a voice from heaven say, "This is my Son, whom I love; with him I am well pleased" (Matthew 3:16-17 NIV).

Despite all this, here John is sending a message to Jesus, asking Him, "Are you the one? Are you really the one – or should we expect somebody else?" Can you imagine how exasperated Jesus must have felt? Pay attention to His response. He told the messenger to report to John "what you hear and see." And what was on that list? Two primary things: Jesus was healing the sick and Jesus was preaching the good news.

Here and in many other accounts Jesus places healing and preaching the good news on equal ground. Believe Him. Trust Him. Hand Him all your doubts, which come from the evil one who is trying to distract you from God's path.

Hold in your heart Jesus' words, "Blessed is he who is not hindered from seeing the Truth." Jesus always beckons us to God's truth – that He loves us, that He proclaims He is Jehovah-rapha, and that He is ever faithful to us.

Wonderful Jehovah-rapha, take my doubts. I stand on Your Word where it is written that Your Son healed the sick and preached Your gospel of love and repentance. Protect me from the evil one. Let me stand fully in Your truth and follow Your guidance for my health and my life. Thank You for healing me, Father. Thank You. In the name of Your Son, Jesus Christ, my Savior and my Redeemer, I pray, Amen.

Day 187

In you, O Lord, do I put my trust and confidently take refuge; let me never be put to shame or confusion! (Psalm 71:1 AMP)

Whom do you trust? And whom do you believe? In whose advice do you take refuge? These are critical questions that must be answered. As Christians, we often answer quickly, "Oh, I believe in God the Father Almighty and in Jesus Christ His Son."

If this is really true, why is it that, when we get sick, we usually do one of two things – either we ignore the problem and hope it will go away or we run to the doctor for relief of our symptoms? When it comes to health issues, many of us actually put our trust almost entirely in earthly physicians and ask God for assistance only when medical science has run out of answers.

We must turn to God *first*. Get guidance first; *then* act. Confusion stirs our mind and it provides satan with fertile ground to get control of us. We must still our mind, offer our health problem up to God, and be willing to hear whatever God has to say to us. We may hear to make changes in our diet or to use herbs and essential oils to assist our bodies to heal or to go to an earthly physician for advice or treatment. We must then have the faith and the courage to act on the guidance we have received.

What is critical to understand is that the guidance isn't over! At each tiny step along the way, we must ask for more instruction. If we seek a natural health professional, we must check with God to see if the recommendations we got from him or her are right for us. If we seek a medical physician, we must do likewise.

We must keep our faith centered in God and put the guidance of the Great Physician first and foremost in our lives. God can and does work through people, but remember it is *the Lord* who is our refuge. It is *the Lord* who is the authority in our lives. It is *the Lord's* advice that should determine the exact path for our healing.

O, Lord, You are my refuge. I proclaim my trust in You. I proclaim my faith in You as my Great Physician. Sometimes I feel like David, O God, and I get confused. Sometimes I seem to have so many ailments. I hear the warnings from dedicated physicians and I see the test results and all this seems so definite. I make a commitment today, Lord, to seek Your wisdom and guidance – no matter what it is. Give me strength to walk the path You mark for me – no matter what it is. I stand on your Holy Word that You are the God who heals me. In Jesus' name, I pray, Amen.

Day 188

Finally, be strong in the Lord and in his mighty power. (Ephesians 6:10 NIV)

Sickness diminishes our strength. When we experience severe illness or injury, we are forced to change our focus. The daily activities that we thought were so important are often interrupted. Our whole perspective changes.

For these reasons many people think that God causes the illness or accident in order to make us change. However, what they forget is that such a lesson is useful only if it works. The fact is that many people who are stricken physically become angry and bitter, and they stay that way. They have been snared by satan and they can't shake loose from his grip. For the rest of their days they scream at God's injustice and blame God for making them sick.

It isn't God who is the creator of illness. It is satan who wills it and who wreaks havoc on our bodies. But supreme power does not belong to the evil one. When we feel ill, can we still do mighty works for the Lord? Of course we can. When we feel sick, can we still be a powerful witness for God's love? Of course we can. When we are hurt, can we still be useful to God? Of course we can. But God wants more for us and He can always make lemonade from the devil's lemons.

There is no power greater than God's. Claim God's mighty strength. Acknowledge the places where your faith is weak and the issues where satan creates confusion in your mind about God's will for your health. Take these concerns to God in prayer and meditation. Get to the core of your truth and determine if you are ready and willing to be healthy. If you aren't sure whether God wants you to be well, talk to God about your doubt. Listen to God's answer. Claim God's strength and wear it as your armor.

Almighty God, You know there are times when I get confused by satan's whispers and I feel despair about my illness. I even wonder if You really have made me sick for some purpose I don't understand. Help me to say firmly as Your Son showed me, "Get behind me, satan." You could crush satan beneath Your feet, but instead You ask me to choose whether to listen to the voice of the evil one and his lies or whether to listen to Your Holy voice and Your Holy Word. I choose to follow You, God, and only You. I claim Your strength, Your awesome power, and Your truth that you are Jehovah-rapha, the God who heals me. In the name of Jesus, my Savior and my Redeemer, I pray, Amen.

Day 189

Jesus, once more deeply moved, came to the tomb. It was a cave with a stone laid across the entrance. "Take away the stone," he said. "But Lord," said Martha, the sister of the dead man, "by this time there is a bad odor, for he has been there four days." Then Jesus said, "Did I not tell you that if you believed, you would see the glory of God?" . . . Jesus called in a loud voice, "Lazarus, come out!" The dead man came out, his hands and feet wrapped with strips of linen and a cloth around his face. Jesus said to them, "Take off the grave clothes and let him go." (John 11:38-40, 43-44 NIV)

Lazarus was a dear friend of Jesus and he had died before his time. So what seems impossible to us occurred – Lazarus was raised from the dead by Jesus. This isn't an isolated example; there are a number of instances of people being raised from the dead in the Scriptures. In fact, when Jesus sent out His disciples He instructed them not only to heal the sick but also to raise the dead.

Why raise the dead? Because they had died before their time. Their lifespan had been altered by the evil one. Notice as you read God's Word that those who are raised from the dead are young people rather than elderly people who have lived their days.

God wants us to live a long life that is productive for Him. Can He make even a short life glorify Him? Of course, He can. But He can do so much more when a person's days are fulfilled.

Having a person's life cut short by a disease that eats away his body and fills him with pain does not glorify God. However, it pleases satan enormously. Once more he subverts God's plan and he causes great suffering for God's people – just as he whipped people into a frenzy so that they would throw early Christians into a pit of lions.

We are called by Jesus to believe and see the glory of God. Focus all your heart and mind and soul on the words, "I am the God who heals you." Allow those words to fill every cell in your body. Ask the Holy Spirit to transform every cell to a healthy state. Command every cell to function normally, according to God's Holy will and plan.

Awesome Lord, no mighty act is beyond Your power – even raising people from the dead. Sometimes I almost feel lifeless, God, as energy slips away from me. Forgive my sins. Remove my doubt. Heal my body. Let me live as a witness for Your love and healing grace. In Jesus' name, I pray, Amen.

Day 190

Be well balanced (temperate, sober of mind), be vigilant and cautious at all times; for that enemy of yours, the devil, roams around like a lion roaring [in fierce hunger], seeking someone to seize upon and devour. (1 Peter 5:8 AMP)

What a vivid picture of how the devil works! He stalks around like a lion on the prowl, looking for someone to seize and devour. If only he always came in the form of a lion, we probably wouldn't fall into his traps so easily. But he is usually a disguised lion and hopes to catch us unaware.

Sometimes satan seems to devour us in one big gulp, but usually he nibbles and nibbles and nibbles at us. He chips away at our health through one tiny decision after another. Just one order of French fries even though we know they are filled with harmful grease. Just more day with our feet up, even though we know our bodies need some exercise. Just one more night of staying up past midnight, even though we know our bodies need rest in order to heal. Just one more . . . The list goes on and on. One unhealthy decision occasionally won't harm us. But we have a way of forgetting how many of them we make.

What does Peter say we must do to avoid being caught by the devil? Be well balanced; be vigilant; be cautious. These recommendations are especially important when we feel sick. At the same time they are often harder to follow then because we usually have less energy. Too often it seems that when we don't feel well, it is much easier to make an unhealthy choice than a healthy one.

Ask God for His constant guidance and protection. Also bring people into your life who will support you, help you, and encourage you. Ask them to give you feedback to alert you when they see your vigilance waning. Have them join you in prayer that you will resist the evil one.

Almighty God, I know the devil exists and wants to entrap me. You are the Lord God Almighty and in You I trust. Protect me, Father, from the temptations of the evil one. There are consequences to my actions, and I need You to keep me centered, grounded, and focused on You, Lord, so that I will make wise decisions that will contribute to my health and recovery. Keep me balanced, God, so that I can recognize when I begin to stray from the path You want me to take. You are Jehovah-Rapha. You are my healer and You are my Protector. In Jesus' name, I pray, Amen.

Day 191

Accept him whose faith is weak, without passing judgment on disputable matters. One man's faith allows him to eat everything, but another man, whose faith is weak, eats only vegetables. The man who eats everything must not look down on him who does not, and the man who does not eat everything must not condemn the man who does, for God has accepted him. Who are you to judge someone else's servant? To his own master he stands or falls. And he will stand, for the Lord is able to make him stand. . . . He who eats meat, eats to the Lord, for he gives thanks to God; and he who abstains, does so to the Lord and gives thanks to God. For none of us lives to himself alone and none of us dies to himself alone. If we live, we live to the Lord; and if we die, we die to the Lord. So, whether we live or die, we belong to the Lord. (Romans 14:1-4, 6-8 NIV)

A great deal of debate rages whether it is "best" to be a vegetarian or whether it is best to eat some meat. Many theories have been offered and most are confusing. To follow them all would be impossible. According to the Holy Scriptures, the Genesis 1:29 instruction for eating was one based on fruits, vegetables, seeds, and nuts. Later in Genesis, meat is introduced and further specific instructions are given in Exodus and Leviticus. When we look at the life of Jesus, we see that He ate fish and lamb. All these references in the Scripture offer guidelines for us.

What are you supposed to do? Study the Holy Scriptures to see what God tells you about healthy foods. Be open to hearing the opinions of health professionals in both the natural health and conventional medical fields, yet at the same time do not feel *compelled* to follow any of them. Pray with them and then also go in prayer alone.

God created your body and God knows better than any living person (including you!) exactly how it is functioning and what type of nutrients it needs. Ask the Holy Spirit to reveal to you what you should eat, including specifics such as frequency, method of cooking, etc. And don't forget that God's instructions for you for one particular day may not be the same for another day. Jehovah-rapha wants you to be well and He will show you the proper nutrition for your body.

Wonderful Jehovah-rapha, I want to be healthy and I know that what I eat is a major factor in creating the wellness I seek. I come to You, God, asking for specific instructions about the foods You want me to eat. I am willing to do as You instruct. Give me the self-discipline to make the changes You ask of me so that I may be Your full partner in my healing. In the name of Your Son, Jesus Christ, I pray, Amen.

Day 192

When Jesus came to the region of Caesarea Philippi, he asked his disciples, "Who do people say the Son of Man is?" They replied, "Some say John the Baptist; others say Elijah; and still others, Jeremiah or one of the prophets." "But what about you?" he asked. "Who do you say I am?" Simon Peter answered, "You are the Christ, the Son of the living God." Jesus replied, "Blessed are you, Simon son of Jonah, for this was not revealed to you by man, but by my Father in heaven." (Matthew 16:13-17 NIV)

Who do *you* say Jesus is? Just as He asked His disciples this question, He also asks you today. Every one of us has to answer that question and the answer will determine the course of our lives. When Peter calls Jesus the Christ, the Son of God, Jesus' reply is very interesting. "Ah, Peter, you have received revelation knowledge. You were *told* this information by the Father."

As a society, we have a rather schizophrenic response to Divine revelations. When in a church setting, we accept the notion of praying to God and having Him provide answers although we aren't very specific how this will happen. Yet if someone is outside of church and he says, "God told me to do such-and-such a thing" we often feel uneasy and sometimes we send them for psychiatric help.

Peter was willing to listen to God's voice. And because this was so crucial Jesus told him that he was blessed and that upon his shoulders He would build His church.

Receiving Divine revelation is as critical for you as it was for Peter. It is especially vital for your healing process and recovery. You have to be able to receive specific instructions and guidance for the precise path you are to follow in your healing. You also have to be able to discern the voice of God which guides you to healing from the whispers of the evil one which lead you to destruction.

Do not underestimate the ability of the evil one to deceive you and get you off God's path. So stand firm on God's Word. Put on the armor of the Lord and listen for His revelation knowledge for your healing.

Almighty God, let me hear Your voice – and Yours alone. Let me always be willing to hear Your Word and to follow Your perfect will and guidance. Show me everything you want me to do, Jehovah-rapha, for my healing. With grateful thanks and in the name of Your Son, Jesus Christ, I pray, Amen.

Day 193

The crowd joined in the attack against Paul and Silas, and the magistrates ordered them to be stripped and beaten. After they had been severely flogged, they were thrown into prison, and the jailer was commanded to guard them carefully. Upon receiving such orders, he put them in the inner cell and fastened their feet in the stocks. About midnight Paul and Silas were praying and singing hymns to God, and the other prisoners were listening to them. Suddenly there was such a violent earthquake that the foundations of the prison were shaken. At once all the prison doors flew open, and everybody's chains came loose. (Acts 16:22-26 NIV)

Over and over again we are given stories of the ways that God frees His people. Here we see Paul and Silas being brutally beaten and then thrown into prison unjustly. What was their response? To plot revenge or escape? To curse the people who had wronged them? No. What they did was to sing! There they were – wounded and hurting – and they were sitting in the jail cell singing hymns.

And they were praying. Stop for a minute and imagine what they might have been praying for. Healing? Deliverance? Forgiveness for those who had wronged them? Guidance for what they were to do now? Perhaps all of these. In their case God answered dramatically and clearly. A great earthquake came, the prison walls were shaken and damaged, the prison doors flew open, and everybody's chains came loose. What a mighty God!

Now let us consider a situation that occurred many, many years before. Daniel, too, was wrongly imprisoned. He was sealed up in a den of lions. But look what happened. "Daniel answered, '. . . My God sent his angel, and he shut the mouths of the lions. They have not hurt me, because I was found innocent in his sight' " (Daniel 6:21-22 NIV)

Know that no matter what your situation, you are the beloved child of the Lord God Almighty. Nothing is too hard for Him. There is no situation too hopeless for Him to change. We must accept our responsibility for being vigilant and for taking wise action. If we seek His guidance, we will get it. And it is written that with His help we can overcome anything.

Lord God Almighty, You are my strength and my salvation. No power is greater than You. Like Paul and Silas and Daniel I pray to you in the face of my difficulties and tribulations. You are my great Redeemer and I thank You for my deliverance. In Jesus' name, I pray, Amen.

Day 194

And whatsoever ye shall ask in my name, that will I do, that the Father may be glorified in the Son. If ye shall ask any thing in my name, I will do it. (John 14:13-14 KJV)

Once again, we are told to ask and it will be done as we request. Ask anything, Jesus says. But ask it in My name, He cautions us. Why in His name? Because that provides the underpinning for the asking. When we ask in the name of Jesus, we are asking as a representative and as a follower of Jesus. Therefore, our asking has to be in line with the way Jesus would ask.

What does this mean? It means we must ask believing. And we must believe not only that God can do what we ask but that God wants to do what we ask. Jesus always stayed aligned with God's will. He never asked God for something that He knew to be outside of God's will. He forgave people's sins and he healed all who received Him. Jesus did not turn some away because God did not want a particular person to be forgiven or a particular person to be healed. Jesus knew that God wanted them *all* forgiven and God wanted them *all* healed.

God was glorified because His Son faithfully performed the works of the Father. And God will be glorified when each of us acts as a vessel for Jesus to continue to do the works of the Father. The Amplified Bible reads, "And I will do [I Myself will grant] whatever you ask in my name [as presenting all that I AM], so that the Father may be glorified and extolled in (through) the Son."

Don't let satan talk you into believing God is glorified by your diseases. Instead, listen carefully to the words of Jesus. God is glorified when we choose to walk with Him as He intended in the Garden of Eden. God is glorified when we choose to follow His Son and when we choose to carry on the work and instructions of His Son.

Claim God's Word. Go to God in prayer and make your requests in the name of Jesus Christ. Seek to be a vessel for letting God's glory shine through to all who meet you.

Lord God Almighty, I glorify Your Holy name. I seek to glorify You with the words of my mouth and in my daily actions. You sent Your Son to be an example for me. In the name of Jesus Christ, I ask for healing – of my soul, of my emotional wounds, and of my physical ailments and infirmities. In the name of Jesus Christ, I ask to be a channel for the healing of others. In the name of Jesus Christ, I ask to walk in Your perfect will. In the name of the Jesus Christ, I pray, Amen.

Day 195

. . . for I, the Lord your God, am a jealous God, visiting the iniquity of the fathers upon the children to the third and fourth generations of those who hate Me. (Deuteronomy 5:9 AMP)

The sins of the fathers are visited upon the sons. This is a generational curse that is apparent in matters of health, being scientifically explained in terms of genetic coding. Unwise life choices of parents – including poor nutrition and promiscuous sexual activity – result in physical changes and DNA changes which are inherited by children. Today a great deal of attention is being given to the genetic basis of disease, and many people, upon understanding their genetic inheritance, become very fatalistic. It is as though they feel doomed by their genes. For most of them, fear takes hold, and the belief locks into place that they will probably get the condition that has been identified.

Having a genetic predisposition to a disease does not mean that you have to manifest it. Look positively at the information you have. By acknowledging your genetics, you have identified your weakest links in your health chain. Now, nourish and support the body systems that are involved. Find the herbs and essential oils that God provided for that purpose. Learn about the foods and nutrients that you need. Examine homeopathic remedies that have been used to help the body re-program itself and even, some believe, facilitate a change in DNA coding. Pray for guidance for the precise steps you are to take in your journey to health. As you receive God's instructions, follow them completely and wholeheartedly.

Jesus Christ healed many who had been ill from birth. Surely, some of them had genetic conditions. Jesus overcame *everything* on the Cross, including the curse and all your infirmities. "Be ye transformed," Jesus said. That begins with the renewal of your mind and spirit so pray for it. "With God all things are possible." Believe in His healing power and His healing grace.

Almighty God, You have told me very clearly to have no other gods before me and that includes the god of science. Sometimes I feel trapped and afraid of my own genes. But I know that fear does not come from You. You sent Your Son Jesus Christ to redeem me and to make me whole. Take my fears, Lord. Transform every part of me that is not exactly as You want it to be. Show me what You want me to do to be well and whole. Show me Your path and I will follow. With grateful thanks, in Jesus' name, I pray, Amen.

Day 196

Very early in the morning, while it was still dark, Jesus got up, left the house and went off to a solitary place, where he prayed. (Mark 1:35 NIV)

Immediately Jesus made his disciples get into the boat and go on ahead of him to Bethsaida, while he dismissed the crowd. After leaving them, he went up on a mountainside to pray. (Mark 6:45-46 NIV)

Do you allow yourself time alone for spiritual renewal? Do you take the time to get away from your family, your friends, and your responsibilities so that you can pray and talk things over with God?

Jesus is our perfect model, and we can draw great comfort from that. He was constantly besieged by people. The Scriptures often describe Jesus "withdrawing" and yet the people streamed after Him and pressed around Him. Most of us are not famous and don't have crowds following us. Nevertheless, we, too, have the pressure of daily duties that sometimes seem to be a relentless burden instead of a joyous service to God.

When that happens, we must learn to "get in the boat" by ourselves and go to a solitary place. Maybe it means getting in the car and going off for an overnight respite. Or maybe it means sending family away for a day, taking the telephone off the hook, setting aside all the laundry and the cleaning and the yard work – then simply resting, praying, and meditating.

It takes courage to take a time out. You can always think of a thousand reasons why you can't do it right now. Maybe in a week – or a month. The fact is that the father of lies deceives you by making you think you "can't" stop. Everyone needs to stop for revitalization and to reaffirm and restore priorities. Jesus was not sick and yet He needed time alone.

When you *do* feel sick or are involved in any form of physical recovery, you need this time even more. Time alone is critical for rest, renewal, and rejuvenation. Turn your mind off and set your worries aside. Allow every cell of your body to relax and allow your mind and your soul to float in God's peace and God's love.

Almighty God, give me the courage to take some time to rest and to focus on You. I get tangled in my daily activities and I push through them even when I feel so tired. Help me to find a quiet place where I can hear You speak to me and show me my purpose and Your plan. In the name of Your Son Christ Jesus, my Savior and my Redeemer, I pray, Amen.

Day 197

Therefore shall they eat of the fruit of their own way, and be filled with their own de-vices. . . . But whoso hearkeneth unto me shall dwell safely and shall be quiet from fear of evil. (Proverbs 1:31, 33 KJV)

How often fear of evil traps us. As a small child, the strongest desire of your heart was probably to feel loved and safe and secure. This issue of safety is one that permeates almost every part of our being yet we rarely acknowledge it as adults except when we think of having enough locks on our doors. Fear can paralyze us and keep us stuck. It keeps us from sending our love out into the world and fulfilling God's purpose for us. As the devil's work, fear pulls us inward.

What is the solution? Get close to God, listen, and then follow through. All these are involved in the act of hearkening. How does this relate to our healing? Is it safe to be well or is it sometimes safer to be sick? Sickness can provide a hiding place that feels safe. Yes, there may be physical pain and suffering. But for those with emotional pain that goes very deep, the trauma of dealing with those wounds can be overwhelming. The pain of sickness is easier to bear. And since it seems beyond our control, we think we are absolved from responsibility.

When we feel sick, we often are "eating the fruit of our own way." And we stay sick because we are "filled with our own devices." We have to "let go and let God." We have to put aside the "way things have always been done" and dare to let God direct our treatment.

Jesus asked the fishermen to go into deep water in the light of day when they believed that the "right" way to fish was to drag their nets at night in the shallow areas around the rocks. Maybe God wants you to use His remedies – either along with man's medicine or perhaps in place of it. Are you going to insist that your way is best? Or will you have the trust of the fishermen and do it God's way?

Those who follow God shall dwell safely and shall be quiet from fear of evil.

Lord God Almighty, sometimes I am stubborn and think I know better than You how to accomplish my healing. Help me to harken unto You and to let go of my attachment to "my own desires." I draw close to You now, God, and I am listening. I want to dwell safely and I want to be free from the fear of evil. Heal me, Lord. Shelter me and protect me. In the name of Your Son, Jesus Christ, my Savior and my Redeemer, I pray, Amen.

Day 198

Later Jesus appeared to the Eleven as they were eating; he rebuked them for their lack of faith and their stubborn refusal to believe those who had seen him after he had rise. He said to them, "Go into all the world and preach the good news to all creation. Whoever believes and is baptized will be saved, but whoever does not believe will be condemned. And these signs will accompany those who believe: In my name they will drive out demons; they will speak in new tongues; they will pick up snakes with their hands; and when they drink deadly poison, it will not hurt them at all; they will place their hands on sick people, and they will get well." After the Lord Jesus had spoken to them, he was taken up into heaven and he sat at the right hand of God. Then the disciples went out and preached everywhere, and the Lord worked with them and confirmed his word by the signs that accompanied it. (Mark 16:14-20 NIV)

The Lord Jesus Christ promised "Lo, I am with you always, even to the end of the world" and He kept His promise. Holy Scripture tells us that He worked with His disciples, and He confirmed His Word by the signs that He promised.

The word of Christ Jesus applies to us as much as it did to the disciples. We are His disciples, too. We are His ambassadors. We are His living witnesses. We are to present ourselves to others as testimony that God's Word is true and holy and to be honored. We are to carry out the directives of Christ Jesus and to continue His work on earth. We are to speak His words of salvation and healing with authority and are to reflect their power and their truth in our lives.

The spoken word is very powerful, but only when actions flow forth naturally that are consistent with the word. We are not only to proclaim God's healing power, but we are to manifest God's healing power.

The Lord Jesus Christ sits at the right hand of the Father and works with us every minute, helping, supporting, and strengthening us. He is depending on us to believe in Him fully and to carry on His work to spread the good news of God's love and redemption and to heal the sick.

Wonderful Jehovah-rapha, thank You for sending Your Son Christ Jesus to save me from my sins and to carry my infirmities to the Cross. I accept the mission to carry on His work and I know that He is with me always, supporting, strengthening, and healing. Thank You for Your eternal love and Your gracious healing hand on my body. In Jesus' name, I pray, Amen.

Day 199

Hezekiah had asked Isaiah, "What will be the sign that the Lord will heal me and that I will go up to the temple of the Lord on the third day from now?" Isaiah answered, "This is the Lord's sign to you that the Lord will do what he has promised: Shall the shadow go forward ten steps, or shall it go back ten steps?" "It is a simple matter for the shadow to go forward ten steps," said Hezekiah. "Rather, have it go back ten steps." Then the prophet Isaiah called upon the Lord, and the Lord made the shadow go back the ten steps it had gone down on the stairway of Ahaz. (2 Kings 20:8-11 NIV)

We return to the story of Hezekiah, king of Judah. Having become ill to the point of death, he had prayed to God and been told by the prophet Isaiah that God promised to heal him in three days. What would you do if God told you that you would be healed in three days? Would you trust in God's message? Or would you want something more, some proof that you could see or touch that God would keep His promise? Hezekiah wanted proof.

Most of us, if we are honest, would also like a sign. We live in a physical body in a physical world. Yes, there is a very real spiritual world beyond what we can see and touch. But it requires great faith to stay grounded in that unseen abode of the Almighty.

Before you beat yourself up for wanting a sign, take a look at the kind of man that Hezekiah was. Here was a man who said to God, "Remember, O Lord, how I have walked before you faithfully and with wholehearted devotion and have done what is good in your eyes." This was a remarkable man.

How many of us can say what Hezekiah said? Not many of us. Yet even as remarkable as he was, Hezekiah still had doubt. He still had fear. And he still wanted something to hold onto while God was working the healing of His promise.

God understands our needs and He knows our weaknesses. He already knows your heart. If your faith is weak, you may ask God for help.

Merciful Father, there are times when my faith is weak. I sin and fall short of what I know I should be; I can't truthfully pray all the words that Hezekiah said to You. But God, You know the innermost places of my heart. I need Your healing. I know You are healing me now. But I hunger for a sign, O Lord, something to hang onto while You are working Your way in me. I wait obediently for it. In Jesus' name, I pray, Amen.

Day 200

Be still and know that I am God. (Psalm 46:10 KJV)

Everyone needs focused time with God. For most people this takes the form of prayer, which is a vital part of our spiritual life. It is a time for us to offer up our fears and our hurts. It is a time for us to intercede for others. It is a time for us to express our gratitude for God's many blessings.

However, when we pray, we are busy talking to God. If we spend all our focused time with God in the act of praying to Him, we do not allow God to speak to us. Hearing God's voice is critical because we cannot align ourselves with God's will for us if we don't listen to Him. It is interesting that most of us were taught as children to pray, but few of us were taught to listen.

Most people find it difficult to "find the time" to listen to God. They may say their morning or evening prayers and some find time for daily reading of the Scripture. But quiet, focused listening is rare. Why is that? Perhaps it is due to the fact that we are often afraid of what we will hear. There isn't much point in taking the time to listen to God, if we don't intend to act on the guidance that we are given. But to do so often takes great trust and great boldness. Frequently, God's guidance does not seem logical or realistic and is not in accord with the opinions of people we trust.

Turn to God's Word. The Bible is filled with accounts of people who listened, who heard, and who acted. Often, they endured great ridicule when they did so. Can you *really* imagine what Noah went through while he was building the ark?

Get still in your mind. Open yourself to God and the Holy Spirit. Ask for specific guidance for your health. Ask to hear only the voice of God, only the voice of the Holy Spirit – and no other. Ask for clarity so that you know exactly what it is that God wants you to do. "Ask and you shall receive." Dare to listen. Dare to follow your guidance. Know that God is the Great Physician.

Almighty God, You are the Great Physician. I still my mind. I set aside all the voices of my family, friends, and advisors and open my heart to You. Let me hear only Your voice, O Lord. Only Yours. I need to know what to do. Take my fears and hold me in Your loving arms so I can hear You clearly. I am willing to hear You. I am willing to act on Your guidance. Thank you, God. And now, I end my prayer and listen to You, O Lord. In Jesus' name, I pray, Amen.

Day 201

Let your eyes look straight ahead, fix your gaze directly before you. Make level paths for your feet and take only ways that are firm. Do not swerve to the right or the left; keep your foot from evil. (Proverbs 4:25-27 NIV)

Just as the spiritual path is narrow and straight, so is the path to physical recovery. There are so many options and paths to take, how can you find the right one? How can you keep from swerving to the right or the left? The answer comes by determining the final authority for your health decisions. You must be clear in your mind who has the last word. Is it God? Or is it medical doctors? Or health professionals? Or your family?

Make the decision to have God as your final authority. Now keep your eyes fixed straight ahead at Him. This means going to Him for guidance in every single decision you must make in your treatment and recovery. Every single one. It takes only one wrong step to move you onto shaky ground where you are vulnerable and easy prey for the evil one.

Think of the myriad of decisions you make. Should I go to the members of the church for them to pray for me for the health problem I am having now? Should I seek assistance at the physical level as well as at the spiritual level? Should I see a doctor? If so, which one? Are the recommendations of this particular doctor right for me and my recovery? Should I use any natural remedies? If so, which ones? Exactly how much of a particular herb or essential oil should I use? Should I see a natural health professional? If so, which one? Are the recommendations of this particular health professional right for me and my recovery? The choices go on and on.

God is always available to you. At the request of Jesus, He has sent the Holy Spirit to you to reveal the truth. God has done everything He can to say to you, "Here I am. Come to Me. Let Me guide your way."

Almighty God, You are Jehovah-rapha, and I affirm that You are my final authority for every single health decision that I make. I keep my eyes straight ahead, fixed only on You, Lord. Make the path level for my feet. Keep me walking on firm ground. Guide me, God, so that I do not swerve to the right or the left and do not fall prey to the evil one. Thank You for sending the Holy Spirit to reveal the truth to me in all the many decisions I must make each day. Show me exactly what you want me to do at the physical level to join in partnership with You for my healing. In Jesus' name, I pray, Amen.

Day 202

The Lord is my light and my salvation; whom shall I fear? The Lord is the strength of my life; of whom shall I be afraid? When the wicked, even mine enemies and my foes, came upon me to eat up my flesh, they stumbled and fell. Though an host should encamp against me, my heart shall not fear: though war should rise against me, in this will I be confident. One thing have I desired of the Lord, that will I seek after; that I may dwell in the house of the Lord all the days of my life, to behold the beauty of the Lord, and to enquire in his temple. (Psalm 27:1-4 KJV)

There is no reason to be fearful. No matter what circumstance you find yourself in. No matter what disease or medical condition you may have. You are fully protected.

How beautifully Psalm 27 expresses the protection of the Lord. When you are plunged into darkness, the Lord is your light. When you feel confused and overwhelmed, the Lord is your salvation, your deliverer. When you seem weak, the Lord is your strength. When you feel besieged by the evil one, the Lord is your protector.

Even though your foes come upon you to eat up your flesh, they will stumble and fall. Does this graphic picture not describe the action of many diseases – to eat up your flesh, to crumble your bones, to destroy your cells? But the evil one cannot prevail if the Lord is your leader. Even if you have a *host* of ailments, the evil one cannot prevail. Not even then. You can remain confident and sure, having unshakable trust that the Lord God Almighty will prevail.

The Psalmist asks you to do only one thing: to dwell in the house of the Lord all the days of your life, gazing upon the beauty of the Lord and seeking Him in his temple. Put Jehovah-rapha first, above everything else. Put His guidance first, above all other opinions and recommendations. Stay focused on God and only on God. As you make the choice to dwell in His house forever, offer your body to Him as a temple to His glory and honor.

Almighty God, You are my protector. There are times when I feel confused, but at this moment I feel confident and unafraid. You are my stronghold and I will fear no disease. Even though I am experiencing a host of ailments, I know that You are more powerful than all of them. I seek to dwell with You forever, God. You are my light and my guide. I chart my course by Your directions. I come to You and offer my body as Your Holy temple. I worship and praise You. In Jesus' name, I pray, Amen.

Day 203

This is what the Lord says: "In the time of my favor I will answer you, and in the day of salvation I will help you; I will keep you and will make you to be a covenant for the people, to restore the land and to reassign its desolate inheritances, to say to the captives, 'Come out,' and to those in darkness, 'Be free!'" (Isaiah 49:8-9 NIV)

From the beginning God gave us liberty. We always had the free choice to walk with Him as part of His family or to reject Him. Without that free choice our relationship would be meaningless.

Adam exercised his free choice option when he chose to eat the forbidden fruit and to know evil. Unfortunately, that choice made him and all of the rest of us subjects of satan. We became imprisoned by our sin and vulnerable to all the things are part of satan's handiwork.

God so loved us that He sent His Son Christ Jesus who calls to us, "Come out. Be free." Jesus calls us to move out from the darkness and to stand with us in God's light as free people once again. He brings us Divine liberty. He has loosed the bonds of our sin. He has loosed the bonds of disease.

You who feel sick understand what it is like to be a captive. Your energy is low and you feel bound by the effects of your illness or injury. Too often you may despair that you will ever feel well again. Your future may appear dark. At those moments you allow satan to triumph because you forget God's covenant to bring you into liberty. God claims you. God frees you. God restores you. God wants you well.

Speak God's Word to every cell in your body. Identify the body parts which are weak and command them to receive the strength, freedom, and healing of the Lord God Almighty. Accept God's Word and be filled with God's Holy light of freedom.

Lord God Almighty, I have felt trapped by my health problem for too long. I understand what it is to feel like a captive. I know that I am allowing satan to triumph in my life because I am forgetting Your covenant with me to bring me into liberty. Restore me, God. Restore my freedom. I resist the evil one and I stand firmly on Your Holy Word. You sent Your Son Jesus Christ to set me free once and for all. Thank You, Heavenly Father. In the name of Your Son, Jesus Christ, I pray, Amen.

Day 204

Light is sweet, and it pleases the eyes to see the sun. (Ecclesiastes 11:7 NIV)

Light. It was the first thing God created and it was also the way Jesus described Himself. It is essential both for our spirit and for a healthy body.

Light actually has healing properties. Through exposure to the sun our bodies manufacture vitamin D. Unfortunately, many of us spend almost no time in the sun during the day, and our bodies consequently suffer from lack of exposure to God's natural light. It is healthy to spend a minimum of twenty to forty minutes a day in the sunshine, provided we are using appropriate sunscreen. Those people with abundant nutrient intake from their food rarely experience skin problems from reasonable exposure to the sun.

When indoors, we need to use the proper type of light. Most people use incandescent lamps which emit light rays from only part of the full spectrum of the sun. The most harmful light source is fluorescent lights, which sap your strength and your energy. Change the bulbs in your home and your workplace to full spectrum lighting. You will notice that your eyes do not become as fatigued and that your energy level increases. It is amazing the results we experience when we return to God's plan for our health instead of using artificial methods that are not in synchronization with the way that our bodies function.

Jesus told us, "I am the light of the world." Close your eyes and feel His light beam down on you. Feel it cover you like a warm blanket. Breathe deeply and breathe the Christ light into your body. Let it fill your lungs and mix with the oxygen. Now feel it travel through your blood vessels and go into every organ. Feel it energize every gland. See a little star of the light of Jesus Christ in every cell in your body. Watch it twinkle there sending out His love, His peace, and His healing.

Your light has come. No matter what your situation at this very moment, "let your light shine before men." Your faith is a great light that can be a beacon to others. In spite of your difficulties, shine, shine, shine.

God of Glory, I will take the time to enjoy Your sunshine in a wise and healthy manner. I want to spend more time in the light of the sun outside and to spend more time in the light of the Son inside. I want my light to shine before others so that they will come to praise You as I do. In Jesus' name, I pray, Amen.

Day 205

Restore to me the joy of your salvation and grant me a willing spirit, to sustain me. (Psalm 51:12 NIV)

God never forces us. From the beginning He wanted His children to love Him, be obedient, and live as His family – all voluntarily and with joy in their hearts. So He set up the system under which we have always lived – we know the rules, we have free will to make our own decisions, and we experience the consequences of our choices.

This is true for our spiritual selves and also for our physical selves. Let us look at what this means for our health. Illness can't take hold in your body unless the environment exists for it to grow. God designed your body to survive and to heal itself. If you have become ill, you must be willing to examine what happened to create the situation you are in. And then you must be willing to make some changes and do things differently.

Doing what you did got you where you are. Are you willing to accept that statement? It is the essence of taking responsibility for your health. Satan attacks you where you are most vulnerable. He knows your weaknesses and exploits them. Most often it is only one tiny decision after another over a period of months and years that finally culminate in your illness.

For example, do you really believe that it is all right to pop anti-acids in your mouth so that you won't feel the pain of eating foods that your body can no longer digest? Do you really believe that carrying deep anger toward your brother will have no effect on your health? Do you really believe that gallbladder surgery is an easy solution to remove your pain and still allow you to eat what you used to eat?

Remember that Jesus asked, "Do you want to be well?" He knew that He could heal a person but that he would be sick again soon if he were not willing to make changes in his life. How willing are you to make healthy choices in your life? How willing are you to change?

Dear Heavenly Father, grant to me a willing spirit. Restore to me the joy of Your salvation. I want to be well, God. I accept responsibility for my decisions, and I am willing to examine my life and my choices to see what I need to do differently. Guide me, Lord. Show me the path You want me to take for my recovery. I am willing to listen. I am willing to follow. I am willing to act as You tell me. In Jesus' name, I pray, Amen.

Day 206

There is a time for everything and a season for every activity under heaven: a time to be born and a time to die, a time to plant and a time to uproot, a time to kill and a time to heal, a time to tear down and a time to build, a time to weep and a time to laugh, a time to mourn and a time to dance, a time to scatter stones and a time to gather them, a time to embrace and a time to refrain, a time to search and a time to give up, a time to keep and a time to throw away, a time to tear and a time to mend, a time to be silent and a time to speak, a time to love and a time to hate, a time for war and a time for peace. (Ecclesiastes 3:1-8 NIV)

Often the emotional baggage that you carry makes you sick. You must be willing to deal with your emotional issues if you really want to be well. Too many people do not want to change. They want to take a pill or have some surgery and then be able to continue doing exactly what they were doing. They want not only to continue to eat the same foods, but they also want to continue behaving the same way.

Unless you are willing to look within at your emotions, your motivations, and your desires, you are not likely to recover in your physical body. Your emotions and your body dance together, each affecting the other and each being affected by the other.

There is a time to search and a time to give up. Are you willing to take the time to search for your wounds? You know many of them but others may be so deeply hidden that you may need assistance from a counselor to get to them. The search is likely to be painful. However, make no mistake about it; to leave the wound inside is to leave a festering pocket of poison that will eventually affect your physical body and will make you sick.

Certainly not all illnesses come from emotional wounds inside, but many do. If you have asked for healing and have not received it, perhaps the reason is due to the emotional wound inside.

Once you have found the wounds and claimed them, there is a time to give them up and to throw them away. Are you willing to do that? Or have you gotten used to being victim to them? Have you gotten used to using them to manipulate others? When you are ready, hand them to God and ask Him to fill you instead with His healing love.

Almighty God, it is time for me to search for my emotional wounds and it is time for me to let them go. I am ready, Lord, and I am willing. Walk with me through the pain and then bring me Your peace. In the name of Christ Jesus, my Savior and my Redeemer, I pray, Amen.

Day 207

Let the word of Christ dwell in you richly as you teach and admonish one another with all wisdom, and as you sing psalms, hymns and spiritual songs with gratitude in your hearts to God. (Colossians 3:16 NIV)

One of the best ways to promote your healing is to fill your life with music. Paul very wisely exhorted the Colossians to "sing psalms, hymns, and spiritual songs." Interestingly, he told them something even more important, something about their attitude. They were to sing with gratitude in their hearts to God.

When you feel discouraged or are in pain or just feel out of sorts with your life, few things can restore you more quickly than music that fills your spirit. Create a library of cassettes and compact discs that have hymns and spiritual songs which bring joy to your heart and peace to your soul. Make listening to these hymns a part of your daily activities. Play them while you are in the car or doing household chores. In some cases, it is feasible to play them as background music while you are working – and you accomplish your tasks much more quickly and efficiently.

The more you listen, the more the message penetrates within. The vibrations of the sound waves actually create healthy vibrations within the cells of your body. Every organ and every gland get a little energy boost from the music and facilitate your healing. The words and the music join to create a unique method for healing. Think of every song as a healing treatment.

Join in with the music and sing along. Don't judge your musical ability. Just let go and sing. When you do so, breathe deeply from your abdomen and let your lungs expand. Feel your vocal cords vibrate and then feel that vibration resonate in every cell of your body. Move, dance, or sway to the music.

Let your whole body become an instrument glorifying the Lord your Creator. Sometimes you may become so attuned that tears suddenly start to flow as you are overwhelmed by the grace and love that stream from heaven to surround you and fill you.

These moments are special gifts. Treasure them. Go in song to God often with gratitude on your lips and in your heart.

Gracious Father, I am delighted to be able to worship You with psalms and hymns and songs. Music fills me with a feeling of awe and joy and energy. It calms my fears and bolsters my faith. I sing my praise. In the name of Christ Jesus, my Savior and my Redeemer, I pray, Amen.

Day 208

But as it is written, "Eye hath not seen, nor ear heard, neither have entered into the heart of man, the things which God hath prepared for them that love him." (1 Corinthians 2:9 KJV)

In your wildest imagination you can't picture all the wondrous things which your Heavenly Father wants to give you. One of the blessings that God wants His children to have is good health. When He created the Garden of Eden, He provided that Adam and Eve should be healthy, strong, and vital. There was no sickness and disease that could harm them. Another place that God works His perfect will is heaven. There is no sickness and disease there either. Jesus came to show us exactly what God's will for us is because He did only those things that were according to God's will. And Jesus healed everyone who came to Him to be made well.

There is one requirement: that we love God. Love isn't simply an emotion that we feel. Love consists of hundred of thousands of actions minute by minute, based on our decisions and intent. Love is what you *do*. To love God means that you trust God with your entire being. To love God means that you ask Him for guidance in your life. To love God means that you obey the instructions that you are given.

Most Christians think that they love, trust, and obey God – at least most of the time. However, when they feel sick, the pattern is often to follow conventional methods of dealing with illness automatically. As long as the treatments are working or are not life-threatening, they rarely involve God in their recovery. It is only when surgery is pending or the treatments aren't working, that they go to God in prayer.

God doesn't want to be an afterthought. He wants to be your *first* consultation. To love God is to trust Him with your life and to be willing to seek His advice first. To love God is to be willing to obey His directives for your healing. His instructions may be for you to follow conventional methods or they may be a different way.

Stand fast in your love for Him. Stand fast in your trust that your eye has not seen and your ear has not heard nor has it entered into your heart the things which God has prepared for you.

Wonderful Jehovah-rapha, it is written that, if I remain faithful in love to You, You will take care of me. I believe Your Word, Lord. I trust You. I act on my faith and I seek Your advice and instruction. I obey Your voice and I thank You for my healing. In the name of Your Son, Jesus Christ, I pray, Amen.

Day 209

A man . . . fell into the hands of robbers. They stripped him of his clothes, beat him and went away, leaving him half dead. . . . But a Samaritan . . . saw him . . . [and] took pity on him. He went to him and bandaged his wounds, pouring on oil and wine. Then he put the man on his own donkey, took him to an inn and took care of him. . . . Which . . . was a neighbor? . . . Go and do likewise. (Luke 10:30, 33-34, 36-37 NIV)

Isn't it interesting that when Jesus wanted to illustrate how to be a good neighbor, he chose to use an example of one person being an instrument of healing for another person? The story of the good Samaritan is just a story that Jesus made up, yet look at the details He put in. The Samaritan used natural substances (wine and oil) to help to heal the wound; he bandaged the injury; he took him to shelter; and he cared for him.

Jesus could have used an example of being spiritually helpful to a neighbor. But He didn't. One more time Jesus emphasized the importance of the healing of the body. Even though our soul is our "real" essence and the Divine part of us that is eternal, our body is important as a temporary vessel. It is the temple that houses our soul and the Holy Spirit. Since the body is a temple, its health is vital.

There is one important point that isn't mentioned, but it is implied. It is that the wounded man accepted the help of the good Samaritan. He was willing to receive what the Samaritan had to offer. As we extend our help to our neighbors, we must remember, however, that not everyone may be ready or able to receive our message or methods of healing and no one should be pushed. Our offering should be gentle and light, giving our neighbor a graceful way to accept or decline it.

God wants us to be a good neighbor and to help others who are in distress. We may not be doctors or medical professionals, but we can share God's message of healing and our personal testimony of using God's remedies in our recovery to those who want to hear it. The interesting thing is that, as we help others to heal, we find our own healing is accelerated. The giving and receiving spin around in a circle, magnifying God's healing grace.

Merciful God, Your Son Jesus Christ taught us how to be a good neighbor. You have so graciously blessed me with Your healing. Help me to follow the instructions of Jesus and to pass along all that I have received. Use me, O God, in Your work and according to Your plan for my life. In the name of the Father, Son, and Holy Spirit, I pray, Amen.

Day 210

Then Peter came to Jesus and asked, "Lord, how many times shall I forgive my brother when he sins against me? Up to seven times?" Jesus answered, "I tell you, not seven times, but seventy-seven times." (Matthew 18:21-22 NIV)

Are you carrying hurts or anger toward someone? If so, these negative feelings are taking a heavy toll on the health of your physical body, in addition to the toll on your spirit.

Many people struggle with forgiveness because they confuse it with the concept of pardon. Forgiveness really means to stop carrying resentment against someone who has offended or hurt you. It *may* also mean to excuse them without requiring a penalty or punishment for the offense. Do you see the difference? Forgiveness is really about the person who was hurt and pardoning is more about the person who did the offending. Forgiveness does not require you to pardon anyone or to include an abusive offender in your life again. You may still hold others accountable for their actions.

Jesus tells you to forgive so many times that you lose count in the process. Why? Because He knows that the issue is that you must let go of the resentment smoldering inside you. That resentment isn't hurting the person who offended you at all. It isn't affecting *him,* but it is killing *you.* It is destroying your spirit and sapping your energy. By holding on to resentment, you become the offender against yourself. You recreate the offense over and over again and re-wound yourself. The new offender is you, *yourself,* and not the other person.

You cannot heal when you are filled with resentment toward anyone – whether it is someone else or whether it is yourself. You must reach the point where you are willing to forgive others and, *just as important,* to forgive *yourself* of all things you regret doing or not doing. Let the past go. As the resentment leaves, God's healing power will fill you.

Dear Gracious Lord, I realize that I have been carrying some old hurts inside for a long time. I know now that I have been the one hurting myself by keeping my resentment alive. Help me to let go, God. I now choose to forgive those who have hurt me, and I give my wounds and my resentments to You, Heavenly Father. I'm tired of carrying them. Take them. Cleanse me; free me; heal me. In Jesus' name, I pray, Amen.

Day 211

Therefore, if anyone is in Christ, he is a new creation; the old has gone, the new has come! All this is from God, who reconciled us to himself through Christ and gave us the ministry of reconciliation: that God was reconciling the world to himself in Christ, not counting men's sins against them. (2 Corinthians 5:17-19 NIV)

If anyone is in Christ, he is a new creation. We have been born again. We have been saved and redeemed. How comforting that is for us.

When we feel sick or have an injury, this knowledge is important for us. God created our bodies to regenerate every minute of every day, thus making them perpetually new creations. The various cells in our bodies have different lifespans and then they are replaced by new ones. The old has gone and the new has come. This cycle of replacement was intended as a constant renewal within us. God designed us with the intent that we be healthy.

If sick and dying cells are replaced, why don't we get well automatically? In many cases we do. It is estimated that over 80 percent of all health problems for which we seek medical care would have resulted in recovery without any medical attention. The body already had inherently within itself the mechanism from God for healing. What about the other health problems?

When we allow our body to get out of balance and to stay out of balance, the message control center (the DNA) of the cells changes. Instead of a pattern for a healthy cell being transmitted to the next generation of cells, we find a pattern for an unhealthy cell being transmitted. Then we need some sort of intervention in order to restore ourselves to health.

There are many options – herbs, essential oils, pharmaceuticals, the touch of God – just to name a few. Enter into prayer with your requests and your questions. Then listen for the Holy Spirit to speak to you and follow the guidance that you are given.

Almighty God, through Jesus Christ You have redeemed me from my sins and You have restored me. I shout with joy that I am a new creation! Thank You for touching my body, God, and transforming every cell that needs healing. Thank You for bringing each cell to its perfect functioning according to Your intent and will. Thank You, Lord. In Jesus' name, I pray, Amen.

But when he saw the multitudes, he was moved with compassion on them, because they fainted, and were scattered abroad, as sheep having no shepherd. Then saith he unto his disciples, "The harvest truly is plenteous, but the labourers are few; Pray ye therefore the Lord of the harvest, that he will send forth labourers into his harvest." And when he had called unto him his twelve disciples, he gave them power against unclean spirits, to cast them out, and to heal all manner of sickness and all manner of disease. . . . These twelve Jesus sent forth. (Matthew 9:36-38, 10:1, 5 KJV)

Multitudes of people kept coming to Jesus. Everywhere He went they came to Him, seeking His words, His hope, His encouragement. They were drawn to Him as sheep come to the shepherd for food. Jesus was filled with compassion for them and here He expresses His frustration by His own limitations. There are so many people, He says. So many. And all are in need. They are ready to receive what I have to offer. They are ripe for my Word, like a harvest ready to be picked. But I need help to reach them. I need laborers in the field.

Who are the laborers? People who have already heard and who believe. The laborers are the believers who are willing to take action on their beliefs. What did Jesus do after He recognized that He couldn't do everything Himself, that He needed help? He called His twelve disciples around Him, He gave them power over the evil one so that they could heal, and He sent them out to feed His flock.

You are called to be a laborer for the Lord also. There are still multitudes who are hurting. Many do not know the Lord at all. Others have heard only half of the message – they believe in salvation of the soul but not salvation from their illnesses.

Be willing to be one of God's laborers. Don't be hesitant to step forward. Don't wait until your own healing is fully manifested before telling others the wonderful news of the gospel: You have been redeemed in soul and in body.

Heavenly Father, I want to be one of Your laborers. I know what it is like to be hurting and afraid, to be confused and wandering around looking for help and for hope. Part of me wants to wait until my own healing is fully manifested, but I know it is evidence of a greater faith for me to step forward now. Let me be an example to others of Your love, Your healing grace, and Your power. Thank You, Lord, for Your many blessings on me. Help me to pass them on to others. In Jesus' name, I pray, Amen.

Day 213

And I will ask the Father, and he will give you another Counselor to be with you forever – the Spirit of truth. (John 14:16-17 NIV)

Jesus is our gentle, caring Lord, who wants us to be protected always. Before He left the earth in His physical form, He told His disciples that He was asking the Father to send a counselor to be with His followers forever. Think for a moment of the magnitude of what He was saying.

Jesus said that the Father "will give you another Counselor." The Holy Spirit is a gift from a God who desires that we live in abundance. We already had the Lord God Almighty to call on and we already had Jesus Christ His Son. Yet the Son was asking the Father for yet *another* counselor and comforter for us.

And what is the purpose of the Holy Spirit? It is the "Spirit of truth" – to show the way for us. Like a compass which always turns to the north even in the darkest night, the Holy Spirit always points us to the truth.

When we are ill, we need the truth more than ever. It is easy to be deceived by the appearance of our illness and by the numerous opinions from the people around us. We need to be clear about God's purpose in our life and God's will for us. Therefore, we need to call on the Holy Spirit, the voice of truth, who provides a major support for us. Having the Holy Spirit indwell us keeps us centered and grounded in God's purpose and guides us always along the path that is for our highest good.

Ask for the Holy Spirit to fill you whenever you have any decision to make. Receive this Counselor in gratitude as a vital part of your healing.

Dear Heavenly Father, thank You for Your gracious gift to me of the Holy Spirit. Sometimes I forget to call for this Counselor in my daily life and in my healing process. I often get caught up in making my own decisions and I sometimes blindly follow the opinions of others. I need to know Your truth, O God, even when I am reluctant to hear it. The Holy Spirit always points the way for me and I am grateful. When the Holy Spirit fills me, God, I feel Your Holy presence in my soul and in every cell of my body. When the Holy Spirit fills me, I feel Your peace within. When the Holy Spirit fills me, I hear Your guidance and directions. Thank You, thank You, thank You. In the name of the Father, Son, and Holy Spirit, I pray, Amen.

Day 214

There some people brought to him [Jesus] a man who was deaf and could hardly talk, and they begged him to place his hand on the man. After he took him aside, away from the crowd, Jesus put his fingers into the man's ears. Then he spit and touched the man's tongue. He looked up to heaven and with a deep sigh said to him, "Ephphatha!" (which means, "Be opened!"). At this, the man's ears were opened, his tongue was loosened and he began to speak plainly. Jesus commanded them not to tell anyone. But the more he did so, the more they kept talking about it. People were overwhelmed with amazement. "He has done everything well," they said, "He even makes the deaf hear and the mute speak." (Mark 7:32-37 NIV)

Again and again and again we are told of the love, compassion, and healing of Jesus. No matter what the affliction, He healed it. Interestingly, He used different methods at different times. In this passage in Mark He uses His spittle to heal a deaf man while at other times he uses mud. Notice that in the following passages He heals simply by the touch of His hand:

A large crowd of his disciples was there and a great number of people from all over Judea, from Jerusalem, and from the coast of Tyre and Sidon, who had come to hear him and to be healed of their diseases. Those troubled by evil spirits were cured, and the people all tried to touch him, because power was coming from him and healing them all. (Luke 6:17-19 NIV)

But the Pharisees went out and plotted how they might kill Jesus. Aware of this, Jesus withdrew from that place. Many followed him, and he healed all their sick, warning them not to tell who he was. (Matthew 12:14-16 NIV)

Fill your soul with the Holy Word telling of Jesus' healing touch. Claim this healing in your body. Jesus took your sins and your infirmities to the Cross, so stand on the promises of God's Word. Give God all your praise and thanksgiving.

Wonderful Jehovah-rapha, there are times when I become discouraged. Let me turn to Your Holy Word and immerse myself in these wonderful stories of the compassionate healing of Your Son Jesus Christ. By His stripes I am healed today. In the name of Jesus Christ, my Savior, Amen.

Day 215

With long life will I satisfy him and show him my salvation. (Psalm 91:16 NIV)

Who is responsible for long life? Some people may answer "God" but actually most people credit modern medical science with giving us long life. They point to statistics as their proof. The life expectancy of a person born in the United States in 1900 was about 45. The life expectancy of a person born one hundred years later in 2000 is over 75. Most people hail drugs, surgery, complicated machinery, organ transplants, and massive treatment modalities for this extension of life.

The truth is that this difference in life expectancy is almost entirely due to improvements in keeping infants alive. When deaths for children up to the age of 2 are removed, statistics reveal that a person born in the year 2000 will live, on average, only 3 years longer than a person born in 1900. Over and over again the real truth is that the drugs, treatments, and massive medical interventions do not result in people living longer lives. They may not die of the disease they were treated for, but another disease often results from the treatment and that will be the cause of death.

A key problem is that the very definition of science *forbids* any involvement by God. How tragic. God must surely weep for us. We are to be ever mindful that we are not God and that we have very few answers about life. When we exalt ourselves to the status of God and proclaim that something will happen or not happen based on a set of test results or scientific experiments, we have fallen into the trap of the evil one.

We are supposed to think and to create, and we are supposed to use the minds that God gave us. But we are to make our explorations under the revelation knowledge and guidance of God. We are to draw our conclusions with the caveat that our understanding is always very limited when compared to the understanding of God. This allows us to put the appearance of things into perspective while looking beyond to God's Divine reality and truth.

Lord God, You are the author of all life, ALL life. You have declared it is Your desire to satisfy me with long life and to show me Your salvation. I come, God, with a grateful heart and with a commitment to fulfill Your purpose in my life. Show me the way. Prevent me from being misled by the appearance of things, and keep me always attuned to Your perfect truth. In the name of the Father, Son, and Holy Spirit, I pray, Amen.

Day 216

People were bringing little children to Jesus to have him touch them, but the disciples rebuked them. When Jesus saw this, he was indignant. He said to them, "Let the little children come to me, and do not hinder them, for the kingdom of God belongs to such as these. I tell you the truth, anyone who will not receive the kingdom of God like a little child will never enter it." And he took the children in his arms, put his hands on them and blessed them. (Mark 10:13-16 NIV)

We are all children of God, but we often lose sight of that identity because we take ourselves so seriously as adults. Children, unless they are burdened early in life, have a light-hearted way of looking at their world. They know how to play and how to have fun.

It is time for you to lighten up! Illness can weigh you down with problems, worries, and fatigue. Little by little, every task becomes heavy, and you smile less and less. Your face develops worry lines and the twinkle leaves your eyes. Make the decision to lighten up and brighten up. Cast your cares on the Lord and decide to make a joyful noise to Him instead.

Find some outlet for play in your life. Do you like jokes? Find someone to be your "laugh partner" to share funny stories that tickle your funny bone. Do you like to play sports? Find a team and join it. Do you like board games? Ask a couple of friends to have a weekly game with you. Do you like to swing? "Adopt" a neighbor's child and take him to the park.

When at all possible, have some play activities that you do with adults and other play activities that you do with children. You will respond differently emotionally to children from the way you respond to adults and, therefore, the physiological effects will be slightly different. The more joy, silly giggles, and belly laughter you experience when you play, the healthier you will become. Your glands release many beneficial substances during happy play, and you will feel your body and your emotions becoming lighter and brighter.

Dear Heavenly Father, You are my all-loving parent who will never fail me or let me down. Teach me to come to you as a little child. Teach me to play at Your feet in the safety and security of Your love. Let joy and laughter fill my body and my spirit and be part of my healing. In the name of Your Son, Jesus Christ, my Savior and my Redeemer, I pray, Amen.

Day 217

And the God of all grace, who called you to his eternal glory in Christ, after you have suffered a little while, will himself restore you and make you strong, firm and steadfast. To him be the power forever and ever. (1 Peter 5:10-11 NIV)

The God of all grace will restore you and make you strong, firm, and steadfast. You have suffered and now is the time to receive the power of God, the strength of God, and the restoration of God.

God *wants* to restore you and to make you whole, complete, and well. His will for you has never changed. God intended for us to walk with Him in the Garden as members of His family. God wanted us to be His free companions so we were given free will. We made a horrible choice to know evil and, ever since, God has focused on our redemption. God extends His grace directly to You, and He has already accomplished your total redemption through the blood of His Son, Jesus Christ.

Close your eyes, take a deep breath, and feel the grace of God fill you. Feel Him restoring you. Feel His power strengthening you – your spirit, your mind, and every cell in your body. Feel yourself becoming firmly focused on God's will for your life, and make a commitment to remain steadfast to His purpose for you.

When temptations come to mislead you to follow the patterns of the world that you know are unhealthy ones, remember to stay focused on your commitment. The evil one wants to get you off God's path, and he comes in many guises that may not seem obvious to you. Remain steadfast and accept no person's recommendations for your health until you have gone to your Father for His guidance.

God wants you to be well. He wants you to walk whole in the Garden and to be a glorious witness to His grace and power.

Almighty God of infinite grace, I come to You as Your child. Hold me in Your loving arms. Fill me with Your Holy love and grace and restore me. Make me what I ought to be – what You want me to be – because I truly want to fulfill Your purpose for my life. Your Son, Jesus, sent His followers to tell others of Your love and to heal the sick. Help me to be one of the followers who fulfills that mission. Make me strong, firm, and steadfast, O God. Thank You for protecting me, guiding me, and healing me. In Jesus' name, I pray, Amen.

Day 218

No good tree bears bad fruit, nor does a bad tree bear good fruit. Each tree is recognized by its own fruit. People do not pick figs from thornbushes, or grapes from briers. The good man brings good things out of the good stored up in his heart, and the evil man brings evil things out of the evil stored up in his heart. For out of the overflow of his heart his mouth speaks. (Luke 6:43-45 NIV)

For out of the overflow of the heart the mouth speaks. The good man brings good things out the good stored up in him, and the evil man brings evil things out of the evil stored up in him. (Matthew 12:34-35 NIV)

The seed contains the potential of the mature plant. What you plant is what you will harvest, if you nurture it to maturity. Jesus describes a truth that is almost ridiculous when viewed in the physical world. If you plant a briar bush, you cannot harvest grapes from it. Yet people constantly sow negative seeds with their words by speaking their ailments and problems and still foolishly expect that they can reap a harvest of healing from it.

Whatever is in our hearts is what will flow out of our mouth in our general conversation. "My thyroid doesn't work anymore; I'll have to take medication for the rest of my life," we say – and we plant a briar bush. How can we utter those words and expect to receive healing? Instead, we must sow the correct seed that will mature into the outcome we seek. For example, we can change our words to this: "No matter what the appearance is, no disease can stay in my body. By His stripes I am healed. I am following guidance from the Holy Spirit to use natural thyroid hormone medication, essential oils, and herbs at the present time. I enforce the Word on my thyroid and I thank God for healing me." What a glorious grape vine those words plant!

Remember that every word you speak is a seed that determines what kind of result you will have. Immerse yourself in God's Word. Every time you are tempted to speak negative words about your health, quote the Scripture instead.

By changing your word-seeds, you will bear good fruit and will be in alignment with God's purpose for your life.

Heavenly Father, I want to bear good fruit. I know that my mouth speaks out of the overflow of my heart. I want to bring forth good things out of the good stored up in me. Teach me Your ways, O Lord. Thank You for healing me. In Jesus' name, I pray, Amen.

Day 219

He also said, "This is what the kingdom of God is like. A man scatters seed on the ground. Night and day, whether he sleeps or gets up, the seed sprouts and grows, though he does not know how. All by itself the soil produces grain – first the stalk, then the head, then the full kernel in the head. As soon as the grain is ripe, he puts the sickle to it, because the harvest has come." (Mark 4:26-29 NIV)

In His teachings, Jesus used numerous illustrations of a farmer planting seeds because that metaphor was perfect to describe the way that God's Word operates and the way that faith grows.

God's Word is the living, perfect seed of God's Divine truth. "Faith comes by hearing and hearing by the Word of God," we are told in Romans 10:17. Without the Word of God, there is no faith. We must hear it, receive it, and plant it in our hearts.

Is a planted seed the same thing as a mature plant? Of course not. The seed has the potential to be a mature plant, but it needs time and the proper environment in order to grow, strengthen, and develop. Likewise, the Word of God needs time and the proper environment in order to grow within us.

Too often healing never manifests itself for people because they fail to view the Word of God and their faith as a seed that must be nurtured. They pray for healing and then look the next day for an instant improvement in their symptoms. The truth is that they are basing their faith on the things they can witness with their five senses even though God's Word is very clear that faith is based on things that are *unseen*. What would happen if a farmer dug up his seed every morning to try to find out if his seed was growing? The answer is so obvious that it is ridiculous. Yet, when we do the same thing with our health, we think we are being sensible.

Stop judging your healing by analyzing the symptoms that you see. Take the actions for your healing that you are instructed by the Holy Spirit, and then stand on your faith that God is healing you according to His Word.

Blessed Creator, watch over Your Holy Word which I have planted in my heart. I join You in nurturing these seeds as they develop into a strong, unshakable harvest of faith. I receive Your Word and I fill my heart with Your love. I speak Your Word and declare that You are the God who heals me. I live Your Word and follow Your Son Jesus Christ. Thank You, God, for Your abundant blessings in my life. In Jesus' name, I pray, Amen.

Day 220

Heal me, O Lord, and I shall be healed; save me, and I shall be saved; for thou art my praise. (Jeremiah 17:14 KJV)

What does the word "heal" mean to you? We ask for healing, yet oddly enough, many people aren't sure what that means.

Let's consider two different scenarios, both assuming that you are living two thousand years ago at the time of Jesus. In the first one you have just fallen and broken your arm when someone comes running by and shouts that Jesus is coming down the street! You have heard stories that Jesus has healed people, so, despite your pain, you grab your arm and move as quickly as possible to find Him. When you get to Him, you ask Him to heal you. He looks at you, smiles, and touches your arm. It is instantaneously healed.

In the second scenario, you have also fallen and broken your arm. You do not know who Jesus is because He has never visited your village. However, there is a person who often helps people who are injured and ill. In great pain, you manage to pick yourself up and you find this man. He sets your arm, puts it in a splint, and binds it up. He gives you some wild lettuce, wood betony, and willow for pain relief, and he also gives you some oatstraw, dulse, and knitbone to help the bones heal. In a few weeks, your arm heals beautifully and you can use it just as well as you did before you broke it.

Is one healing greater than the other? One was due to the miraculous intervention of Jesus Christ. The other was due to the miracle God imbued in each living creature – an inborn ability to regenerate and to heal – combined with God's remedies and man's own treatment skills. The latter method is rarely viewed as a miracle, yet it is.

There are many paths to healing and many forms that healing takes. Do not make assumptions about the way that God wants your healing to occur. Pray. Invite Jesus Christ to be a part of your healing. Ask the Holy Spirit every step of the way for guidance and then follow it.

Wonderful Jehovah-rapha, You are the God who heals me. You breathed into my body the breath of life and with it the miracle of regeneration. You also sent Your Son to die on the Cross for my sins and for my infirmities. Thank You for creating so many ways for me to be healed. Help me to walk the path of recovery that You want for me. In Jesus' name, I pray, Amen.

Day 221

When they had crossed over, they landed at Gennesaret. And when the men of that place recognized Jesus, they sent word to all the surrounding country. People brought all their sick to him and begged him to let the sick just touch the edge of his cloak, and all who touched him were healed. (Matthew 14:34-36 NIV)

All who touched Him were healed. All who touched even just the edge of His garment were healed. Were they healed miraculously in a single moment? In many cases, yes. Too many people read the Scriptures, see the numerous times that Jesus healed instantaneously, and then let their own faith depend on whether they, too, receive a speedy healing.

For many of us healing comes as part of a longer process of recovery. It is no less a healing. And it is a miracle in its own way. It just isn't an instantaneous miracle. Of course, we'd all rather have the instant cure. Done! It would be so much easier that way.

Healing usually does not last unless we comprehend our part in it and make changes. Otherwise, as fast as God heals us, we create more illness in other areas. For example, we have our gallbladder removed, and then we actually take pride in resuming eating everything we ate before we got sick. We delude ourselves into thinking we are healed when we have made no change in what caused the problem in the first place.

Imagine having a clogged fuel filter in your car and deciding the solution was to remove the entire fuel pump rather than to clean out the filter and stop using contaminated gas. Many of our health "solutions" are just as foolish. We fail to see the long-term effect of our actions because the consequences may occur years or even decades later.

Don't tell God how He must heal you. Allow God to work His will in His own way. Be open to instruction. The Holy Spirit will show you every step you must take. You must be willing to take action. And you must be persistent in standing on God's Word and hold onto your faith no matter what the appearance is – until your healing is manifested.

Wonderful Jehovah-rapha, I know You are healing me according to Your Divine will and in the way that is right for me. Teach me patience and help me to stand firm in my faith as I stand on Your Word. I accept my responsibility for acting on Your guidance, and I will be diligent and faithful in following Your Word. In Jesus' name, I pray, Amen.

Day 222

Forgive us our sins, for we also forgive everyone who sins against us. (Luke 11:4 NIV)

Jesus included forgiveness in the prayer that He taught us because He knew how critical it is to our spiritual, emotional, and physical health for us to receive God's forgiving grace and to stop carrying around resentments toward others.

Resentment requires a lot of energy – both spiritual and physical – to keep it alive. When you feel sick, you need all your energy for healing, for rebuilding, and for positive activity. So you simply can't afford to carry resentment.

How do you get rid of it? How do you forgive? Begin by taking some time to write down the name of every person who has hurt you. Bring the hurt into your mind and see whether you still feel some emotion with it – whether anger, resentment, or sorrow. If you feel no emotion at all, be honest with yourself to determine if the reason is due to the fact that you have accomplished forgiveness or if the reason is due to the fact that you have buried your feelings so deeply that you don't feel them. Allow several days to make your list. Make sure that you have included every resentment you are aware of on it.

Now you must ask yourself if you are ready to let these resentments go. If so, say each name on the list and then tell that person that you forgive him and that you are giving your resentment toward him to God. Forgive yourself for carrying the resentment all this time. Turn it all over to God. Pray the Lord's prayer. Ask God to forgive you and ask for His help in letting go of the resentments you are carrying inside.

It often helps to tear up your list or to burn it as a symbol of your letting go. If you become aware of feelings of resentment sneaking back in, just keep turning them over to God. Continue to ask God for help until you are cleansed and free from your old burdens.

Almighty God, I am tired of carrying resentments inside. I am tired of feeling sick. I am tired of being frustrated. I am tired of watching other people live active lives when I feel limited. I give my resentments to You, God – every one of them. I lay them down at your feet. I am willing to let go of the past. I want to live cleansed, free, and healed. I am truly repentant of my transgressions. Forgive me of my sins, Father, as I forgive everyone who has sinned against me. In Your loving name, I pray, Amen.

Day 223

"I have seen his ways, but I will heal him; I will guide him and restore comfort to him, creating praise on the lips of the mourners in Israel. Peace, peace, to those far and near," says the Lord. "And I will heal them." (Isaiah 57:18-19 NIV)

"Peace, peace," God tells us. Those of us who feel sick often have trouble finding peace. We are filled with aches of the heart and aches of the body and are restless by day and sleepless by night.

"Peace," God says. "Peace. I will heal." Do you live in the security of God's peace? Or are you sidetracked by your aches and pains and worries? If you are, you are like most of us. But God tells us there is another way.

A major source of our problem is the words we speak. Just as God's words are powerful, so are our own. Look at what God says He is going to do: He is going to "create praise on the lips of the mourners in Israel." God is going to change his people's language from negative words of mourning to positive ones of praise.

How do we destroy our peace with words? One way is by using words of harsh judgment, such as "That person is really stupid." Another is by hurling emotional words of pain and anger, such as, "I hate you!" or "I wish you were dead."

Sometimes we plant seeds for our own health problems when we accuse someone, "You are a real pain in the neck." Other times we create our own health situation by complaining, using the powerful words "I am." We say, "I am so sick" or "I am never going to be able to see." We even set up problems when we think we are joking or are trying to be dramatic. For example, we say, "That comedian just kills me." And "I'd die for a soft drink."

Allow God to cleanse your heart and to bring praise to your lips. Sing glorious thanks to Him for His mighty works in your life. He is the God who heals you and who brings you peace.

Almighty God, just for today I am going to pay special attention to all the words that I speak. Help me to watch the words of my mouth and create on my lips words of praise for You and for all Your blessings on me. You are awesome and wonderful, and I sing Your praise. Nothing is too hard for You and I give You my total trust. Guide me, restore comfort to me, heal me. Bring me Your wonderful peace, Lord. In the name of Your Son, Jesus Christ, I pray, Amen.

Day 224

Simon, Simon, Satan has asked to sift you as wheat. But I have prayed for you, Simon, that your faith may not fail. And when you have turned back, strengthen your brothers. (Luke 22:31-32 NIV)

We find Jesus with His disciples in the Upper Room just after He has celebrated what we now call the Lord's Supper with them. He has told them that one of them will betray Him. At that point the disciples get into an argument over who the traitor is. That discussion leads to another issue – who among them is the greatest. Jesus speaks up and tells them that "the greatest among you should be like the youngest, and the one who rules like the one who serves."

Jesus then calls Simon Peter by name and tells him that satan wants to pulverize him, "to sift you as wheat." Jesus knows that satan's method is to prowl the earth, looking to devour God's people – so Peter was a prime target.

Jesus said, "But I have prayed for you, Simon, that your faith may not fail. And when you have turned back, strengthen your brothers." Peter protests that he will never fail Jesus, but Jesus tells him he will betray him three times in the coming hours.

Take a moment to make these words of Jesus live for you. Hear Jesus saying to you, "I have prayed for you that your faith may not fail." Say it out loud and use your own name. Feel Jesus standing beside you, supporting you. Isn't it both awesome and humbling to think of Jesus praying for you? In those moments when you feel your faith slipping and when you begin to wonder if you will ever feel well, tell the evil one to leave you and to take his lies with him.

Call upon Jesus and see Jesus praying that your faith will not fail. Know that He bore your sins and your illnesses on the Cross for you. There is nothing you and Jesus cannot face together. There is nothing you and Jesus cannot overcome because He has already done it in sacrifice for you.

Gracious Lord, You loved me so much that You sent Your Son into the world to die for my sins and my infirmities. I am awed to know that Christ Jesus is praying for me so that my faith will not fail. In His name, I resist the evil one and I command him to leave my body and my entire being. I stand on Your Holy Word and enforce it on every cell in my body. I seek to fulfill Your will, Lord, and Your purpose for my life. In Jesus' name, I pray, Amen.

Day 225

Whoever obeys his command will come to no harm, and the wise heart will know the proper time and procedure. For there is a proper time and procedure for every matter, though a man's misery weighs heavily upon him. (Ecclesiastes 8:5-6 NIV)

Isn't this a wonderful Scripture? And how comforting it is. We can certainly relate to being weighed down by our misery. Yet if we follow God's guidance in every step of the way for our healing, we will come to no harm. The wise heart will know the proper time and procedure because the Holy Spirit will tell us exactly what that timing is and what those procedures are. All we have to do is to ask.

We are blessed in having many procedures available to help us in our recovery. It helps to have some idea of what choices exist that might be useful in our healing. The one which most people use is conventional medical treatment. In addition, there are many others: herbs, essential oils and aromatherapy, chelation therapy, hydrotherapy, acupuncture, massage, homeopathy, vitamins and supplements, flower essences, chiropractic, orthobionomy, magnetic therapy, naturopathy, photoluminescence, music and sound therapy, and body work therapies.

Explore these and other options, gathering knowledge about what they are and how they work. As you investigate options for particular diseases, you will discover the variety of methods that have been successful. For example, for cancer there is the antineoplaston therapy of Dr. Stanislaw Burzynski, Issel's whole-body therapy, essiac tea, Gerson therapy, oxygen therapy, hyperthermia, and bioelectric therapy.

You will find that there are many approaches which have been used for whatever health problem you are facing. Some of them have official government sanction and some do not. Let the Holy Spirit be your final authority rather than some person or governmental body. Be vigilant to guard your right to follow God's guidance without governmental intervention.

Go into prayer with the information you have learned. Make no assumptions about the form that your healing "should" take. Ask the Holy Spirit to reveal your path to you. Know that whoever obeys the command of the Lord will come to no harm.

Merciful God, my misery weighs heavily on me, but I strive to obey Your commands always. Give me wisdom through the Holy Spirit and show me the proper time and procedure for each step on my path to my recovery. In the name of Your Son, Jesus Christ, I pray, Amen.

Day 226

Cleanse me with hyssop, and I will be clean; wash me, and I will be whiter than snow.
(Psalm 51:7 NIV)

If the person has been healed of his infectious skin disease, the priest shall order that two live clean birds and some cedar wood, scarlet yarn and hyssop be brought for the one to be cleansed. (Leviticus 14:3-4 NIV)

Just as spiritual cleansing is necessary to wash our souls clean from our sins, so is internal cleansing necessary to wash our bodies clean from toxins.

When you feel sick, you must examine your body systems to see if it is appropriate to begin a program for cleansing. Particular attention needs to be given to the colon and the liver. Depending on your individual situation, you may need to build rather than to cleanse initially. There are many herbs which have been used historically for their effectiveness and there are numerous preparations available. Ask the Holy Spirit what you need to do at this time and follow the guidance that you are given.

These particular verses from the Holy Scripture mention hyssop as an herb that was used in Biblical times for internal cleansing. Other herbs are used more widely now for general cleansing purposes. Hyssop lubricates internal tissue fluids and removes debris from the surface of all body parts, such as the lungs, stomach, and blood vessels. This action results in great improvement of absorption and elimination.

As an expectorant, hyssop has been used for generations for removing lung congestion and for coughs, colds, and asthma. It has been used historically to improve sluggish circulation. It has been helpful for digestion, especially to expel gas, and for the promotion of sweating to reduce fevers. It may be useful for diseases affecting the skin, such as smallpox and chicken pox. Hyssop may be used externally as a poultice to help heal cuts and to relieve muscular rheumatism and bruises.

Jehovah-rapha provides us generously with herbs, essential oils, and plants that are to be used for maintaining and recovering our health. Learn about them and then ask the Holy Spirit to guide you as you seek your own recovery.

Mighty Creator, thank You for the abundance of herbs and essential oils which You have provided me. Guide me to teachers who can expand my knowledge of Your healing plants. Show me the path You want me to follow for my healing. In Jesus' name, I pray, Amen.

Day 227

Know ye that the Lord he is God; it is he that hath made us and not we ourselves. (Psalm 100:3 KJV)

There is only one Creator of all life and that is Jehovah. God gives us minds to use; however, God intends that our creative efforts be within the context of a partnership with Him. Our creations are to be the result of revelation knowledge and guidance of God. They are not to be solely for material gain and power, but they are to make the world better, safer, and healthier.

The very definition of science now excludes any belief in or relevance of Jehovah. That leaves it wide open to the influence of satan, and, when we create under the influence of the evil one, we sow the seeds of our own destruction. It is a godless science that leads us to poison our foods with chemicals – and convinces us that there are no health consequences. It is a godless science that genetically alters fruits and vegetables into synthetic food that can sit on the shelf for weeks without rotting – and convinces us that there are no health consequences.

It is a godless science that manipulates plants so that they cannot produce seeds of their own that will germinate – and convinces us that there are no health consequences for our children. It is a godless science that clones animals – and convinces us that there are no health and spiritual consequences.

We need science, but we need a God-guided science. If you agree, do what you can to speak out and express your concerns. On the personal level take full responsibility for your health. Seek out organic food that is grown as God intended the plant to be. You cannot heal without having nourishing food. Learn how your body works. It is much easier to heal when you understand how each organ and cell is intended to function and how it interrelates with all the other organs and cells in your body.

Ask God to lead you to counselors and advisors (both medical and otherwise) who will pray with you and will be willing to consider both God-provided and man-made solutions to your health problems.

Creator God, I declare that You and only You are the Great Creator. It is You who have made me and You alone. Help me always to seek Your advice as I choose my food and as I make decisions on treatments offered by science. I know that You want me to be well and that You will direct my path so that I can make the choices that are best for my recovery. In Jesus' name, I pray, Amen.

Day 228

Isaiah answered, "This is the Lord's sign to you that the Lord will do what he has promised: Shall the shadow go forward ten steps, or shall it go back ten steps?" "It is a simple matter for the shadow to go forward ten steps," said Hezekiah. "Rather, have it go back ten steps." Then the prophet Isaiah called upon the Lord, and the Lord made the shadow go back the ten steps it had gone down on the stairway of Ahaz. (2 Kings 20:9-11 NIV)

Hezekiah, king of Judah, is deathly ill and, even though he has been told that God will heal him in three days, he asks for a sign that he really will be well again. There may be a time when you, like Hezekiah, want a sign from God that you have understood His guidance accurately. Go to the Lord in prayer and meditation to determine the sign to be given to you. Hezekiah was given the choice of a miraculous sign of having a shadow move in the direction opposite to its normal path. Yours will probably be something much less spectacular, but still out of the ordinary. Let the Holy Spirit guide you.

Be clear what your question to God is before you ask for the sign. Notice that Hezekiah's question was simple: "Am I going to be healed?" Questions that can be answered by yes or no are best. For example, ask "Should I have my gall bladder removed?" rather than "Should I have my gall bladder removed or should I try natural cleansing methods to heal it?" Also be clear what the meaning of the sign is. After prayer and meditation you may determine that a red maple leaf in your birdbath within three days means yes. Be sure you are very specific, because, if you are not, you will only be confused in the end.

Signs are not tests for God and they should not be requested often. Jesus was frustrated when people kept wanting signs, signs, and more signs. True faith does not need signs. But God is kind and merciful. He knows our weaknesses. And, like a benevolent Father, He continually supports us and allows us to ask from time to time for concrete evidence of His will.

Dear Lord, I struggle with my doubts. I know You are the God who heals me. I know Your Son Jesus Christ bore my sins and infirmities on the Cross. God, I come now because I want a sign. Like Hezekiah, I need something to hold onto while I wait for You to fulfill Your promise. I believe; help my unbelief. Help me to formulate my question clearly and to understand the meaning of the sign. Strengthen my faith, Lord. Work Your healing wonder in me. Help me to trust and remain faithful to Your Word. In Jesus' name, I pray, Amen.

Day 229

And when he was at the place, he said unto them, "Pray that ye enter not into temptation." And he was withdrawn from them about a stone's cast, and kneeled down, and prayed. Saying, "Father, if thou be willing, remove this cup from me: nevertheless not my will, but thine, be done." And there appeared an angel unto him from heaven, strengthening him. And being in an agony he prayed more earnestly: and his sweat was as it were great drops of blood falling down to the ground. And when he rose up from prayer, and was come to his disciples, he found them sleeping for sorrow. And said unto them, Why sleep ye? Rise and pray, lest ye enter into temptation. (Luke 22:40-46 KJV)

God may choose to heal us with an instantaneous, miraculous recovery; however, more often healing comes as part of a slower process. Much faith, perseverance, and courage are required as we walk that path.

Sometimes we know the options ahead may be painful; some may be risky. Sometimes we have been told we "have" to have a certain medical procedure done or we will die. We know that we have to go to God in prayer to find out if that is God's truth for us. In these times of decision, we understand fully the agony Jesus felt in the Garden of Gethsemane. What do we do? Pray fervently. Any decision is wrong if it is made outside of God's will. Any decision is wrong if it is made without consulting the Lord God Almighty and asking for strength to carry out His plan.

When we have major decisions, satan will do everything he can to interfere with our being connected to God. He will do everything he can to send us the wrong answer so that we make the wrong decision. Be very sure that your fear does not determine your answer. When that happens, satan is always in charge.

We may be told by God and the Holy Spirit to use certain treatments that will cause suffering. For example, it hurts to have a broken bone set. Whatever the pain before us, however, we can handle it with courage if we are sure it is part of God's will for us to endure it. God will send His mighty angels to support us and to strengthen us. Trust in Jehovah-rapha to heal you according to His plan.

Merciful God, help me in my struggles to know Your will as I make my health decisions. Protect me from the subversive whispers of satan. Help me to hear You clearly and to act according to Your guidance. In Jesus' name, I pray, Amen.

Day 230

Dear friend, I pray that you may enjoy good health and that all may go well with you, even as your soul is getting along well. It gave me great joy to have some brothers come and tell about your faithfulness to the truth and how you continue to walk in the truth. I have no greater joy than to hear that my children are walking in the truth. (3 John 2-4 NIV)

In this letter of the Apostle John to Gaius, the leader of one of the early Christian churches, John offers encouragement and support. Around A.D. 85 opposition to the Christians was increasing and certain people who had joined the church were causing trouble. John is eager to remind his friends of Christ's teachings and of their mission to spread the gospel.

Beginning his letter with a prayer for Gaius' good health, John knows that physical vitality is important in doing the work of the Lord. Certainly people can be wonderful witnesses no matter what the state of their health, but obviously a healthy person has more energy and mobility than someone who is ill.

If being sick were to be a model for our service to God, then surely Jesus would have left unhealed some of those who came to Him. Or Jesus Himself might even have suffered some ailment. He shared every other obstacle and difficulty that we face as human beings. Isn't it interesting that illness was the only one that He did not share with us? Perhaps that was due to the fact that He came "that it might be fulfilled which was spoken by Esaias the prophet saying, 'Himself took our infirmities and bare our sicknesses'" (Matthew 8:16-17).

Even as you seek your own healing, give support and encouragement to someone who is struggling with a challenge in his life. It may be a physical illness or it may be some other difficulty. Remind him of God's everlasting love and care. Cheer him on to seek first God's truth and then to walk in it. Pray for him as Jesus prayed for those who believed in Him. Live your own life as an example of what it is to walk minute by minute in God's truth, having the courage to follow God's guidance and to depend on Him totally and completely.

Wonderful Jehovah-rapha, I pray that I may enjoy good health and I pray for the good health of my friends and family. Help me to stay faithful, God, to Your purpose and plan for my life. Keep me faithful to Your truth and help me to walk always in that truth. Show me the path You want me to follow and I will be obedient, Lord. In the name of Your Son, Jesus Christ, I pray, Amen.

Day 231

Take wheat and barley, beans and lentils, millet and spelt; put them in a storage jar and use them to make bread for yourself. You are to eat it during the 390 days you lie on your side. (Ezekiel 4:9 NIV)

Which of you, if his son asks for bread, will give him a stone? Or if he asks for a fish, will give him a snake? If you, then though you are evil, know how to give good gifts to your children, how much more will your Father in heaven give good gifts to those who ask him! (Matthew 7:9-11 NIV)

Then he took the seven loaves and the fish, and when he had given thanks, he broke them and gave them to the disciples, and they in turn to the people. They all ate and were satisfied. (Matthew 15:36-37 NIV)

Grains are one of God's special gifts. They can be cultivated all over the world under a wide variety of growing conditions and they can be stored easily. Their diversity is immense – ranging from wheat to corn to rice to rye to millet and to sesame.

Jesus defined Himself as "the bread of life" (John 6:35) and, when He taught us to pray, He told us to say, "Give us this day our daily bread" (Matthew 6:11). Thus, bread has long been a staple, integral part of a healthy diet.

The bread of the Bible was very different from the bread we have today. The white bread which most people eat has had most of its nutrients stripped from it during refining and processing, with only a few substances artificially replaced. "Real" bread is dense, heavy bread made from whole grains. It is not loaded with preservatives and, therefore, spoils quickly if it is not refrigerated – hence, the phrase "give us this day our *daily* bread." Bread made according the recipe found in Ezekiel is now available commercially and provides a healthy option for bread in our diet.

Eating excessive amounts of grains can make the body too acidic. Ask God what types of grains (and quantities) are healthy for you at the present time. You might also ask if Ezekiel's bread is right for you. Listen carefully and follow the guidance you are given.

Wonderful Jehovah-rapha, thank You for grain and for giving me Your guidance about the healthiest way for me to include bread in my diet. Thank You, God, for showing me the path to my healing. In Jesus' name, I pray, Amen.

Day 232

Do not be wise in your own eyes; fear the Lord and shun evil. This will bring health to your body and nourishment to your bones. (Proverbs 3:7-8 NIV)

One of the worst traps we can fall into when we have a health problem is to make assumptions about what we should do. We compartmentalize our faith and bring it into play in our lives too late. "Things" need to be done so we just forge ahead and do them.

We think that certain actions are obvious, logical, and "right" so we never think to take them to God in prayer and to ask His opinion. When we don't give the power to God, we surely open the door to satan. We are wise in our own eyes and our arrogance often costs us dearly. Sometimes it costs us our lives. And even then, we blame God and moan that it was His will.

Most health problems are a result of numerous poor choices you have made over a long period of time. When you finally have to confront the fact that you have a problem, it is time for a complete re-evaluation of the place you have given God in your life.

For example, consider the matter of prescription drugs. Do you assume all prescriptions are right for you and take them unquestioningly? Understand each one thoroughly – the exact beneficial action it is supposed to have in your body and *all* the undesirable effects (called "side effects") from the package insert provided by the manufacturer.

Having gathered your information, place the decision for this medication squarely in the hands of the Almighty. He created your body and understands it and its needs better than any human being ever will, including you. He wants you to be well and will instruct you for your highest good. Ask your doctor to pray with you and to join in partnership with you and Jehovah-rapha in seeking the best solution for your health problems.

Only God is God. Unless we go to Him first we will never know what His path for our healing is supposed to be.

Almighty God, Help me to worship only You and not to exalt myself or any human before You. Help me to increase my knowledge without becoming arrogant, "wise in my own eyes," and vulnerable to the evil one. Bring health to my body and nourishment to my bones. With humility and thanks, in Jesus' name, I pray, Amen.

Day 233

The Lord God formed the man from the dust of the ground and breathed into his nostrils the breath of life, and the man became a living being. (Genesis 2:7 NIV)

Every time we breathe we affirm the moment of our creation. Of all bodily activities the breath is one of the most essential. Few people can sustain life without breathing for more than three minutes or so. Ironically, most of us develop poor breathing habits that contribute to the improper functioning of our bodies.

Watch an infant while it is sleeping. Notice that the entire abdominal area rises with each inhalation and falls with each exhalation. Babies breathe naturally from their diaphragm, pulling the air deeply into the lungs. As children grow up, they encounter stressful events and gradually tighten various muscle groups. By adulthood, most of us breathe shallowly from the upper parts of our lungs.

Stop for a moment and take a deep breath. Did you raise your shoulders in the process? When your abdominal muscles and diaphragm are relaxed and your breathing habits are healthy, your abdomen will extend as you inhale and your shoulders have no need to move. When your abdominal muscles are tight, your abdomen will remain rigid and your upper chest will be pushed outward as the upper lungs fill with air. You are forced to raise your shoulders.

Every cell of your body desperately needs oxygen. Life cannot exist without it. There is evidence that there was a much higher concentration of oxygen in the air at the time of the creation of Adam and Eve, and the effects of our industrial and chemical pollution is to increase rapidly the depletion of this vital nutrient. Take responsibility in your own life to reduce the chemicals that you use that have a negative impact on your air, your environment, and your body.

Learn to breathe properly. One of the easiest ways to do this is to incorporate proper breathing into your prayer time. Re-live this passage from Genesis every time you pray. Allow yourself to relax in the Lord and to breathe deeply from your abdomen and your diaphragm as you pray. Thus your prayer will be not only a prayer of words, but also a prayer of gratitude for the gift of life with which you have been blessed.

Gracious Lord, thank You for the breath of life. Help me to re-learn the proper breathing techniques I had when I was an infant so that all my cells may receive life-giving oxygen. Fill me every moment with Your Holy, healing breath. In Jesus' name, I pray, Amen.

Day 234

You know what has happened throughout Judea, beginning in Galilee after the baptism that John preached – how God anointed Jesus of Nazareth with the Holy Spirit and power, and how he went around doing good and healing all who were under the power of the devil, because God was with him. (Acts 10:37-38 NIV)

In just one sentence Peter makes an astonishing number of important points that are keys to your healing. He begins by saying that God anointed Jesus. With what? The Holy Spirit and power.

Here again is the Greek word *"dynamis"* meaning power, ability, and miracle. Because of Jesus' sacrifice for you, that anointing is available to you. If you ask, you, too, will be filled with the Holy Spirit and power. This anointing was not just for Jesus. It wasn't just for the early Christians. It was for all those who take up the Cross and follow Him.

Jesus went around among the people. Doing what? Doing good and healing. There is the dual mission again. Doing good and healing. Healing whom? Healing *all*. There is that little word "all" again. See how this message is given over and over and over again?

And what conditions was Jesus healing? He was healing problems resulting from people being under the power of the devil. Once more we are told who the father of disease is. Here Peter makes it clear that the source of illness is the evil one and that Jesus removed the devil's power.

Jesus overcame all sickness, and, when He took your illnesses to the Cross, He banished the devil's power forever. Resist the devil. You are clear that you don't want him to have your soul, aren't you? Be just as clear that he is not to have your body either.

How did Jesus do all this? Because God was with Him. And God is with you if you allow Him full sovereignty in your life.

Heavenly Father, let me be all that You want me to be. I have said yes to the call of Your Son Jesus Christ. Let me now accept the power of the Holy Spirit in my life – transforming my soul and my body for Your glory. I seek to do good, following the example of Your Son. Help me to be an instrument for the healing of others. Help me to share with them my journey of understanding Your Holy, healing power. Help me to resist satan always and to stand up firmly for You and Your Son Jesus Christ. Thank you, God, for Your many mercies and Your healing grace that is made manifest in my body. In Jesus' name, I pray, Amen.

Day 235

The Spirit of the Sovereign Lord is on me, because the Lord has anointed me to preach good news to the poor. He has sent me to bind up the brokenhearted, to proclaim freedom for the captives and release from darkness for the prisoners. (Isaiah 61:1 NIV)

Here is the prophecy in Isaiah of the coming Messiah, the Christ who is anointed by God to preach the good news to us all. Because we are all needy spiritually, He is sent to set us free from everything that binds and imprisons us. He brings us liberty of spirit, mind, emotions, and body.

Take a look at another passage, this one from Jeremiah, in which God connects health and healing to liberty for His people. Let the promise of these words sink into your heart.

Nevertheless, I will bring health and healing to it; I will heal my people and will let them enjoy abundant peace and security. I will bring Judah and Israel back from captivity and will rebuild them as they were before. I will cleanse them from all the sin they have committed against me and will forgive all their sins of rebellion against me. Then this city will bring me renown, joy, praise and honor before all nations on earth that hear of all the good things I do for it; and they will be in awe and will tremble at the abundant prosperity and peace I provide for it. (Jeremiah 33:6-9 NIV)

Think of all the ways you feel trapped today. You may feel stuck in emotions of grief for a loved one, betrayal of a friend, or anger toward an adversary. You may feel bound by illness and disease. You may feel boxed in a job you do not like. You may feel caught in a marriage with an unfaithful spouse.

Jesus has the key to set you free from every difficult situation. Open your heart to Him. Be willing to listen. Be willing to act on the guidance you receive. Believe, trust, and act.

Almighty God, thank You for the gift of Your Son Jesus Christ, whom You sent to set me at liberty. Bind up my wounds, bestow your peace and security upon me, and rebuild me, Lord. Thank You, O merciful God. In Jesus' name, I pray, Amen.

Day 236

In all my prayers for all of you, I always pray with joy because of your partnership in the gospel from the first day until now, being confident of this, that he who began a good work in you will carry it on to completion until the day of Christ Jesus. (Philippians 1:4-6 NIV)

Look at all the positive statements in this one sentence. What a lovely phrase: "pray with joy." No matter what situation we find ourselves in we need to pray with joy. Why? Because there is no situation that is beyond the power of God. Not one.

"Partnership in the gospel." How important it is that we stand on God's Word. God created us to walk in the Garden in partnership with Him. When we chose to know evil, we broke that relationship. But God sent Jesus as His Word to redeem us and bring us back to share fully in His kingdom again. Enter into the partnership of the gospel. Accept that God wants you to be saved – meaning to be delivered, rescued, and *healed*.

"Being confident of this, that He who began a good work in you will carry it on to completion." Remember this and believe it when the road to your healing seems longer than you want it to be. Healing that comes instantaneously is wondrous. But healing that is part of a longer process simply requires more persistent faith and more obedient action on our part.

What we have to remember is that God will be faithful to complete what He starts. If we ask for healing and believe God wants us to be well, we must turn the process over to Him. His way is now our way. We must turn to Him in prayer day by day, hour by hour, and sometimes minute by minute.

Our Heavenly Father is our primary consultant, our only Great Physician. Every recommendation we receive from humans must be taken to Him for the final consultation. He will tell us exactly what to do, in minute detail, if we ask Him. We must believe that He cares about each step in the process and that He knows the right choice for us and for our healing.

Dear God, I am Your creation. I trust that You will be faithful to complete Your work in me. I know that You are healing me now and that You will be faithful to complete it. I hand my doubts to You, God. I enter into joyful partnership with You and I stand on Your Holy Word. In the name of Your Son, Jesus Christ, my Redeemer, I pray, Amen.

Day 237

And when you stand praying, if you hold anything against anyone, forgive him, so that your Father in heaven may forgive you your sins. (Mark 11:25 NIV)

Forgiveness means to cease to feel resentment toward someone. No matter how horrible the offense against us, our decision to carry resentment hurts only us. It does not punish the offender or exact any revenge on them. All it does is to eat away at *us*.

Resentment is a powerful negative emotion that colors everything we do. It triggers responses in us when situations come up that don't even involve the offender. It creates a great deal of stress not only on our emotions but also on our bodies. Often illness – and even injuries from accidents – result from the resentment we nurture inside. Our refusal to forgive – to let go of our resentment – carries a heavy price indeed.

How do you get rid of resentment? What if someone has committed a horrendous act against you? What then? Are you supposed to pretend that it never happened? Of course not. Release comes when you get tired of carrying your wounds around, when you get tired of letting someone who hurt you run your life, and when you get tired of living in the past.

There are no magic answers to letting go, and for many people counseling is a useful tool. You must examine exactly what happened and place responsibility where it belongs. For what events were you responsible and for what events was the other person responsible? Then you must be willing to feel fully all the emotions you have. Not just anger, but grief, fear, perhaps terror. Name it, claim it, and be willing to move on.

Those who forgive find that they experience a wonderful release. They have been imprisoned by the past and now walk freely in the present. Healing happens not only in their soul, their emotions, and their mind but also in their body.

Dear Father, You know I have been holding resentment in my heart. I was hurt badly and I just haven't been able to let it go. I'm ready now, God, to release this resentment because I know it is hurting only me. I choose to face all my emotions honestly and boldly. I choose to name my hurts and to see any part I played in the events that wounded me. I claim my own responsibility for keeping the bitterness alive all this time. I lay my resentment down, Lord. I forgive this person who hurt me. And I ask Your forgiveness for my own transgressions. Thank You, God. In the name of Your Son, Jesus Christ, I pray, Amen.

Day 238

Some time later the son of the woman who owned the house became ill. He grew worse and worse, and finally stopped breathing. She said to Elijah, "What do you have against me, man of God? Did you come to remind me of my sin and kill my son?" "Give me your son," Elijah replied. He took him from her arms, carried him to the upper room where he was staying, and laid him on his bed. Then he cried out to the Lord, "O Lord my God, have you brought tragedy also upon this widow I am staying with, by causing her son to die?" Then he stretched himself out on the boy three times and cried to the Lord, "O Lord my God, let this boy's life return to him!" The Lord heard Elijah's cry, and the boy's life returned to him, and he lived. Elijah picked up the child and carried him down from the room into the house. He gave him to his mother and said, "Look, your son is alive!" Then the woman said to Elijah, "Now I know that you are a man of God and that the word of the Lord from your mouth is the truth." (1 Kings 17:17-24 KJV)

What is interesting about this story is to see whom the woman and Elijah blame for the child's illness and death. The woman blames Elijah. "Did you come to remind me of my sin and kill my son?" She acknowledges that she has sinned but she does not take responsibility for it. Instead, she points the finger at Elijah.

Elijah cries out to God and blames Him. "O Lord my God, have you brought tragedy also upon this widow I am staying with, by causing her son to die?" Isn't it interesting that we have gone from the woman's sin to "It's God's fault" in two quick steps? Despite these accusations, what does God do? He heals the child.

We do the same thing that these two people have done. God established a system in nature where we reap what is sown. Yet often when that happens, we want to blame God instead of taking responsibility for the human factors that have led to the disease.

Satan slips in to find our places of vulnerability and he capitalizes on them, further encouraging us to sow unhealthy habits that have disastrous effects so long afterward that we don't even see the connection. Put the blame for illness where it belongs – on the evil one – and thank God for loving you and healing you.

Wonderful Jehovah-rapha, I, too, am guilty of pointing the finger of blame at You when it is the evil one and often my own actions that have led to my illness. No force of evil is more powerful than Your loving goodness and I enforce Your healing Word on my infirmity. In Jesus' name, I pray, Amen.

Day 239

For this reason, since the day we heard about you, we have not stopped praying for you and asking God to fill you with the knowledge of his will through all spiritual wisdom and understanding. And we pray this in order that you may live a life worthy of the Lord and may please him in every way: bearing fruit in every good work, growing in the knowledge of God, being strengthened with all power according to his glorious might so that you may have great endurance and patience, and joyfully giving thanks to the Father, who has qualified you to share in the inheritance of the saints in the kingdom of light. For he has rescued us from the dominion of darkness and brought us into the kingdom of the Son he loves, in whom we have redemption, the forgiveness of sins. (Colossians 1:9-14 NIV)

Paul packs a lot into these few sentences to the people in Colosse. Pay particular attention to the phrase "being strengthened with all power according to his glorious might so that you may have great endurance and patience." When you feel sick, endurance and patience are vital since most healings come as part of a process. And this process almost always takes longer than you want it to take.

To make it through you must have endurance and patience. You have to be able to hold firm to your faith even when you do not have the evidence of your healing at the physical level. Your symptoms are still present and some days they seem to taunt you. The temptation is to focus on these symptoms and to view them as your total reality. Yes, they exist, but they exist as a product of the father of lies.

Look to a reality beyond them. Look to the reality of the power of the healing of Jehovah-rapha who declares, "I am the God who heals you." Look to the reality of the power of the healing of Christ Jesus who bore your infirmities on the Cross.

Almighty God, fill me with the knowledge of Your will through all spiritual wisdom and understanding. God, I want to please You and to serve You well. I want to bear fruit in my work, to fulfill my purpose in this life. Strengthen me with all power according to Your glorious might so that I may have great endurance and patience. I joyfully give thanks to You, O Lord. Thank You for rescuing me from the dominions of darkness and sickness and for bringing me into the kingdom of Your Son Christ Jesus who has borne my sins and infirmities on the Cross. In the name of Your Son, Jesus Christ, my Savior and my Redeemer, I pray, Amen.

Day 240

Commit to the Lord whatever you do, and your plans will succeed. (Proverbs 16:3 NIV)

Commit your life's work to God and enjoy it. Find your passion. Some people seem to be born knowing the work that they want to do. At an early age they begin walking a path that they feel guided toward. Others of us flounder around, going from one thing to another, often plodding along in jobs we do not like. For one reason or another we allow ourselves to get trapped into occupations that do not stimulate or revitalize us.

Generally, if you feel excited, energized by your work, and motivated by a sense of purpose, you are in the right place. Whatever your current situation is, stop right this moment and check in with God about His mission for you. Ask Him if you are doing what He would have you to do. Then listen for the answer. If the answer doesn't come today, keep asking until you receive your reply.

How does having meaningful work relate to your health? Those who are unhappy in their work often fall prey to illness. If you are not engaged in a career that is part of God's plan for you, you will probably be subjected to many internal stresses. You may feel frustrated or overwhelmed, bored or fatigued, restless or unfulfilled. These negative emotions take a toll on your physical health. Illness often provides a way out – or at least a break from the job that is literally killing you.

No matter what your past, you always have the present moment. Don't play victim to your job. Take responsibility for your part in following God's plan for your life. If you are unhappy, ask God for direction and guidance. Find out if you are in the right field or whether you are best suited for entirely different work. Hand your fears and objections over to God. Don't let thoughts of "I'm too old to go back to school" or "How will I support myself?" stop you from getting on God's path for you. When your spiritual self is in alignment with God, then your mind, body, and emotions follow.

Dear God, today I will take some time to check in with You about my life's work. Am I doing today what You want me to do? Is this the way I can serve You best? I want to live with zest and enthusiasm, acting as a powerful witness to Your glory. I await quietly Your instruction. In the blessed name of Your Son Jesus Christ, my Savior and my Redeemer, I pray, Amen.

Day 241

And we rejoice in the hope of the glory of God. Not only so, but we also rejoice in our sufferings, because we know that suffering produces perseverance; perseverance, character; and character, hope. (Romans 5:2-4 NIV)

These verses are often used as a justification of God-authored illness and of the need to endure our physical ailments. For those who believe that God wants His children to be well, how can we be reconciled to this Scripture? The Greek word in these verses that is translated "sufferings" is *"thlipsis." "Thlipsis"* generally means trouble, distress, oppression, and tribulation – none of which refers automatically to suffering from illness.

Jesus told His followers plainly that they would be subject to trials and tribulations. In Matthew 24:9 He says, "Then you will be handed over to be persecuted and put to death, and you will be hated by all nations because of me." In His own life He encountered many difficulties and He had to overcome many attempts of oppression. He was constantly harassed by those in authority, and they repeatedly sought to plot against Him until they finally were successful in carrying out His arrest, beating, and crucifixion.

Jesus is our perfect example of how to handle life. Jesus knew what it was to suffer and to experience agony. But it is interesting that none of His sufferings involved personal sickness and disease until He bore them on the Cross. Yes, He was the Son of God and therefore not solely human. But He came in a body for a reason. He came in a body precisely to show us how to live in it and how to treat it as a precious temple of the Holy Spirit.

Jesus knew what it was like to be weak from hunger and thirst. He knew what it was like to be so tired that He had to get away from everyone and lie down. If He had not lived in the body, we could not relate to Him so personally and so intensely. God sent Jesus to show us the way. "I *am* the way," He told us. And He was then and still is now.

Almighty God, in handling the tribulations of this life I will follow the example of Jesus and seek You and Your will. I know that You are the God who heals me. I hold to Your Word as the expression of Your will. Your Son Jesus Christ told me that my faith would make me whole. I hold to that, Father. I know that You can help me overcome any suffering that I may experience. I rejoice in knowing that You can overcome anything and that, if I am steadfast in my faith, I will come through it victoriously. In Jesus' name, I pray, Amen.

Day 242

"For my thoughts are not your thoughts, neither are your ways my ways," declares the Lord. "As the heavens are higher than the earth, so are my ways higher than your ways and my thoughts than your thoughts." (Isaiah 55:8-9 NIV)

God's thoughts are higher than ours because God can see the big picture and we cannot. All we see is our own world. All we know is what we have learned. God created everything and everyone so He knows all. That is the reason that His ways are better than our ways, which are based on limited information.

When you feel sick, you must be ever mindful of the limitations of your knowledge and the limitations of those you ask for advice. Doctors can be wonderful assistants in your search for recovery. However, sometimes they may feel that they are certain of your prognosis or of the necessity for a certain treatment.

It is very important to find a Christ-filled doctor who is willing to pray with you and who is both willing and able to hear the Holy Spirit guide him or her in making decisions about your care. Standard medical treatment may be exactly what God desires you to use in your recovery. On the other hand, God may have something else in mind.

A doctor who prays with you will be a great ally and partner in helping you to obey God's command. Remember, it is written, "Whoever obeys his command will come to no harm, and the wise heart will know the proper time and procedure. For there is a proper time and procedure for every matter, though a man's misery weighs heavily upon him" (Ecclesiastes 8:5-6).

How comforting it is to know that God's thoughts for us are healing thoughts. And that God's ways are perfect for us. We can lay down our worries and anxieties and rest in the peace of God, knowing that He is guiding our steps and our recovery. Give grateful thanks to Him today for sending us the right teachers. Give grateful thanks to Him today for all His blessings. Give grateful thanks to Him for His protection and help.

Wonderful Jehovah-rapha, Your ways are indeed higher than my ways. And Your thoughts are higher than my thoughts. Send the Holy Spirit, God, to reveal to me the path that I am to take in my recovery. Send me Spirit-filled teachers, advisors, and health professionals to share their counsel with me. In the name of Your Son, Jesus Christ, I pray, Amen.

Day 243

Jesus entered Jericho and was passing through. A man was there by the name of Zacchaeus; he was a chief tax collector and was wealthy. He wanted to see who Jesus was, but being a short man he could not, because of the crowd. So he ran ahead and climbed a sycamore-fig tree to see him, since Jesus was coming that way. When Jesus reached the spot, he looked up and said to him, "Zacchaeus, come down immediately. I must stay at your house today." So he came down at once and welcomed him gladly. All the people saw this and began to mutter, "He has gone to be the guest of a 'sinner.'" But Zacchaeus stood up and said to the Lord, "Look, Lord! Here and now I give half of my possessions to the poor, and if I have cheated anybody out of anything, I will pay back four times the amount." Jesus said to him, "Today salvation has come to this house, because this man, too, is a son of Abraham. For the Son of Man came to seek and to save what was lost." (Luke 19:1-10 NIV)

Zacchaeus teaches us an important lesson about repentance and about making restitution. Because of his actions, Jesus said to him, "Today salvation has come to this house. The Son of Man came to seek and to save what was lost."

We are a whole unit – soul, mind, emotions, and body. When we have violated someone and have not made restitution, we are damaged spiritually and we are also damaged mentally and emotionally.

If we allow our transgression to fester long enough, it may also create physical damage as well. Why? Because we have become vulnerable to the evil one. This is a chink in the armor described in Ephesians 6 and his arrow can get through and pierce us.

To be healed, we have to get right with God and with our fellow man. Own up to your mistakes and make restitution where it is possible to do so. Ask the Holy Spirit for guidance for each particular situation and act according to the instructions that you are given. You cannot be healed if you are carrying burdens of guilt and ill will.

Be willing to atone for your wrongdoings and allow the Lord's peace to fill your soul.

Almighty God, help me to examine my life honestly and to make a list of wrongs I have committed against others. Give me the courage to atone for my mistakes and to make the best restitution that I can. Where it is no longer possible to do so directly to the people I have wronged, show me what You would have me do. I need healing for my soul as well as my body. Thank You, Lord, for redeeming me. In Jesus' name, I pray, Amen.

Day 244

Therefore, the promise comes by faith, so that it may be by grace and may be guaranteed to all Abraham's offspring – not only to those who are of the law but also to those who are of the faith of Abraham. He is the father of us all. As it is written: "I have made you a father of many nations." He is our father in the sight of God, in whom he believed – the God who gives life to the dead and calls things that are not as though they were. Against all hope, Abraham in hope believed and so became the father of many nations, just as it had been said to him, "So shall your offspring be." Without weakening in his faith, he faced the fact that his body was as good as dead – since he was about a hundred years old – and that Sarah's womb was also dead. Yet he did not waver through unbelief regarding the promise of God, but was strengthened in his faith and gave glory to God, being fully persuaded that God had power to do what he had promised. (Romans 4:16-21 NIV)

The Lord God Almighty is the God of the impossible. Certainly, no person in his right mind would look at an elderly, childless couple and offer the slightest possibility that they could be the parents of many nations. Fortunately, there have been, and still are, people of great faith. It is written that "Abraham in hope believed." He believed what God told Him. It was preposterous. It was ridiculous. It was outrageous. But he believed God anyway.

What did he have to do in order to believe? He had to look beyond the reality that he saw. He had to look beyond the appearance of things. Scripture tells us that without weakening in his faith, Abraham faced the fact that he was nearly one hundred years old and that his wife Sarah was well past her childbearing years. The medical facts were abundantly clear. Can't you hear a doctor pronounce with great authority that there was absolutely no hope?

You are faced with the same choice that Abraham had. You also have a promise – the promise of Jehovah-rapha that He is the God who heals you. Like Abraham, you have to "face the facts" of your situation; however, like Abraham, you are called to give all power to God and not to the appearance of your health situation. Like Abraham, you are called to heed God's Word and His instruction and to obey. Keep the faith.

Wonderful Jehovah-rapha, like Abraham I choose to believe Your Word. I see the appearance of my health situation, but I hold to Your vision for my future. Show me the path You want me to follow. In the name of Jesus Christ, my Savior and my Redeemer, I pray, Amen.

Day 245

If you live in Me [abide vitally united to Me] and My words remain in you and continue to live in your hearts, ask whatever you will, and it shall be done for you. (John 15:7 AMP)

The Gospels are full of statements of the limitless power of God. This is one of them. Jesus has just been telling His disciples that He will not be with them much longer on earth. He is sharing with them precious truths that they must learn and absorb into their very being.

Over and over again Jesus has told His followers not to place limitations on God's love or God's power. Here He says, "Ask whatever you will, and it shall be done for you." Ask whatever you will. Jesus set the example and often His examples were in the realm of healing. He asked God to raise Lazarus and Lazarus came forth. He told the lame to walk and it was so.

Does Jesus give us any restrictions or conditions? Yes, there are two requirements in this Scripture. Notice the "if" part of the sentence. First, "if you live in Me." The Amplified Bible explains that this means to "abide vitally united" to Jesus.

Think about what it means to live vitally united to Jesus. It means that your thoughts, your words, and your deeds will be in alignment with Christ. It means that you declare yourself to be a member of Jesus' family and that you are faithful to Him.

The second requirement is that Jesus' words "remain in you and continue to live in your heart." God repeatedly tells you of the importance of His Word. The words of Jesus, the Son of God, are to fill you completely and to live in your heart. If they are alive in you, then they must be manifested in the things that you do and the things that you say.

Invite Jesus and His Word into your heart. Live in Jesus. Live vitally united with Jesus. Then ask whatsoever you will and it will be done unto you according to the Word of Jesus.

Dear God, I declare my faith in You and in Your Son, Jesus Christ. Come into my heart and into every cell of my body. I seek to live united with my Risen Lord, Jesus Christ, in every aspect of my life. I join with Him at every level and dimension of my being. I ask for forgiveness of my sins and the cleansing of my soul. I ask for healing of my body. As I live united with You and Your Son, guide me and show me any specific steps that I need to take as a partner with You in my healing. With grateful thanks, in Jesus' name, I pray, Amen.

Day 246

For, brethren, ye have been called unto liberty. (Galatians 5:13 KJV)

You have been called to liberty. You! Jesus Christ came to set you free. He broke all the bonds that tie you. He released you from the curse of satan. He redeemed you – soul, mind, and body.

Repeatedly, Jesus liberated God's children from old patterns and old beliefs. "God loves you," He proclaims. "Now love one another." And He brings the message of God's healing power. "Your faith has made you well."

Jesus sent His followers out to tell all the world of these messages of liberty for the people. "Heal the sick . . . and tell them, 'The kingdom of God is near you' " (Luke 10:9). Part of the liberty that Jesus brought was release from illness and disease. Your freedom was bought on the Cross where He bore your infirmities as well as your sins.

Satan wants you sick. He binds you with his own devious schemes, but he also leads you into the dismal situation of binding yourself through your fears, your misguided belief systems, and your hectic lifestyle that make it difficult to make healthy choices for your body.

Close your eyes and imagine your illness as a large chain that wraps around your body, binding you tightly. Now see your Lord Jesus Christ walking up to you. He smiles at you with great love and compassion.

Jesus asks you, "Do you want to be well?" If you are willing to accept responsibility for yourself and your health and to be well, say, "Yes, Lord."

See Him reach out His hand and watch the chain disintegrate, falling to the ground. Jesus says to you, "Your sins are forgiven and you are healed. Rise and walk. Go in peace. Witness for me in your life."

Feel the love of God in every cell of your body. Feel the freedom in each cell to function normally according to God's purpose. Give God grateful thanks and rejoice in your healing.

Almighty God, You sent your Son Jesus Christ to set me at liberty. I am free, God, because You have removed me from bondage. Sometimes I reach down and pick those chains back up myself by what I do and what I think and what I believe. Help me, Heavenly Father. You have called me to liberty and I give my bonds to You. Take them. In the name of Jesus, I pray, Amen.

Day 247

Now there were some present at that time who told Jesus about the Galileans whose blood Pilate had mixed with their sacrifices. Jesus answered, "Do you think that these Galileans were worse sinners than all the other Galileans because they suffered this way? I tell you, no! But unless you repent, you too will all perish. Or those eighteen who died when the tower in Siloam fell on them – do you think they were more guilty than all the others living in Jerusalem? I tell you, no! But unless you repent, you too will all perish." (Luke 13:1-5 NIV)

If you feel sick, you may find yourself wondering, "Do I have this illness or injury because I have done something wrong?" It is natural to raise such questions, but it can be dangerous to spend time judging yourself or others. You are likely to end up in a pit of self-condemnation and self-castigation that will only worsen your situation.

Spending time judging yourself is a false piety and gets you nowhere. Likewise, judging others for being ill is just as futile since it often overlooks the fact that satan chooses to attack most harshly those who walk closest to the Lord.

What is important is not judgment and condemnation, but, as Jesus pointed out, our repentance. Seek always to be aware of the ways that you stray from God's will and ask forgiveness, returning to God's plan for you. Ask God to reveal to you what is at the core of your illness. If there are old emotional hurts to be healed, ask Him to show you. If you are carrying grudges and resentments that must be released, ask Him to show you. If you have committed a wrong which needs to be corrected, ask Him to show you.

God's understanding far surpasses your own, so leave all the judging to Him. Keep your focus on asking for wisdom and revelation knowledge of what you need to do to come into alignment with God's purpose

Almighty God, I know that too often I struggle with problems and issues that I shouldn't. I beat myself up for my imperfections and I let the fear of my transgressions convince me that I am unworthy to be healed. Your Son Jesus Christ tells me to repent or I will perish. Lord, I stand before You and ask Your mercy. Forgive me, Father, where I have failed You. Help me to forgive myself where I have failed myself. Reveal to me issues that lie deep at the core of my health problems, and give me the strength, wisdom, and courage to confront and release them. I give You grateful thanks for being Jehovah-rapha, who loves me, cares for me, and heals me. In Jesus' name, I pray, Amen.

Day 248

I will remain in the world no longer, but they are still in the world, and I am coming to you. Holy Father, protect them by the power of your name – the name you gave me – so that they may be one as we are one. . . . My prayer is not that you take them out of the world but that you protect them from the evil one. (John 17:11, 15 NIV)

The Gospel of John records a lengthy prayer that Jesus made shortly before he was arrested, tried, and crucified. In this prayer He prays for Himself, for His disciples, and for all believers.

Notice that Jesus prays for protection for His disciples. He is fully aware of the attacks of the evil one, and He asks His loving heavenly Father to watch over the people he has chosen to carry on His work. He knows attacks will come, but with the power and protection of Jehovah, satan cannot prevail. Jesus will soon go to the Cross and will vanquish the evil one totally and permanently.

We spend so much time praying to Our Heavenly Father in Jesus' name that we rarely think of Jesus praying for us. Just imagine – Jesus praying for us. Jesus praying for *you*. Praying a prayer of protection from the evil one. No matter what arrows the evil one may aim at you, not one can strike your heart with the protection of the Lord.

No matter what trials and tribulations come to you, Jesus has overcome them all. He strengthens you through the Father, who sets you upon a rock of safety. Despite the potent arrows of sickness and disease that the evil one sends at you, God has a plan for your healing. You are His beloved child. He sent His Son Jesus Christ to die for your sins and for your infirmities. Nothing is too hard for Him.

Almighty God, I am humbled by the very thought that Your Son prayed for me long ago and prays for me still. Protect me, God, by the power of Your Holy Name. Keep me safe from the attacks of the evil one. Your Son overcame satan by His death and resurrection, and in His name, I command satan to leave my body and to get out of my life. I know that You are the God who heals me. I know that Your Son healed every single person who came to Him to be made whole. I claim this healing, God. Show me the path You want me to follow in my recovery and I will be obedient. I seek always to follow Your will in my life. In the name of Your Son, Jesus Christ, I pray, Amen.

Day 249

Make a joyful noise unto the Lord, all ye lands. Serve the Lord with gladness; come before his presence with singing. (Psalm 100:1-2 KJV)

Be joyful! Joy is an important emotion because it fills us with Divine energy, which helps us to spread love, compassion, and happiness to everyone around us. We are able truly to serve the Lord with gladness. God wants us to proclaim His Good News. He needs us to be his messengers of the tidings of great joy – that we have been redeemed in soul, mind, and body.

We are to fill the air with our music, coming before God's presence with singing. Not all music today is worthy to be presented to the Lord. We must be careful what songs and what music we are putting in our minds, bodies, and souls. Why is this important? Because music is filled with its own kind of energy. It can be sublime and born of the Divine. No one listening to the Hallelujah Chorus doubts that it was an inspiration of God. However, other music undermines and destroys the spirit and is born of evil forces that seek to entrap us.

Maintaining a spirit of joyfulness and filling your life with music is some-times difficult when you feel sick. Nevertheless, doing so is essential to the restoration of your health. Find a radio station that plays hymns or purchase some cassettes and CDs.

Connecting with Divine energy through hymns allows healing vibrations to flood every cell in your body. It feeds you at every level – boosting your body's immune system, nourishing your mind with positive thoughts, and af-firming your faith.

Claim the healing power of music in your life. Sing out with joy! Proclaim your faith through your music. The more you *sing* the Word, the easier it is to *live* the Word.

O, wonderful Lord, I sing a joyful song to You. How grateful I am for the inspiration of music and hymns. On those days when I struggle with my ailments, have one of Your angels whisper in my ear to remind me to sing a song of thanksgiving for all Your many blessings. Thank You for Your healing presence in my life. I seek to serve You, Lord. I seek to follow the path You have chosen for me. I sing to You in joyful gratitude for Your love, mercy, compassion, and healing. In the name of the Father, Son, and the Holy Spirit, I pray, Amen.

Day 250

Once safely on shore, we found out that the island was called Malta. The islanders showed us unusual kindness. They built a fire and welcomed us all because it was raining and cold. Paul gathered a pile of brushwood and, as he put it on the fire, a viper, driven out by the heat, fastened itself on his hand. When the islanders saw the snake hanging from his hand, they said to each other, "This man must be a murderer; for though he escaped from the sea, Justice has not allowed him to live." But Paul shook the snake off into the fire and suffered no ill effects. The people expected him to swell up or suddenly fall dead, but after waiting a long time and seeing nothing unusual happen to him, they changed their minds and said he was a god. (Acts 28:1-6 NIV)

Who are we? How do we define ourselves and how do others define us? What the islanders witnessed about Paul defied the laws of nature as they understood them, so they first called Paul a murderer. Actually, earlier in his life Paul had been a murderer, having sent many Christians to be eaten by lions.

However, Paul had been redeemed. Even though Paul had never seen Jesus during His earthly life and ministry, he was called by Christ in a dramatic conversion experience on the road to Damascus and came to believe in Him with all his heart. He accepted the commission that Jesus left to all His followers – to preach and to heal.

In Mark 16:15-18, Jesus said that those who accepted His commission could pick up snakes and not be hurt. He also said that they would lay hands on the sick and heal them. Paul, who had never met Jesus in the flesh, believed Jesus' words and he did as Jesus commanded. All on faith. All because he believed. Paul was not a god. But he had the power of Almighty God within him. So when the snake bit him, he did not die or suffer any ill effects. And when sick people were brought to him, he healed them as Jesus had instructed.

You are no different from Paul. Jesus may not have called you as dramatically, but His call is no less real. Are you Paul's kind of Christian – who was able to believe without allowing doubt to limit and weaken him? Let the signs of being a Christian accompany *you.*

Almighty God, I profess my faith in You and in Your Son Jesus Christ. Neither Paul nor I ever walked with Jesus during His earthly ministry. Let me use Paul's life as an example of what service to You in total faith means. Help me as I strive to be a faithful witness for You. In the name of Your Son, Jesus Christ, I pray, Amen.

Day 251

The thief cometh not, but for to steal, and to kill, and to destroy: I am come that they might have life, and that they might have it more abundantly. I am the good shepherd: the good shepherd giveth his life for the sheep. (John 10:10-11 KJV)

Jesus came to bring us abundant life. Not just life, but *abundant* life! This is particularly good news to remember when we feel sick.

What does abundant life mean? Of course, it means that beyond our life in this world, we will have life eternal with the Father. There is no greater abundance than eternity.

But Jesus meant for us to have life abundantly on this earth as well. Think of all the things that you already have as part of that life abundant. Do you have food to eat? Air to breathe? Sun to shine on you? Friends to support you? God's Word to inspire you?

What about your health? You are very familiar with everything that is wrong with you. Take some time now to focus on everything that is *right!* Focus on the life abundant within you.

Spend some time every day for the next week making a journal of things concerning your health which represent life abundant to you. These are things for which you are grateful. Make sure that you list ten items each day.

For example, you may list: I can breathe air in my lungs. My blood pressure is normal. My blood cells carry oxygen to the cells of my body. My kidneys filter wastes from my body. I can move my hands and fingers in order to write. My ears can hear the birds sing. My nose can smell the fragrance of my favorite roses.

Maybe all of the things mentioned here are not true for you; nevertheless, you will find plenty of items to put on your own personal list.

After each item on your list go back and write, "Thank you, God." Gratitude creates a spirit of joy within you and it encourages your body to heal. Focus on the positive. Concentrate your attention on God's many blessings in your life.

Wonderful Jehovah-rapha, thank You for sending Your Son Jesus Christ to give me life abundant. He overcame the evil one who seeks to destroy me and my body. He bore my sins and my infirmities on the Cross. Thank You, God, for offering Your Son as the Perfect Sacrifice for me. In humble gratitude for Your many blessings, I pray in the name of Your Son, Jesus Christ, my Savior and my Redeemer, Amen.

Day 252

Jesus entered Jericho and was passing through. A man was there by the name of Zacchaeus; he was a chief tax collector and was wealthy. He wanted to see who Jesus was, but being a short man he could not, because of the crowd. So he ran ahead and climbed a sycamore-fig tree to see him, since Jesus was coming that way. When Jesus reached the spot, he looked up and said to him, "Zacchaeus, come down immediately. I must stay at your house today." So he came down at once and welcomed him gladly. (Luke 19:1-6 NIV)

Zacchaeus *really* wanted to see Jesus, but he had a little problem. He was so short that he couldn't see over other people's heads when he was in a crowd. Smart and determined, Zacchaeus decided that his height would not be an obstacle to him if he simply climbed a tree. Jesus got to the tree, looked up, and saw Zacchaeus. "Get down, Zacchaeus," Jesus said. "I'm going home to stay with you today." What was Zacchaeus' response? "He came down at once and welcomed him gladly." We almost miss these words because the point of the story appears to be about repentance and restitution.

Are there obstacles in your path to Jesus? It is a strange paradox that, when we are ill, we often have a love-hate relationship with God. Sometimes we believe that it is His will that we feel sick and yet we ask Him to make us well. We have to move past this block to a higher position so that we have a clear view of God's will for our health.

Jesus called to Zacchaeus, "I'm coming home with you today." Jesus calls you today by name and says the same thing: "I want to come home with you." Will you do as Zacchaeus and welcome Him joyfully? Do you really want Him? Remember, He always asks that you follow Him and that means being willing to change your way of viewing your world. His disciples had to drop their nets (which represented their livelihood) and leave their families. Your path to healing may not require a literal move from your career and home, but you will be asked to follow Him in a way that those around you may not understand. Are you willing to welcome Jesus joyfully and to be obedient to Him?

Heavenly Father, I welcome Your Son Jesus Christ into my home and my heart today. Father, thank You for this story of Zacchaeus which reminds me to invite my Savior Jesus Christ into my life gladly with each new day, overcoming all obstacles in my path that separate me from Him. In Jesus' name, I pray, Amen.

Day 253

And I will ask the Father, and He will give you another Comforter (Counselor, Helper, Intercessor, Advocate, Strengthener, and Standby), that He may remain with you forever – The Spirit of Truth, Whom the world cannot receive (welcome, take to its heart), because it does not see Him or know and recognize Him. But you know and recognize Him, for He lives with you [constantly] and will be in you. (John 14:16-17 AMP)

The Holy Spirit has a vital role to play in our healing. We are desperately in need of the Holy Spirit as a beacon of truth because each minute of each day there are new choices to be made. For this meal, what are my healthiest food choices? For this moment, which of God's remedies will support my healing process in the best way? The healthiest choice for this minute may be different from the healthiest choice for the next minute. We must ask the Holy Spirit to illumine us repeatedly with Divine truth.

For example, each morning ask, "Almighty God, protect me and guide me. Holy Spirit, fill me with your Holy presence. Reveal to me what are the best items of clothing for me to wear today to strengthen my immune system and support my healing." Then touch each garment you intend to wear, hold it close against your body, and listen for the Holy Spirit to speak to you. Sometimes you may "hear" a voice speak in your head saying "yes" or "no." Other times you may *feel* the answer when a "jangly" feeling makes you want to put the garment down or a warm feeling makes you want to draw it closer to you.

This is not the way of the world which relies on things it can see and measure. The world separates God from science and boosts about its "objectivity." The world cannot understand that God must be an integral part in absolutely every decision that we make. The world cannot understand that God wants so much for us to enjoy His abundance that He sent His Son to show us the way and that He gave us the Holy Spirit as our constant guide to Divine truth.

Open your heart and your soul to the Holy Spirit. Let him be your teacher and guide to truth.

Heavenly Father, fill me with Divine love. Flood me with Your Divine truth for every step that I take along the path of my healing. Send the Holy Spirit to teach me, instruct me, guide me. Protect me from the doubts and deceptions of the world. Reveal to me now what I need to do to assist my healing. I will be silent and listen so that I can hear Your voice. In the name of the Father, Son, and Holy Spirit, I pray, Amen.

Day 254

I praise you because I am fearfully and wonderfully made. (Psalm 139:14 NIV)

How right David was! We *are* fearfully and wondrously made. We are awesome in soul, mind, and body. We can choose to believe that we evolved to have the bodies we do or we can choose to believe that God specifically designed our bodies to function according to His Holy design. God's Word says that He created us as human beings. Our scientific knowledge has grown exponentially, yet what we do *not* know about the functioning of our bodies far exceeds what we *do* know.

God designed us to live. He put specific intelligence in each cell so that it can carry out its function and so that we do not have to give any thought to supervising each of these trillions of cells. Some event occurs externally or internally, and our trillions of cells respond. This happens every millisecond of every day of every year.

When we make wise choices and provide our bodies with positive experiences, we become partners with God in creating health. When we make foolish or destructive choices, we become partners with satan in creating illness. Satan works so stealthily that often it is only after months, years, and decades of seemingly inconsequential choices that we begin to manifest disease.

Perhaps we are *too* wondrously made! If we put sugar water in our car's gasoline tank, it doesn't take thirty, forty, or fifty years for us to know we have violated the basic rules for the proper functioning of the car. Yet we can often "get away" with violating God's rules for healthy eating for thirty years before illness begins to manifest.

Who is your partner? Choose Jehovah-Rapha, the God who heals you. Make a decision to glorify Him by keeping your temple strong and healthy. Praise your Heavenly Father for making your body in such a wondrous way.

Dear Heavenly Father, thank You for creating my soul, mind, and body in such a wondrous way. I praise You because I am, indeed, fearfully and wonderfully made. I accept my responsibility for my health choices, and I choose You as my partner, God. I want to participate in my healing by proclaiming my complete faith in Your Divine will and by aligning everything I do according to Your will for me. Teach me; guide me; and show me the path you want me to take. In Jesus' name, I pray, Amen.

The hand of the Lord was upon me, and he brought me out by the Spirit of the Lord and set me in the middle of a valley; it was full of bones. . . . He asked me, "Son of man, can these bones live?" I said, "O Sovereign Lord, you alone know." Then he said to me, "Prophesy to these bones and say to them, 'Dry bones, hear the word of the Lord! This is what the Sovereign Lord says to these bones: I will make breath enter you, and you will come to life. I will attach tendons to you and make flesh come upon you and cover you with skin; I will put breath in you, and you will come to life. Then you will know that I am the Lord.'" So I prophesied as I was commanded. And as I was prophesying, there was a noise, a rattling sound, and the bones came together, bone to bone. I looked, and tendons and flesh appeared on them and skin covered them, but there was no breath in them. Then he said to me, "Prophesy to the breath; prophesy, son of man, and say to it, 'This is what the Sovereign Lord says: Come from the four winds, O breath, and breathe into these slain, that they may live.'" So I prophesied as he commanded me and breath entered them; they came to life and stood up on their feet – a vast army. (Ezekiel 37:1, 3-10 NIV)

There are always moments when we despair that we will be healed. At those times read this passage from God's Word. In this vision Ezekiel is in the midst of a valley of dried up bones and God challenges him with a question, "Can these bones live?" Ezekiel knew that God had the power to transform anything. The question was whether God willed it. So he replied, "O, Sovereign Lord, You alone know."

Now watch what happens. God doesn't just reach down and put flesh on the bones. He uses Ezekiel as His instrument and works through him. "Now Ezekiel," God says. "You speak to these bones. You tell them I will put tendons and flesh on them and will breathe the breath of life into them." God is going to do the healing but Ezekiel is to speak God's truth and to participate in the process. Ezekiel did as he was told and the bones came to life and stood up on their feet.

God's will is that you be healed. Read the passage again and put yourself in the valley among the dry bones. See God telling you exactly what He wants you to do to participate in your healing. Stand on God's Word. Speak God's Word. Allow God to raise you up, strong and healthy.

Mighty Lord, raise me up and breathe into me the breath of life. Touch me as You touched the dry bones. I trust in You. Tell me what to do and I will participate like Ezekiel in my healing process. In Jesus' name, Amen.

Day 256

For the Lord is good; his mercy is everlasting; and his truth endureth to all generations. (Psalm 100:5 KJV)

Do not withhold your mercy from me, O Lord; may your love and your truth always protect me. For troubles without number surround me; my sins have overtaken me, and I cannot see. They are more than the hairs of my head, and my heart fails within me. Be pleased, O Lord, to save me; O Lord, come quickly to help me. May all who seek to take my life be put to shame and confusion; may all who desire my ruin be turned back in disgrace. (Psalm 40:11-14 NIV)

Send forth your light and your truth, let them guide me. (Psalm 43:3 NIV)

God's truth endures as your steady beacon. When you are guided by it, you are always headed in the right direction. God wants you to be well and healthy and living in full, vital service to Him. His truth always provides the answers you need for each minute of each day. It certainly would seem to be simple enough to stay focused on it and to chart your course accordingly.

However, the evil one comes to cloud your vision and to distract your attention. He hits you at your most vulnerable times and in your most vulnerable places. He confuses you when you are tired and discouraged, and he tempts you to deviate from the guidance you have been given by the Holy Spirit. He often interferes with your communication with the Lord so you stay unsure whether a certain path is God's will for you or not. If you are agonizing over a decision and question the guidance you have been given, you can be sure that the evil one is entangling you.

Turn to Ephesians 6:10 and put on your full armor of the Lord. In the name of the blood of Jesus command satan to leave you, and ask again for help from Jehovah-rapha, Christ Jesus, and the Holy Spirit. When you know God's truth, you will feel peace in your soul.

The guidance you receive may be as strange as walking around high walls shouting like Joshua or walking straight to the sea with an army behind you like Moses – yet in your soul you will *know* that you are following the path to healing that God wills for you.

Wonderful Jehovah-rapha, send forth your light and your truth and let them guide me. May your love and your truth always protect me. I know that I can rest in Your truth and I declare my willingness to obey Your instructions for my healing. In Jesus' name, I pray, Amen.

Day 257

Then he got into the boat and his disciples followed him. Without warning, a furious storm came up on the lake, so that the waves swept over the boat. But Jesus was sleeping. The disciples went and woke him, saying, "Lord, save us! We're going to drown!" He replied, "You of little faith, why are you so afraid?" Then he got up and rebuked the winds and the waves, and it was completely calm. (Matthew 8:23-26 NIV)

We can all relate to times in our lives when everything seems to be smooth sailing, and then suddenly, without warning, a furious storm comes up.

Usually illness comes upon us gradually day by day, step by step, as we make decisions that are not wise ones. However, occasionally, the evil one unleashes his attack suddenly and without warning. A car crashes into us or a contaminated blood transfusion infects us or something else happens rapidly and swiftly. One moment we were healthy and the next moment we are wounded or ill.

How do we respond at those times? Probably in ways not so different from Jesus' disciples. When the violent storm came up suddenly, they became terrified as the waves swept over the boat. They were fearful for their lives and they yelled to Jesus to save them. Focused on the outcome they feared, they shouted, "Lord, we're going to drown!"

And what was Jesus doing? He was sleeping through the storm. When He was wakened, He got up and chastised His disciples. Why are you so afraid? Where is your faith? And then He got up, rebuked the wind and the waves, and restored calm in their lives.

When illness or injury happens to you, remember this story. Let Christ Jesus speak to you, saying, "Why are you so afraid? Have faith!" Jesus is our victorious conqueror of anything and everything that the evil one can throw at us. Stop wasting your energy on lamenting your problem and start claiming God's power in your life and in your healing.

Almighty God, shore up my faith when it is weak. Keep me focused on Your Son Christ Jesus who is my Savior and my Healer. Let me hear His voice saying, "You of little faith, why are you so afraid?" and let me see Him smile at me with love and compassion. I give You my fears, Father, and I stand in faith on Your Word. In the name of Your Son, Jesus Christ, my Savior and my Redeemer, I pray, Amen.

Day 258

My son, preserve sound judgment and discernment, do not let them out of your sight; they will be life for you, an ornament to grace your neck. Then you will go on your way in safety, and your foot will not stumble; when you lie down, you will not be afraid; when you lie down, your sleep will be sweet. (Proverbs 3:21-24 NIV)

We are told that sound judgment and discernment will be life for us, but the regrettable fact is that most health problems are a result of numerous poor choices we have made over a long period of time. When we are finally confronted with our illness, then we cry to God for healing.

God has been clear about what foods contribute to our health and which ones do not. God has been clear about what lifestyle habits are healthy and what ones are not. We have to see how we have succumbed to the whispers of the evil one and gotten off the track. Then we have to be willing to make the needed corrections. Otherwise, as fast as God heals us, we willfully create more illness in other areas – and that isn't God's will or God's fault.

Develop sound judgment by learning about the underlying causes of your health condition. It is your responsibility to learn the complexities of your body functions and the myriad of health decisions you made that led to your situation. Then and only then are you in a place where you can use your own discernment about solutions presented to you for recovery.

For example, if you do not understand the connections between your osteoporosis and an acid body pH, your kidney function, vitamin D utilization, and mineral absorption, plus many other factors, you will be easily deluded into thinking one pill is going to solve your problems.

Look at the peace of mind that follows from preserving the sound judgment and discernment that comes from God. This verse in Proverbs speaks of many wonderful benefits: life, safety, freedom from fear, and sound sleep. These are all attributes of someone grounded firmly in the Lord and in His care. Acknowledge God as the source of your life and allow Him to lead you to your recovery.

Dear God, help me preserve sound judgment and discernment. Keep me from stumbling and being misled by the evil one. I want to go my way in safety, to lie down without fear, and to sleep soundly and peacefully. I want to live, Lord. Thank You for healing me and fulfilling Your purpose for my life. In the name of Your Son, Jesus Christ, I pray, Amen.

Day 259

Later Jesus . . . rebuked them for their lack of faith. . . . He said to them, "Go into all the world and preach the good news to all creation. Whoever believes and is baptized will be saved, but whoever does not believe will be condemned. And these signs will accompany those who believe: In my name they will drive out demons; they will speak in new tongues; they will pick up snakes with their hands; and when they drink deadly poison, it will not hurt them at all; they will place their hands on sick people, and they will get well." (Mark 16:14-20 NIV)

This version of The Great Commission lists several "signs of those who believe." Especially troublesome to most people are the items about poisons and snakes.

What could Jesus possibly have meant here? Let's look at Jesus' own life for an answer. When satan took Jesus to the top of the Temple and told Him to jump off because the angels would keep Him from being hurt, Jesus refused. Both He and satan knew that what satan said was true and that He would not have been injured if He had jumped.

Nevertheless, Jesus responded by saying, "It is also written, 'Do not put the Lord your God to the test.' " It is highly unlikely that Jesus would have picked up poisonous snakes just to prove that He would not have been harmed by handling them. Jesus was referring to a situation of a sudden, unexpected encounter such as the one which Paul faced when he was accidentally bitten by a snake on the island of Malta. In that story recounted in Acts 28, Paul suffers no ill effects from the bite.

Your healing must never be part of a test for God. If you ask for healing to "prove" God is Lord, you are on the wrong road. What Jesus is saying to us in the Great Commission is that no matter what happens to you, there is a power that can overcome the limited physical laws of nature – if you believe it is so.

Jesus also emphasized in His last words to us the importance of the laying on of hands as a means for healing the sick. He commanded us to go out to all the world, spreading the gospel and healing those who were ill. God wants you well. And He wants you to be an instrument for the healing of others. Heed the commands of His Son, Your Lord and Savior.

Almighty Lord, I accept The Great Commission of Your Son Jesus Christ and commit myself to share His message with all those who are suffering. I also accept His commandment to lay hands on the sick in His name. Strengthen my faith, O Lord, so that I can fulfill Your purpose and Your mission for my life. In Jesus' name, I pray, Amen.

Day 260

Reckless words pierce like a sword, but the tongue of the wise brings healing. (Proverbs 12:18 NIV)

There is a children's rhyme which says, "Sticks and stones can hurt my bones, but words can never harm them." Nothing could be further from the truth. The wisdom of Proverbs 12:18 warns us of the effects of our speech and reminds us to be ever mindful of the consequences of the intent of our words.

The world is filled with hurting, suffering people who cry out for help. You have Good News which many of them have not heard, and, therefore, you have the privilege of being a wise tongue which brings healing. You can be the messenger pointing the way to God's Word, declaring the truth that The Lord God Almighty is the God who heals us. You can proclaim the Word which says of Christ Jesus that "by His stripes I am healed." You can announce the Word which says that "Whatever you ask for in prayer, believe that you have received it, and it will be yours."

Your words will be healing caresses for all who hear them. Many of those who hear you will bless you for being an instrument for change in their lives. They are the ones who are ready. They are the ones who have been praying for help in a spirit of openness and willingness to accept responsibility for their thoughts and actions.

However, not everyone is ready to receive the message you have to offer. You do not have to be defensive nor do you have to persuade the other person to accept your viewpoint. Simply speak the words the Holy Spirit gives you and God will handle the rest.

Remember that God always allows every person free will and the right to choose his own path. Jesus never attempted to force anyone to receive Him. Instead, listen to Him tell you (just as He told His disciples so long ago) to bless the one who cannot hear you, "shake the dust off your feet," and move on to someone who is ready to receive your healing words.

Wonderful Jehovah-rapha, help me to guard my tongue and to refrain from speaking or thinking reckless words which pierce like a sword. These are the words of the evil one. They are words that harm me and everyone around me. Teach me, Lord, instead to have the tongue of the wise which brings healing. I want to be an instrument of healing, God, not only for myself but for others also. Send the Holy Spirit to speak through me as I share the Good News. In Jesus' name, I pray, Amen.

Day 261

Who has woe? Who has sorrow? Who has strife? Who has complaints? Who has needless bruises? Who has bloodshot eye? Those who linger over wine, who go to sample bowls of mixed wine. Do not gaze at wine when it is red, when it sparkles in the cup, when it goes down smoothly! In the end it bites like a snake and poisons like a viper. Your eyes will see strange sights and your mind imagine confusing things. You will be like one sleeping on the high seas, lying on top of the rigging. "They hit me," you will say, "but I'm not hurt! They beat me, but I don't feel it! When will I wake up so I can find another drink?"
(Proverbs 23:29-35 NIV)

Some of those who are physically ill also have to deal with the issue of addiction. This may be an addiction to alcohol, to mind-altering drugs, to certain prescription drugs, to tobacco, to caffeine, or to sugar. There are many substances which can take control in our lives and upon which we become dependent.

At the bottom of all addictions is emotional pain. The substance or activity to which we are addicted gives us a momentary feeling of power or control and deadens our vulnerable feelings. Deep inside we are feeling afraid or lonely or rejected or grief-stricken. The inner pain is one we are afraid to face, and we find that the addictive substance blunts the pain and allows us to hide. As long as we stay actively involved in our addiction, we can pretend to be a helpless victim, and we can avoid taking responsibility for our lives.

Many addictions have disastrous effects on our health because old emotional wounds fester within and have a major impact at the physical level. To be well in our bodies, we will also have to be healed in our souls and our emotions and our minds. The pain has to be confronted, owned, experienced, and then released.

God is ever faithful and helps us to release us from the old pain. Ours is a God who brings us liberty. He wants us to be set free from all bondage so that we can walk the joyous path of health and liberty that He intended.

Loving Father, give me the courage to face my addictions. Give me the courage to look at the inner wounds that I carry. Help me to bring them into Your light, to embrace them, and then to let them go. Give me the strength to put aside my role of victim and to accept boldly my responsibilities in making wise choices for my life. Stand with me, God, and help me to stay on the path You want me to follow. In the name of Your Son, Jesus Christ, my Savior and my Redeemer, I pray, Amen.

Day 262

If the owner of the house had known at what time of night the thief was coming, he would have kept watch and would not have let his house be broken into. (Matthew 24:43 NIV)

This statement of Jesus is given in his warning to the people that they must remain alert for His return because "the Son of Man will come at an hour when you do not expect him."

But there is another message here as well. We need to remain vigilant not only for the return of Christ but also for the daily assaults of the evil one. Satan wants to destroy our health and he does this with guerrilla warfare-type attacks. They come little bits at a time, chipping slowly away at our health. Since most of us have not learned to be aware of our bodies and our health, we often fail to notice the subtle changes that are occurring. Usually what changes we notice, we rationalize away. The Prince of Darkness begins to take residence in us and we aren't paying attention. Inch by inch, we allow satan to move in and take over our temple.

We are exhorted to be vigilant and aware. We must pay attention. Notice the small changes in your body. By doing so, you can forbid satan from taking over your temple.

What do you do when you notice small changes? First, give thanks to God for helping you to be aware and ask that He help you to grow in this awareness. Second, go immediately into prayer. Describe to God what you have noticed. God knows already, of course, but the point is that *you* need to be clear. Third, ask God for guidance as to the path you are to take for your healing. Fourth, be quiet and meditate. Listen for the Holy Spirit to speak to you. Fifth, follow the guidance that you heard. Do not let any person turn you from obeying clear guidance you receive from God. Sixth, say "thank You" to God for your healing.

O, powerful Almighty Father, guard me and guide me every minute of every day. I lose focus too often, and I miss signals that I am under attack from the enemy who seeks to separate me from You. Too often I let my health get out of control because I don't pay attention. Sometimes I just feel too overwhelmed or afraid or angry or despondent. Cleanse my soul, O Lord. Remove these patterns and habits from the very core of my being. Raise me up. Send Your Holy angels to keep me aware and to help me to act on Your guidance. I fling myself into Your loving arms and I rest in Your strength. In the blessed name of Jesus Christ, I pray, Amen.

Day 263

Put your finger here; see my hands. Reach out your hand and put it into my side. Stop doubting and believe. (John 20:27 NIV)

Doubt keeps us in confusion. When we have health decisions to make, we can be so bombarded with opinions that we don't know what to do. This is particularly true if we feel victimized by being ill or injured. Why not stay victim and allow others to dictate our path of recovery? God calls us to a position of responsibility. He calls us to receive all pertinent input but then to turn to Him for the final decision.

How do we find out what God's choice is for us? We find out through prayer followed by silent listening. Some of us have learned how to do this, but many of us struggle for clarity in hearing God's voice. Satan certainly will try to confuse us anyway he can because he wants us to stay sick and powerless.

One technique we can use from time to time is to ask for concrete assistance. We need the same thing that Thomas needed. He was filled with doubt and needed something concrete. Jesus didn't tell him he was stupid or bad or wrong. He gently put Thomas' hand in the wound to let him feel for himself. It is okay to do likewise.

Suppose you are in doubt whether it is God's will for you to have particular medical procedure. You have prayed and meditated, but you haven't heard God's voice clearly. Ask God for some concrete help. For example, you might ask for two feathers in a certain area of your yard if you are supposed to have the treatment or three feathers if you are to choose a different path. Be creative in selecting your concrete guide. In general, you will find it is best to choose some sign from nature since that is so close to God.

Make sure you are humble and clear in your purpose. You are not trying to test God. And you are not demanding that God "perform." You are admitting your fear and are humbly seeking clarity – like Thomas – and an end to your confusion and doubt so that you can stay on the path.

Dear Gracious Lord, you know all my weaknesses better than I do. You know that there are times when I feel frightened and confused, and I feel compelled to follow some treatment that everybody else uses. I believe that You want me to be well. I believe that You have specific plans for my healing. In your great mercy, show me in a real way that I can see or touch Your plan for me. I choose to follow You, Lord. Help me to make the right decision in alignment with Your Divine plan for me. In the name of Jesus Christ, my Savior and my Redeemer, I pray, Amen.

Day 264

Nevertheless, more and more men and women believed in the Lord and were added to their number. As a result, people brought the sick into the streets and laid them on beds and mats so that at least Peter's shadow might fall on some of them as he passed by. Crowds gathered also from the towns around Jerusalem, bringing their sick and those tormented by evil spirits, and all of them were healed. (Acts 5:14-16 NIV)

Peter worked to follow Jesus' instructions and to carry on Jesus' mission. Most of us are aware of Peter's work to carry the gospel, but usually little attention is paid to repeated references in the Scriptures to the healing that was also part of Peter's mission.

Here we see Peter winning many converts to Christ and, *as a result,* scores of people who were physically and mentally ill were brought to him for healing. Why "as a result?" Because part of the message of Christ that Peter delivered was that they had been redeemed from their sins *and* from their infirmities. If Peter had preached the way most messages are delivered in churches today, no one would have even thought of the idea of bringing the sick for healing.

Yet in this passage we see many, many people coming to Peter as a result of Peter's message. And how many of those who came were healed? All of them. There is that word again – *all.* There were no exceptions, no rejections. No one was turned away because it was God's will that he was sick. No one was excluded because he needed to learn an important lesson. Not a single person was left to be ill. All were healed. All.

People were even healed when Peter's shadow passed over them. None of this came from Peter, of course. This was the working of Jehovah-rapha through the power of the Holy Spirit. Jesus promised that the Holy Spirit would baptize His followers with power.

Accept the message that healing is meant for *you.* Accept the power of the Holy Spirit in *your* life. Accept the dual mission that Jesus gives to *you* just as He gave it to Peter – to spread the gospel of salvation of soul and of body.

Gracious Lord, thank You for Your Holy Scriptures which show me over and over again the patterns You want for me to follow. Help me to be like Peter, an instrument for Jesus, who spread the Word of healing of soul and body. Fill me with the power of Your Holy Spirit, God, so that I may do likewise. It is my joy to do Your will, Lord. In the name of Jesus Christ, my Savior and my Redeemer, I pray, Amen.

Day 265

A merry heart doeth good like a medicine. (Proverbs 17:22 KJV)

Laugh. Smile. Joy is an essential ingredient for your healing.

This can be hard to do when you are feeling physical pain, when your energy feels depleted, and when you feel bad all over. The problem is that the sadness inside stunts your healing.

Solomon understood this because the rest of verse 22 in Proverbs 17 reads, "But a broken spirit drieth the bones." Illness often drags us down and saps our spirit. When this happens, our healing is slowed and sometimes halted. How vivid a picture this is: a broken spirit drying up the bones. When you succumb to despair, this is exactly what happens to all the cells in your body.

It is critical to change the internal environment. As Christians, we learn to act outrageously. We learn to sing when we are hurting, to give thanks when we feel ill, and to laugh when we are feeling despair. A merry heart is its own medicine. Scientists have discovered that laughter releases substances which reduce pain and help the body in its healing process. People have actually overcome illness through a type of laughter therapy. They watched funny movies, read jokes, and spent a large amount of time each day laughing.

The Holy Scriptures are an excellent source of joyful messages. When Jesus was born, the angels proclaimed, "We bring tidings of great joy!" Find joyful music and play it. Immerse your entire being in the healing vibrations of "Joyful, Joyful, We Adore Thee." Notice how your body actually feels different after you allow the music and the message to penetrate your entire being – physical, mental, and spiritual.

The Psalms are filled with praise and joy and gratitude. Read them out loud and share them with others. Make it a practice to laugh often during the day. Be sure to give and receive your quota of hugs and smiles. Praise God with joyful thanks for His healing power.

Heavenly Father, there are many times when I feel bad. At those time I want to hide under the covers and yell with anger or cry with despair. Instead, Lord, I stand on Your Word and I choose to sing, "Joyful, joyful, I adore thee." I come before Your presence with joy and gratitude and thanksgiving in my heart. You are the source of all healing, and You are my rock. In You I place all my faith and trust. In the name of Christ Jesus, my Savior and my Redeemer, I pray, Amen.

Day 266

Those who trust in the Lord are like Mount Zion, which cannot be shaken but endures forever. (Psalm 125:1 NIV)

O, to have unshakable trust! Trusting God "ought" to be the easiest thing in the world to do. Often it is easy enough to *say* we trust. But our thoughts and our actions bear the fingerprints of the lack of the trust we proclaim.

Satan seeks to undermine our trust at every opportunity. One excellent means to do this is by attacking our health. If the medical news is bad, we react in a myriad of ways. Sometimes we get angry and wonder why God "let" it happen. Sometimes we become depressed and surrender to despair. Sometimes we panic and become overwhelmed at the scientific opinions which are presented to us as absolute fact. Sometimes we sob with fear. Other times we shut down our emotions and refuse to feel or confront our situation.

Emotions are gifts from our Creator and they need to be acknowledged. But no matter what the challenge, we must trust God. Why? Because without trust, guidance is meaningless. We have to be in a place of spiritual trust before the Holy Spirit can talk to us and show us the path we need to take. We have to be in a place of spiritual trust before we can actually take the actions we are directed to take. We have to be in a place of spiritual trust before we can continue to hold to that path in spite of people and events that would be obstacles to us.

Trust is the foundation of our relationship with God. When it comes to our health, the appearance of trust is easy. The reality of putting trust in God before putting trust in any human being (including family, friends, and medical personnel) is sometimes quite difficult.

Trusting God does not mean that you disregard the opinions and advice of others, but it does mean that you allow God's guidance to determine the choices you make. Take a deep breath now and declare your faith in your Creator.

O, Mighty Father, I seek to live in trust with every breath I take. But I struggle sometimes, God. I get lost. I get scared. And I realize that I have wandered off the path you mean for me to walk. Hold me close, God. Bring me back. Help me to keep my focus on trusting You. You are my Creator and I trust You to guide me. I trust You to heal my soul and my spirit, and I trust You to heal my body according to the methods You feel are best for me. In the name of the Father, Son, and the Holy Spirit, I pray, Amen.

Day 267

Be not deceived; God is not mocked: for whatsoever a man soweth, that shall he also reap.
(Galatians 6:7 KJV)

God set up a world that has simple operating principles. One of the most important is that what we sow determines what we reap. Whatever we do has an effect; it has consequences. The interesting thing is that for the most part these consequences are not unexpected. Yet time and again we claim surprise because we want to blame someone or something other than ourselves for the situation in which we find ourselves.

If you want to be well, you must understand this principle. God will not be mocked. You can't violate His laws of good health and then moan and pretend to be innocent. If you poison the soil with chemicals and spray your food with pesticides, you can expect to reap the deadly results. If you sit all day and do not move your body, you can expect to reap the crippling results. If you stress yourself by working at a job you do not love, then you can expect to reap the depleting results.

You reap not only what you sow yourself, but you also reap what your parents and your grandparents have sown. As each generation does things which weakens them, they pass along DNA that is a little weaker to each succeeding generation.

God has given *us* authority here to have dominion. We forget this fact although it is clearly written in God's Word. We tend to blame God in times of disaster and even hold Him responsible for making us sick. "It's God's will," we claim. We fail to look at all the ways that the seeds of illness were sown by us and our parents and do not want to accept the responsibility of reaping the consequences.

God will not be mocked. But the incredible truth is that He is willing to extend His grace to you and to heal you in spite of what you have done. He forgives you of your sins and He heals you of your diseases. He loves you beyond your imagination.

Dear God, I know I am reaping what I have sown. I am truly sorry for the mistakes that I have made that have contributed to my current health situation. Being sorry doesn't mean anything unless I take action to do things differently. I know many of the things to do and I am doing them. Guide me, God, and lead me according to Your plan and design. In the name of Your Son, Jesus Christ, I pray, Amen.

Day 268

Worship the Lord your God, and his blessing will be on your food and water. (Exodus 23:25 NIV)

Let every breath and every action be joyful worship of the Lord God Almighty, the Great I AM. Worshipping God means going to Him with honor and with reverence and giving Him an exalted place in your soul and in your life. When you do this, what will happen?

This passage gives us a bit of a surprise for an answer. It tells us that God's blessing will be on your food and water. That certainly seems to take us from the sublime to the mundane, doesn't it? Let's see now, when you honor God, He will bless your food and water. Why does God care about those things?

For that matter, why do Christians ask a blessing on their food and water before every meal? Part of it is to remind ourselves of God's sovereignty and grace in our lives. But the other part is that God's blessing on our food and water is integral to our physical vitality.

Food and water provide the basic nutrition that we need in order for our bodies to be healthy. Since God wants us to be healthy, He needs for us to eat the proper foods that will nourish and sustain us. When we sit down to eat, God *wants* to bless our food. He *wants* to keep us healthy and strong.

When God blesses our food, He fills it with His power and presence, and therefore there is no room for the evil one to exist in it. The blessing on your food actually changes the vibrations in it. God's power of transformation is loosed on each item on your plate to make it healthier to eat than it was before the blessing.

At your next meal, bow your head and ask God to bless your food and water. Don't say your blessing mechanically, but instead say it with conviction and purpose. Feel the Holy Spirit fill you and your food. Eat slowly and know that you are receiving not only nutritious food for your body but also the energy and healing love of God.

Loving God, thank You for the abundance of the foods that You have provided for me. I do my best to locate pure, wholesome, organic food as You designed it because I understand the importance of unadulterated food for the health of my body. I worship You, Jehovah-rapha, as my God and my Creator. Let Your blessing always be on my food and my water so that I may be strong in fulfilling Your purpose for my life. In Jesus' name, I pray, Amen.

Day 269

He himself bore our sins in his body on the tree, so that we might die to sins and live for righteousness; by his wounds you have been healed. For you were like sheep going astray, but now you have returned to the Shepherd and Overseer of your souls. (1 Peter 2:24-25 NIV)

"By His wounds you have been healed." Hallelujah!

Repeat out loud three times, "By His wounds I have been healed." "By His wounds I have been healed." "By His wounds I have been healed." It has already been done. Claim it, because it has already been done. What you are seeking now is the manifestation of that healing.

Healing of the body alone means nothing if your soul is in jeopardy. That is the reason that Jesus came to bear both our sins and our infirmities. The healing of both body and soul was part of Jesus' mission. He said to the teachers of the law who opposed Him, "Which is easier to say, 'Your sins are forgiven,' or to say, 'Get up and walk'?" When He spoke both the words of forgiveness *and* the words of healing to a paralytic, the paralytic was healed.

Jesus bore our sins in his body on the tree. Ask God's forgiveness for your sins. Sometimes "sin" is a word that we use to mean doing great wrongs such as stealing or killing. But what about those little actions in life when we break in a line or cut someone off in our car or are rude to someone on the phone. Or what about the times when we fail to do certain things that we know we should – such as failing to pay attention that it was someone's birthday, not doing household chores that need to be done, or not calling someone who is lonely.

Sins are really anything that misses the mark. Whatever yours are, ask God to forgive you. The sense of relief and release frees you to focus your energy on healing your body instead of defending your mistakes.

We have been claimed by our Shepherd. See yourself standing peacefully and contentedly in His shadow as He stands by watching you, caring for you, and loving you.

Lord God Almighty, thank You for sending Your Son Jesus Christ to bear my sins in his body on the tree, so that I might die to my sins and live for righteousness. By His wounds I have been healed! I was like a sheep going astray, but now I have been returned to You, my shepherd and overseer of my soul. Thank You, Lord, for redeeming me. I come willingly to You. I was lost but now I am found. In the name of Your Son, Jesus Christ, I pray, Amen.

Day 270

It is the Spirit who testifies, because the Spirit is the truth. (1 John 5:6 NIV)

Jesus asked the Father to send us the Holy Spirit as our beacon of truth. What does that mean to us when we feel sick? It means that, before we take any action with regard to our health, we ask the Holy Spirit to reveal to us the course of action that is in alignment with God's will.

Let's take a concrete example. Suppose you notice a problem with your vision. You go to God in prayer with the question, "Should I see an ophthalmologist?" You hear a "yes." The doctor diagnoses macular degeneration, telling you that there is no medical cure, but that a new laser procedure might help. What do you do now? Do you have the new treatment? Or do you start researching large print books and aids for the blind? Or do you pretend that somehow everything will be all right and do nothing? How do you find God's truth for you?

Learn as much as you can about your condition by asking the Holy Spirit to guide you in your search for information. For example, you find a supplement and herbal treatment protocol that a doctor has used to reverse the early stages of your disease; you discover the testimony of some people who have reversed their condition with magnetic therapy; and you discover that sometimes people's vision has gotten worse after the new laser procedure.

Now you ask one question at a time. Phrasing questions that require only a yes or no response make it much easier to discern the answer. Ask, "God, do you want me to use some form of herbal support for my eyes?" Then listen for the answer. "Do you want me to use magnet therapy?" Then listen. "God, do you want me to have the laser treatment?" And listen again. Slowly, one at a time proceed down your entire list of possibilities. Be sure your answer has come from the Holy Spirit and only the Holy Spirit, remembering that the evil one will try to deceive you. At the end ask if there is another option that you should consider that you haven't mentioned.

Now you know what to do for today. Each new day brings more questions so keep asking. As you heal and move forward with your recovery, both the questions and the answers change.

Almighty God, help me to follow always your wonderful Counselor, the Holy Spirit. My life is in Your loving hands. I will do Your will. In the name of Christ Jesus, my Savior and my Redeemer, I pray, Amen.

Day 271

On his arrival, Jesus found that Lazarus had already been in the tomb for four days. . . .
"Lord," Martha said to Jesus, "if you had been here, my brother would not have died. But
I know that even now God will give you whatever you ask." . . . Jesus, once more deeply
moved, came to the tomb. It was a cave with a stone laid across the entrance. "Take away the
stone," he said. "But Lord," said Martha, the sister of the dead man, "by this time there is a
bad odor, for he has been there four days." Then Jesus said, "Did I not tell you that if you
believed, you would see the glory of God?" . . . Jesus called in a loud voice, "Lazarus,
come out!" The dead man came out, his hands and feet wrapped with strips of linen, and a
cloth around his face. Jesus said to them, "Take off the grave clothes and let him go."
(John 11:17, 21-22, 38-40, 43-44 NIV)

Have you ever wondered why Jesus asked the mourners at Lazarus' tomb to take away the stone? Surely it would have been just as easy for Jesus to have rolled the stone away as to raise Lazarus from the dead. Jesus was teaching both the mourners and us a very important lesson: it is up to us to do our part as we participate in our healing.

We have to be willing to listen, and we have to be willing to act on the guidance that we hear. Since Jesus was standing beside Martha, talking to her, it was very easy for her to hear Him with her ears. She knew Him; she trusted Him; she loved Him; she had seen Him heal other people. Yet when He gave her the first instruction, she objected. The first word out of her mouth was "But . . ." She was being asked to trust, to have faith, and to take action according to the guidance that she was given – even if it didn't make sense to her.

We have not seen Jesus in the flesh as Martha did. Nevertheless, we are called to obedience in exactly the same way that she was. When illness struck her brother, she sent for Jesus. Likewise, when the evil one attacks us with illness, we are to call on Christ immediately.

We are to go to Him in prayer. Then we ask the Holy Spirit to reveal to us what we are to do for our healing. We may be healed instantly. More likely, we will be told the first step to take, the first stone to roll away. Sometimes it makes no sense to us.

Nevertheless, we are required to have faith, to be obedient, and to take action.

Wonderful Jehovah-rapha, show me the stone to roll away and I will do it. I will obey Your
guidance because I trust in Your healing. Raise me up, Lord, and set me free. In the name
of Your Son, Jesus Christ, Amen.

Day 272

And let the peace (soul harmony which comes) from Christ rule (act as umpire continually) in your hearts [deciding and settling with finality all questions that arise in your minds, in that peaceful state] to which as [members of Christ's] one body you were also called [to live]. And be thankful (appreciative), [giving praise to God always]. (Colossians 3:15 AMP)

Is your heart filled with peace and soul-harmony? Peace is a pool of tranquility that reflects your connection to your Creator. It is one of the things that people value most and yet rarely have.

There is no peace if we are filled with bitterness about our health condition. There is no peace if we are filled with loneliness and despair. There is no peace if we are angry with our family and friends. There is no peace if we are terrified about our future. There is no peace if we are afraid to die. And there is no peace if we are afraid to live.

The expansion of this Scripture that is provided by The Amplified Bible helps us to understand the intent of Paul's words. He so beautifully explains how it is that we can have peace in our hearts. It is through letting Christ and the Holy Spirit rule in our hearts and settle *with finality* all questions that arise in our minds. All questions!

When we feel sick, there are many, many decisions to be made, and the choices seem endless. If we use our *own* wisdom or that of other people only, we are often burdened with doubts about whether we have done the "right" thing or the "wrong" thing.

Instead of struggling with these decisions, we need to turn them over to God and let Christ rule in our hearts. We are then guided to the right path for us, and the result is peace in our soul. We are called to *live*, not merely to survive in a desperate struggle from one day to the next.

Take your concerns to God in prayer now. Breathe deeply and listen for your guidance. Feel the peace of Christ come upon you. And give thanks.

Gracious God, I let myself get caught in a trap of confusion and I feel overwhelmed. I want You and Your Son Jesus Christ to settle with finality all my questions and concerns. I come to You, Jehovah-rapha. You are the God who heals me. I choose to live, Lord, and I offer myself to You. Rule my heart; rule my life; direct my path and I will follow. Bless me with Your peace. Thank You, merciful Lord. In Jesus' name, I pray, Amen.

Day 273

O Lord, how manifold are thy works! In wisdom hast thou made them all: the earth is full of thy riches. (Psalm 104:24 KJV)

It is regrettable that we fail to educate ourselves about the riches of the earth and sources of good nutrition that exist around us. One primary example is the lowly dandelion, a treasure house of nutrition and healing properties. Think of the amount of money that is spent each year by people buying pesticides that kill the dandelion and poison our earth and water supply in the process. Where yards have been sprayed with pesticides, the dandelions cannot be eaten for several years after the spraying has stopped.

It is quite likely that, if there are dandelions growing in your yard, you need them! You can even put the lovely yellow flower petals in your salad for potassium, iron, and vitamin A. The dandelion leaf has high levels of beta-carotene which provides a safe source of vitamin A for the body, and it is also a good source of potassium for muscular strength. Dandelion leaves are beneficial to the skin and eyes, help keep hollow organs free from mucus build-up and infection, strengthen the immune system, and assist those with low blood sugar to stabilize their blood sugar level.

Dandelion roots are a wonderful source of sodium, one of the primary minerals needed for the body to balance pH levels internally. Most people think of sodium in the form of salt or sodium chloride. It is very difficult for the human body to break the sodium chloride bond; consequently, there can be unhealthy complications from consuming large amounts of salt. Interestingly, when you eat vegetable sources with high organic sodium content, you can actually drive out old inorganic sodium deposits from the body. Dandelion root extracts have historically been used for such health problems as muscle and joint stiffness, ulcers, stomach disorders, liver cleansing, and blood cleansing. It is a very valuable blood builder.

It is no accident that we have dandelions in our yards. They were put there *in wisdom* and were meant to be used for our nourishment and healing.

Almighty God, forgive me for being uninformed about Your creations. Forgive me for destroying what You created in wisdom. Help me to protect this earth and build my health. I want to learn, Lord. In Jesus' name, I pray, Amen.

Day 274

There is a way that seems right to a man and appears straight before him, but at the end of it is the way of death. (Proverbs 16:25 AMP)

It is interesting that this same verse appears twice in Proverbs. It is repeated here and in Proverbs 14:12. Often when our health problems hit us hard, we find we are on "the way of death" even though we had thought we were doing the "right" thing. The root of the problem is our failure to include God as a full partner in each of our decisions. We hand over responsibility for our health to scientists and to government "authorities" and follow their pronouncements instead of taking their recommendations to God before acting.

Edward Jenner believed he was doing something beneficial for mankind when he discovered the technique of vaccinations for smallpox. At first glance it would seem that only positive things have resulted since smallpox has almost been eradicated throughout the world. Repeatedly, a new vaccine is hailed as the solution to a current health problem. It is particularly seductive because having a simple shot means no one has to change what he is doing – or ask God for guidance. We now have a great proliferation of vaccines that are administered to our children. By the age of six most American children have received more than twenty-five. Unfortunately, no one really knows all of the effects of these vaccines. We know that larger and larger numbers of children are experiencing asthma, allergies, ear infections, and other problems. And many reputable scientists believe that "new" diseases afflicting adults in their forties, fifties, and sixties are a result of mutated viruses received from childhood vaccinations.

We now eat genetically engineered foods – most without our knowledge or consent. Do we really believe that we know more about making a healthy tomato than God? What arrogance! What roads to death are we paving for ourselves and for our children?

The point of God's Word in Proverbs is that you must not follow any human being *unquestioningly*. Ask questions. Seek the "facts." Then take this information to God in prayer and follow only Him.

Almighty God, I pray for scientists and ask that they be filled with Your Holy Spirit so that their discoveries will benefit us. Let me not be complaisant, Lord, so that my right to follow Your guidance is taken away from me by an unwise government. Keep me ever mindful of the deceptions of the evil one, and, as Your Son Jesus taught me to pray, deliver me from him. In Jesus' name, I pray, Amen.

Day 275

If your brother sins against you, go and show him his fault, just between the two of you. If he listens to you, you have won your brother over. But if he will not listen, take one or two others along, so that 'every matter may be established by the testimony of two or three witnesses.' If he refuses to listen to them, tell it to the church; and if he refuses to listen even to the church, treat him as you would a pagan or a tax collector. (Matthew 18:15-17 NIV)

Your physical health is integrally connected to your emotional and spiritual health. If you are carrying bitterness, anger, sorrow, or grief for a family member or friend or acquaintance, whether living or dead, that inner pain is affecting your health in a negative way. You cannot carry negative feelings without paying a price.

Jesus gives us an important lesson here in how to handle the situation. Even though in this particular passage He is talking about a situation in which your brother has wronged you, it certainly applies to any situation involving relationships, including those in which there may be wrongs on your part as well. Jesus shows us how to do what we can to work things out.

Notice that you must be heard. You are to be persistent in trying to work things out only up to a point. You are not supposed to keep trying to force things to be amenable because in doing so you violate both yourself and the other person.

Remember that God forces no one to love Him; you must allow others the same freedom – the right *not* to love you. Also remember that Jesus said that His family was those who shared His journey and followed God's will, not simply those into whose family He was born.

Ask God for the courage to shake the dust of those who do not choose to receive you off your feet. Trust Him to bring new family into your life. You will experience a new freedom, and you will open your soul and your body up for God's love to heal not only your spirit but also every cell in your body.

Loving Father, I have been to my brother and I have not been received. Hold him in Your loving arms and give me courage to let go in love and to stop replaying the relationship I have missed. Wipe my tears that flow; I offer them in behalf of someone who is also hurting today. I choose to sing a song of praise to You and I thank You for healing my spirit and my body. Love me, Lord. In Jesus' name, I pray, Amen.

Day 276

Do not overwork to be rich; because of your own understanding, cease! Will you set your eyes on that which is not? For riches certainly make themselves wings; they fly away like an eagle toward heaven. (Proverbs 23:4-5 NKJV)

Money is certainly useful and there is nothing wrong with having it. God created a world of great abundance and we are to enjoy that world. Jesus sometimes used money as illustrations in his parables, and His examples emphasized the importance of multiplication of money as well as its wise and prudent use.

Yet the pursuit of riches as its own goal is a deceptive path. Working day and night for the power or security of money in the end depletes you and leaves you with nothing of value. Feeling driven to work has a disastrous effect on your health.

The sense of never having enough time and of needing to do more and more in less and less time creates enormous stress in the body that eventually weakens the immune system and many organ systems. This kind of overwork reflects an inner lack of faith in God's timing and God's plan at work in your life.

Take some "time out" to get connected to God. Take an afternoon off or a day off and create a mini-retreat for yourself. Find a place where you can be contemplative and worshipful. If you stay at home, take the phone off the hook and arrange for a private, quiet time alone. Release your concerns to God. Ask Him to set your timetables and to establish your work schedule. Trust Him with your work.

Do not be deceived by the illusion that rich people "have it all." Ask God for His guidance in showing you how you are to meet your financial needs. And when you are blessed with financial abundance, ask God for ways that you can share it with others.

Almighty God, help me to keep my perspectives straight in life. It is easy to get caught up in the struggle for money. Money seems so important, and sometimes I believe that having it will solve all of my problems. Show me, God, the purpose You have for my life. I trust that, as I stay faithful to follow Your plan for me, all my needs will be met. Help me to be ever mindful of the needs of others and to share what I have – whether it is from the scarcity of the widow's mite or from great abundance. Teach me to work for You, God, and not for earthly wealth. In Jesus' name, I pray, Amen.

Day 277

They will be like a well-watered garden, and they will sorrow no more. Then maidens will dance and be glad, young men and old as well. I will turn their mourning into gladness; I will give them comfort and joy instead of sorrow. (Jeremiah 31:12-13 NIV)

How do you handle disappointment, sadness, and regrets? Some people stay locked in their grief and bound by their sorrow all their life. The wound in their soul and their emotions remains unhealed, and they never engage fully with life again. Instead, they live with a piece of themselves that is dead and lifeless. Frequently, this leads to illness and disease. Grief can actually depress the immune system; sorrow can cause constrictions in blood vessels decreasing blood flow to organs and cells. There are often cases of spouses who have lived many years together and who die within months of each other. The grief of the surviving spouse was so overwhelming as to have a catastrophic effect on both body and spirit.

Take a look at your life. Are you carrying some sorrow or grief? It may be for a person you loved and who has died. Or it may be a sorrow for something you missed when you were growing up. It is very common for people growing up in seriously dysfunctional families to carry grief for not being loved as they needed to be loved. There is also grief for a life situation that you missed. You may have longed to be married and grieve over never having found a spouse – or you may have longed to be a parent and grieve over never having had children.

When we suffer a great loss, there is a time to mourn and to grieve. A strong love deserves strong grief. But at some point we have to offer our grief to God. Grief can provide a hiding place and give us an excuse to withdraw from life. It takes courage to give our grief to God, to let go of the past, and to become fully engaged in the present. God has a mission and a purpose for us, and we cannot fulfill it if we are looking backward to the way things were and are bemoaning the way things might have been.

Are you willing to let go of your grief? God promises to turn your mourning into gladness and to give you comfort and joy instead of sorrow. God is always with you and He wants you to live and to fulfill His purpose for your life.

Almighty God, I have grieved long enough. Turn my mourning into gladness. Give me comfort and joy. Fill my body with Your healing blessing. In the name of Your Son, Jesus Christ, I pray, Amen.

Day 278

Delight thyself also in the Lord; and he shall give thee the desires of thine heart.
(Psalm 37:4 KJV)

Most people like to quote this passage but few really believe it is true. The reason that people don't "get" this proverb is that they don't realize that they often have hidden agendas buried deeply within their heart and soul.

You may say you want prosperity. Is your work also your joy or are you doing it simply because you have calculated its monetary reward?

You may say you desire a life mate. Do you have the qualities you are seeking in someone else? You attract who you are, not who you want to be.

You may say you want to be healthy. Are you willing to let *God*, and not some human being, make the final decision in every step along your path to recovery? Are you willing to let go of the benefits of being ill, such as getting support and attention? Are you willing to stop being angry with God for things that have happened – or things that didn't happen – to you in your life?

You must be brave enough to look deeply within at the *true* desires of your heart because these are what God sees. Which ones are desires of a little child who was hurt many years ago but who still holds onto those hurts and those fears? And which ones are desires of an adult, angry with God for seeming to have let him or her down in the past? These subterranean desires are powerful, protective mechanisms that control your life until you reveal and transform them.

Ferret out your true desires for your health. If you desire to be well, examine your heart for your hidden desires that block you from it. Find the things that hinder your faith and undermine your trust. Remove them from your heart and offer them to God. Make the desire of your heart for health clear and pure before the Lord.

Dear God, give me the courage to look deeply within my heart. Give me the courage to find all my hidden agendas and to bring each one into the light. Give me the courage to examine each one, keep the ones I want, and throw the rest away. I choose to remove all impediments to my healing, giving You all my emotional crutches, all my anger, and all my fear. Create in me a new heart with a clear desire to be well. Thank you, Jehovah-rapha, for healing me. In the name of Your Son, Jesus Christ, my Savior and my Redeemer, I pray, Amen.

Day 279

Do not be quick with your mouth, do not be hasty in your heart to utter anything before God. God is in heaven and you are on earth, so let your words be few. (Ecclesiastes 5:2 NIV)

But when ye pray, use not vain repetitions, as the heathen do: for they think that they shall be heard for their much speaking. Be not ye therefore like unto them: for your Father knoweth what things ye have need of, before ye ask him. (Matthew 6:7-8 KJV)

Don't keep begging God to heal you. State your need clearly one time, remembering that "the Father knows what you need before you ask Him." When you ask for your healing, do so simply and without giving a detailed list of all your woes. Jesus tells us "not to keep on babbling like pagans, for they think they will be heard because of their many words."

Why is Jesus saying this? Because He wants you to understand that the way you pray reflects the quality of your faith. If you keep going on and on, wallowing in your problem, you are exhibiting a lack of faith in the willingness of Jehovah to be your healer and deliverer. If you pray over and over and over again for healing, you are proving that either you do not believe you have been heard or that you do not believe God has taken action in your behalf. For example, suppose a friend asks for a loan and you tell him that you will give it to him at the end of the week when you get paid. If your friend doubts you, he will keep asking you about the loan; if he trusts you, he will say nothing more until he receives the money.

So what is the best way to pray for healing? Ask once for healing for a particular problem. Then until that healing is manifested, be like Jonah and offer prayers of thanksgiving for being heard and for being delivered. Praise God for your healing. And ask Him to reveal to you if there is anything that you need to do in order to participate in your healing. If you receive instructions, follow them. If you do not, then stand firm on God's Word, keep praising Jehovah-rapha, and wait patiently.

Dear Father, teach me to speak to You simply and without vain repetitions. Sometimes my faith weakens and I find myself asking You again for healing. Forgive me, Father, for doubting Your Word and Your will for my healing. I thank You, Jehovah-rapha, for hearing me. In Jesus' name, I pray, Amen.

Day 280

In the same way, the Spirit helps us in our weakness. We do not know what we ought to pray for, but the Spirit himself intercedes for us with groans that words cannot express. And he who searches our hearts knows the mind of the Spirit, because the Spirit intercedes for the saints in accordance with God's will. (Romans 8:26-27 NIV)

Isn't this an interesting statement of Paul – "we do not know what we ought to pray for"? Usually we think we are sure exactly what we should pray for.

When we feel sick, most of us pray to "be well." But if we leave our prayer vague and broadly worded, we absolve ourselves of the responsibility to take action, having left our healing up to "God's will" which many of us are not even sure includes our healing. The other end of the spectrum is to seek medical advice, to begin treatment, and *then* to pray for a successful outcome of the particular treatment we have begun. Again, we have absolved ourselves of the responsibility for our own actions, having handed it over to medical authorities.

Be clear in your own mind that it is God's will for you to be well. Then ask the Holy Spirit to help you in your weakness. Ask the Holy Spirit to intercede for you before Jehovah-rapha. Ask the Holy Spirit to guide you in every step along your path to your healing. Offer each option for healing that you can think of to God in prayer.

But remember the advice that we may "not know what to pray for." So ask the Holy Spirit to reveal to you all appropriate revelation knowledge for your healing. Then be quiet and listen.

Give grateful thanks that the Holy Spirit will intercede for you. Stand firm on God's Word and trust that you will be directed along your own particular pathway to healing.

Merciful God, I realize that there are times when I don't know what I should pray for. Thank You for sending the Holy Spirit to help me and intercede for me. It is my desire that everything I do be in accordance with Your Holy will just as everything that Your Son Christ Jesus did was in accordance with Your Holy will. He healed all who came to Him. I come to Your Son. I come, O Lord. Help me in my weakness. Guide me. Show me the path You want me to take today for my healing. In the name of Your Son, Jesus Christ, I pray, Amen.

Day 281

And there he found a certain man named Aeneas, which had kept his bed eight years, and was sick of the palsy. And Peter said unto him, "Aeneas, Jesus Christ maketh thee whole: arise, and make thy bed." And he arose immediately. (Acts 9:33-34 KJV)

Peter wasn't anyone "special." He was a fisherman, not a learned medical person of science. When the going got really tough, he even denied that he knew Jesus. Yet here he is, having repented of betraying Christ and doing exactly what Jesus told him to do – going into the world sharing the gospel and healing the sick.

Peter said to Aeneas, "Jesus Christ maketh thee whole." Jesus Christ makes *you* whole, too. Do you believe that statement? *Can* you believe it?

It would seem strange not to believe it, yet few really do. We allow ourselves to be caught up in doubts, in shame, and in confusion. We find it hard to shake many church traditions which tell us that God has a purpose for making us sick – and, if that is so, then we can't be sure whether God wants us to be well. We find it hard to believe that God would want to save, rescue, and heal *us*.

We also find it hard to believe that God can speak to us to tell us the tiny details necessary for our recovery. For example, God can tell us which essential oils to use in our healing. God can tell us what herbs to take and exactly how much. God can tell us which foods to eat and when. God can tell us which fabrics are healthiest for us to wear. God can advise us about man-made medications also. Every element of our health is important to God, and He is there to help and guide us.

God calls us to rise and make our bed. Put away the thoughts and actions of cultivating illness. Get up and get on with the business of living. Visualize this as your reality. See yourself being a living witness for the glory of God. Keep your eyes focused on your Risen Lord and take action.

Almighty Father, thank You for message of love, redemption, and healing as it is revealed in Your Holy Scripture. I am filled with hope and inspiration by reading the accounts of the early church in action. When I see Peter healing those who suffer, I know that I, too, can be healed. Thank you, Lord, for your great mercies on me. Help me to grow in faith and to be a witness to others of Your glorious healing power. In the name of Your Son, Jesus Christ, who makes me whole, I pray, Amen.

Day 282

. . . If we are being called to account today for an act of kindness shown to a cripple and are asked how he was healed, then know this, you and all the people of Israel: It is by the name of Jesus Christ of Nazareth, whom you crucified but whom God raised from the dead, that this man stands before you healed. He [Jesus] is the stone you builders rejected, which has become the capstone. Salvation is found in no one else, for there is no other name under heaven given to men by which we must be saved. (Acts 4:9-12 NIV)

Peter healed a crippled man and he got into trouble for it. The rulers, elders, and teachers of the law called Peter before them for questioning. They wanted to stop this from happening again, and they wanted to know the source of his power. Peter told them plainly that his power came from Jesus, whom God had raised from the dead.

Verse 12 is an important one. "Salvation is found in no one else, for there is no other name under heaven given to men by which we must be saved." The first word in the sentence is "soteria," a Greek word which means salvation, rescue, and deliverance. The last word in the sentence is "sozo," a Greek word which means save, rescue, deliver, and *heal*. Notice that being saved and being healed are bound together in the meaning of the word just as Jesus repeatedly bound them together in his description of His mission and purpose and in His instructions to all His followers for *their* mission and *their* purpose.

Accept the salvation that God has offered to you. Praise God that you have been given salvation for your soul, your precious eternal self. But recognize, accept, and believe that this salvation is for your *entire* being – for your mind and your body as well. No more can satan have the power to torment you, depress you, discourage you. No more can satan have the power to fill your body with diseases, ailments, and sicknesses. Satan can have this power only if you allow him to have it. Give your complete, focused faith to Jesus Christ, who has redeemed, saved, and healed you.

Dear God, I am saved. I am healed. Your Holy Word proclaims it. Your Son Jesus Christ proclaims it. My wholeness of spirit and body is Your Divine will. You sent Your Son to redeem me. Two thousand years ago You redeemed me. Salvation is found in no one but You, God. I accept Your salvation, Your rescue, Your deliverance, and Your healing. Thank you, God, for Your mercy and Your blessings. In the name of Jesus Christ, my Savior and my Redeemer, I pray, Amen.

Day 283

These all look to you to give them their food at the proper time. When you give it to them, they gather it up; when you open your hand, they are satisfied with good things. When you hide your face, they are terrified; when you take away their breath, they die and return to the dust. (Psalm 104:27-29 NIV)

In this psalm David speaks of death. "When You take away their breath, they die and return to the dust." This depiction of death is interesting because it shows the way we are really supposed to die. The psalmist has just told us that God gives us food to nourish us and that He satisfies us with good things. Among those good things is a life lived in service to the Lord. God breathed in Adam the breath of life. He wants us to fulfill the number of our days and then, when it is time, He will simply "take away our breath" and we will die.

We should live a long, healthy life in service to God and for His glory. There is no reason why we should die a long and agonizing death. That is part of satan's plan, not God's. Jesus would certainly not have worked so hard and so consistently to heal people – without one single exception – if it were not God's will for us to be well.

What happens when God's plan is subverted by the evil one? We die early before our time. Take a look at every account in the Scriptures of someone being raised from the dead either in the Old Testament or the New Testament. It was never a person who had already fulfilled his years; it was always someone who had died prematurely. Satan delights in interfering with God's plans. Nevertheless, satan can never prevail in the end, because God will always bring His children to Himself.

If we live in partnership with God and accept responsibility for our health, we will take the actions we need to take for being well. We then affirm to God our desire to live and to receive God's blessings, including good health.

When we have fulfilled our days and it is time to be welcomed to our heavenly home, we simply let God take back the breath of life and move it – and us – to the place Jesus has prepared for us, according to His word and His promise.

Lord God Almighty, I want to fulfill my days in this bodily temple in good health and in total service to You. When the time comes and I am old, I look forward to Your taking my earthly breath as gently as You gave it and then to being with You in my heavenly home. In the name of Your Son, Jesus Christ, I pray, Amen.

Day 284

Blessed are those who mourn, for they will be comforted. (Matthew 5:4 NIV)

What are your inner wounds? Loneliness? Rejection? Betrayal? What are your deepest unfulfilled longings? For your family to love you? To feel secure and safe in the lives of the people you love? Every person wants to be loved, just as he is. It seems such a simple desire. Yet we are often insecure and hurting, driven by our fear into behaviors that only deepen our pain and compound our problem. We keep knocking on the wrong door, begging to be let in and pushing the grief of rejection deeper and deeper into our soul.

Jesus tells us the way out. Blessed are they who mourn for they shall be comforted. You must mourn your inner child who suffered pain, fear, and loneliness. You must mourn your inner child who looked at the world with the freshness of a young soul and who could not comprehend what was happening. You must mourn your inner child who handled the pain in the best way he knew how. As you grieve, offer your pain and your suffering up for the ones who hurt you. Offer it up for *their* pain. And offer it up for the pain and suffering of someone you don't even know.

Hand your pain and your grief to God. Ask Him to take it and to heal the holes in your soul. Ask Jesus to come in and to fill you with His Christ-light so that you will shine with His love. In the process you will release your resentment toward those who are the source of this pain. You may also choose to communicate directly with the person or through prayer if the person does not want to receive you or has died.

Remember that Jesus admonished us to love others as ourselves, so if you allow others to act abusively to you and to treat you with disrespect, you are simply creating more pain. And you will have to acknowledge that this new pain is a consequence of your own actions and *you* are the one responsible for it. You cannot fix or change others. You can fix only yourself with the help of God.

Mourn your pain and release it to God. You will be comforted by knowing that you are a beloved child of God and always have a home in His loving arms. You will receive healing for your soul and for your body as well.

Loving Father, I have faced the pains of my past and I give them to You. Take them, Lord. Heal my wounds. I rest in Your loving arms. In Jesus' name, I pray, Amen.

Day 285

Ask, and it shall be given you; seek, and ye shall find; knock, and it shall be opened unto you: for every one that asketh receiveth; and he that seeketh findeth; and to him that knocketh it shall be opened. (Matthew 7:7-8 KJV)

Jesus tells us here how to be well. Ask, seek, and knock. Go to God, Jesus tells us. Go to your Creator.

God does not intrude on us. He does not force Himself in our lives or in our hearts. God created us as His family but He allows us to run away as rebellious children. He could lock us up, but He doesn't. Satan is the one who seeks to imprison us, not God. So God says, "You must come looking for me." But He also says, "I am here!"

All of us have times when we have strayed away from God's presence. We have gotten off the track. Jesus tells you that you have to make the journey toward God on your own. You must go to Him. This is not a journey to be made in fear, however, because Jesus' message was clear and consistent: God loves you. God loves you all the more because you are trying so hard to find Him.

Ask, seek, and knock. Why would Jesus have made such a sweeping statement as this? Isn't it interesting that He didn't give us a list of exceptions? He didn't say, "But don't ask to be healed, because it is God's will for you to be sick." Jesus simply said, "Ask." This isn't like a child wishing for a pony. This is telling God the deepest desires of our heart.

All of these words are action words that require you to do something. All of these things have an underlying foundation of faith and trust. You must ask, *believing* that it will be given. You must seek, *believing* that you will find. You must knock, *believing* that the door will be opened. Stand on the Word of God and trust in your healing.

Gracious Lord, I come to You willingly. Your Precious Son Jesus taught me to ask, seek, and knock. I am asking, God. Guide my steps so that I find my path to my healing. Open the door so that I may step into Your loving arms. Enfold me, God, in Your healing wings. I choose to have the faith to trust even when I don't see evidence of my healing at the physical level. I trust that You are manifesting it in Your own way. In the name of Your Son, Jesus Christ, my Savior and my Redeemer, I pray, Amen.

Day 286

Which of you fathers, if your son asks for a fish, will give him a snake instead? Or if he asks for an egg, will give him a scorpion? If you then though you are evil, know how to give good gifts to your children, how much more will your Father in heaven give the Holy Spirit to those who ask him! (Luke 11:11-13 NIV)

Controversy abounds about the advisability of eating eggs. One day the media reports on studies that warn us of the hazards from substances in eggs and another day the media reports on contradicting studies that report that eggs are good for us after all. For years we have been told that eggs were loaded with cholesterol and, therefore, we should avoid eating them. Then we were told that eggs also have high levels of lecithin which emulsifies cholesterol – so maybe eggs aren't really so bad. In the confusion we become more and more frustrated.

The egg is a very nutritious food. It is rich in essential fatty acids (especially omega-3) and half the fat in it is monounsaturated (like olive oil). Since it contains all eight essential amino acids, it is a very high-quality protein food. The problems appear to come either when eggs are eaten in excess, or when they are consumed in processed forms – such as powdered egg yolk. Also hens are now caged, drugged with hormones and antibiotics, and generally live miserable, stressed lives. Therefore, we experience problems from eating the chemically contaminated eggs laid by these hens.

The Holy Scriptures offer basic guidelines. Jesus describes an organic, free-range egg as a "good gift" that a father would give his child. Jesus was the One who was sent to redeem us from our sins and our infirmities and to bear our diseases on the Cross. Surely He would not tell us to eat a food that would be universally harmful to our bodies.

God also knows better than any person alive, better than any medical professional, better than any natural health advisor, better than any nutritionist, exactly what your particular nutritional needs are. Ask Him to reveal to you if you are to eat eggs. If you receive an affirmative answer, then ask for information on the precise quantity, frequency, cooking methods, and all the other details you need to know. Give grateful thanks to God for His guidance as you join with Him to restore your temple.

Wonderful Jehovah-rapha, thank You for the gift of the egg. Show me if I am to eat it at this time in my recovery. If so, teach me the ways to use it for my health and nutrition. In Jesus' name, I pray, Amen.

Day 287

May the God of hope fill you with all joy and peace as you trust in him, so that you may overflow with hope by the power of the Holy Spirit. (Romans 15:13 NIV)

Paul describes God as the "God of hope." Sometimes the English meaning of words is a little misleading and that is true here. When we "hope" for something, we aren't sure whether it will happen or not. Hoping and wishing are somewhat similar. We can hope we win the lottery and have no actual belief that we will at all. We are just hoping.

Although Paul speaks of hope, he also uses the phrase, "as you trust in him." Trust is very different from hope. Trust is based on a definite belief in something or someone. Trust between two people has to be developed over time to allow a time of testing to see if each party will be faithful to his word. To hope that you will keep your word and to trust that you will keep your word are two very different things.

God is much more than the God of hope as we usually use that term. Jehovah-rapha is the God of His Word. When you stand on God's Word, you do more than hope. You expect God to fulfill His Word. You don't hope that He will or wonder if He can or guess whether He wants to help you. You *know.* You believe. You trust.

Think of the word "hope" as *inspiration.* "May the God of *inspiration* fill you with all joy and peace as you trust in Him, so that you may overflow with *inspiration* by the power of the Holy Spirit." With God's inspiration we are encouraged to see beyond appearances and to look at our challenges through the eyes of God. We are bolstered and lifted to declare that "I can do all things through Christ who strengthens me."

We are bold to stand on God's Word that He is the God who heals us. We are filled with the knowledge that nothing is too hard for God and that He reigns supreme over everything and everyone, including the evil one.

Be filled with the spirit of the Lord. Let your life radiate the joy and peace of knowing that God keeps His Word.

Wonderful Jehovah-rapha, let Your spirit fill me so that I will overflow with Your inspiration, love, joy, and peace. I do more than overflow with hope, Lord; I overflow with absolute trust that You keep Your Word. You have declared Yourself as the God who heals me. I stand on Your Word and I claim it. Thank You for healing me, Father. You are mighty and awesome and I sing my gratitude and praise to You. In Jesus' name, I pray, Amen.

Day 288

The Lord is [rigidly] righteous in all His ways and gracious and merciful in all His works. The Lord is near to all who call upon Him, to all who call upon Him sincerely and in truth. He will fulfill the desires of those who reverently and worshipfully fear Him; He also will hear their cry and will save them. (Psalm 145:17-19 AMP)

David tells us that God is near to all who call upon Him sincerely and in truth. Notice those qualifying words – "sincerely" and "in truth." Some people call on the Lord in a state of perpetual pouting and childish whining. They have a huge laundry list of all the things that are wrong with them and often accuse God of failing to take all their problems away. They moan and groan and cry, "Why? Why?"

David tells us we can freely call upon the Lord over and over again *as long as we are doing so sincerely and in truth.* What does that mean? That we are willing to be open to what God reveals to us.

How often are we blessed with Divine guidance and then we fail to act on it because we decide that it "won't work" or doesn't follow conventional healing methods? How often do we miss out on our healing because we don't want to take the time to apply herbs or essential oils or other healing substances night after night or day after day? How often do we seal our own fate when we rebel against the path we are shown for being healthy?

We too often want our healing to be quick, simple, and easy. We especially want to be relieved of all responsibility for it. We want someone else to make the decisions, someone else to give us the pills, and someone else to do the work.

If the results are successful, we are delighted and we thank God. If they aren't, we sit back and play the part of the valiant victim who "did everything" and then blame God, saying it was His will that we not be healed.

Call upon God sincerely and in truth. Have the courage to take full responsibility for your actions. Make sure that every single one of those actions is based on specific guidance from the Lord your God.

Dear Father Almighty, I call upon You sincerely and in truth, and I know You are near to me. Give me the courage to face my responsibilities to seek Your guidance and to follow it without question or hesitation. I trust that You want me to be well and that You will show me the path You want me to follow. In Jesus' name, I pray, Amen.

Day 289

By faith Moses' parents hid him for three months after he was born, because they saw he was no ordinary child, and they were not afraid of the king's edict. By faith Moses, when he had grown up, refused to be known as the son of Pharaoh's daughter. He chose to be mistreated along with the people of God rather than to enjoy the pleasures of sin for a short time. He regarded disgrace for the sake of Christ as of greater value than the treasures of Egypt, because he was looking ahead to his reward. By faith he left Egypt, not fearing the king's anger; he persevered because he saw him who is invisible. By faith he kept the Passover and the sprinkling of blood, so that the destroyer of the firstborn would not touch the firstborn of Israel. (Hebrews 11:23-28 NIV)

Faith is the foundation upon which we stand. Like Moses, we declare our faith in Jehovah-rapha and in Christ Jesus in each decision we make and in each action we take. Nonbelievers scoff at the faith of Christians – yet they, too, live lives of faith. The difference is what they put their faith in. Some choose to put their faith in money, some in science, some in political power.

Faith is "the evidence of things not seen" (Hebrews 11:1). We so stubbornly insist on defining reality by our five senses. If we can't see it or touch it, then it isn't real – and conversely, if we can see it and we can touch it, then it must be exactly as it appears to be. This belief system keeps us mired in illness and disease. We insist on focusing on the symptoms that we can see and feel, and we declare that to be our total reality. We begin to define ourselves by the disease we manifest. "I am a diabetic," we say. Or "I am an epileptic." We claim our diseases as a part of us: "I have cancer" and "I have arthritis." As long as we "have" it, it surely "has" us.

What about realities we cannot see with our eyes or touch with our hands? Is God's Word real when it declares that Jehovah-rapha is the God who heals us? Did Christ Jesus "take our infirmities and bear our sicknesses" on Calvary's Cross? To see this reality we must look with the eyes of our soul. We must connect with our Creator through the spirit and be led by our faith to act upon Holy reality. Do not be deceived by the appearance of your illness. Stand on faith in God's reality and Word.

Wonderful Jehovah-rapha, I remain steadfast in my faith in Your healing power. Christ Jesus took my infirmities to Calvary's Cross and He overcame all disease. Thank You, God, for healing me. In Jesus' name, I pray, Amen.

Day 290

Such confidence as this is ours through Christ before God. Not that we are competent in ourselves to claim anything for ourselves, but our competence comes from God. He has made us competent as ministers of a new covenant – not of the letter but of the Spirit; for the letter kills, but the Spirit gives life. . . . Therefore, since we have such a hope, we are very bold. We are not like Moses, who would put a veil over his face to keep the Israelites from gazing at it while the radiance was fading away. But their minds were made dull, for to this day the same veil remains when the old covenant is read. It has not been removed, because only in Christ is it taken away. Even to this day when Moses is read, a veil covers their hearts. But whenever anyone turns to the Lord, the veil is taken away. Now the Lord is the Spirit, and where the Spirit of the Lord is, there is freedom. And we, who with unveiled faces all reflect the Lord's glory, are being transformed into his likeness with ever-increasing glory, which comes from the Lord, who is the Spirit. (2 Corinthians 3:4-6, 12-18 NIV)

We are all ministers of a new covenant, the covenant bought for us with the blood of Christ Jesus. With this covenant we are released from all bondage and step into the world in freedom. Who is it that has overcome the world? Only those who believe that Jesus is the Son of God. Paul tells us that our foundation is not the letter of the law (the traditions of man) but it is the new Spirit of life abundant in Jesus Christ. We are to be transformed into the likeness of Christ by being faithful ministers of this new covenant.

Enforce God's Word on every cell in your body. In the name of Jesus command the evil one to leave your presence. In the name of Jesus command your organs and body systems to function according to God's design and plan. Ask believing that it is already happening and allow the transformation to bring you into wholeness.

As followers of Christ, we are called to put His Words into practice. He repeatedly told his followers to have faith in what they ask. He repeatedly healed all the sick who came to Him. He repeatedly sent His followers out with a dual mission – to preach the gospel of love and repentance and to heal the sick. Accept the command to be a minister of the new covenant. Be a living witness of God's redemptive power – in body and in soul.

Almighty Lord, help me to be a minister of the new covenant, sharing Your message of life, redemption, and healing to all I meet. In the name of Your Son, Christ Jesus, my Savior and my Redeemer, I pray, Amen.

Day 291

For ye have need of patience, that, after ye have done the will of God, ye might receive the promise. (Hebrews 10:36 KJV)

Sometimes your healing doesn't come as quickly as you want. Healing can happen in an instant – but often it comes as part of a process. While God works at His Divine spiritual level, you are to work at the physical level.

Whenever you are dealing with illness, it is important to include in your solutions natural, God-given remedies. It most cases you will find they provide complete solutions for you without having to seek additional man-made assistance.

Determining the proper natural remedies requires commitment on your part to search for information. You must invest some time in order to learn about the astounding variety of remedies God has provided to help His people heal.

Pray for guidance. Always pray for guidance. And then remember the passage in Hebrews and have patience. If you follow the guidance you receive in prayer, you will be following the will of God. If your healing is to be part of a process, then you must persevere patiently in using the remedies you are instructed to use for your healing.

What you must believe in your heart and soul is that, if you keep the faith, you will indeed "receive the promise." Jesus repeatedly told those who came to Him that their faith was an integral part of their healing. "Your faith has made you well," He said.

Faith is the element that keeps you focused on God's promise. It fills every cell in your body with the positive healing energy of God. It provides the environment that is essential for God to fulfill His promise.

Glorious God, I believe. I believe Your Holy Word. I believe Your Holy promises. You have declared that You are the God who heals me. I seek Your guidance always. Keep me on the path that You want me to follow for my healing. I commit myself to follow with patience and perseverance. I know that it is Your will that I be well because Your Holy Scriptures proclaim that message, and I know that Your Son Jesus Christ healed all who came to Him. I also know that Jesus bore my sins and my infirmities on the Cross. Your promise was fulfilled in the blood of Your Precious Son. I will be patient for the manifestation of Your healing. In the name of Christ Jesus, my Savior and my Redeemer, I pray, Amen.

Day 292

Casting the whole of your care [all your anxieties, all your worries, all your concerns, once and for all] on Him, for He cares for you affectionately and cares about you watchfully.
(1 Peter 5:7 AMP)

If you ask a rational person if he would rather be loaded down with worries or if he would rather be literally "care-free," he would undoubtedly tell you that he would prefer to have no burdens.

We know that Jesus specifically told us to give Him our burdens. In fact, we know that Jesus has already carried our heaviest burdens to the Cross. He has already atoned for our sins and he has already borne our sicknesses. It has already been done.

Yet here almost all of us are – steeped in worry, especially when we feel sick. How worry consumes us! It saps our energy, depletes our emotional and physical reserves, and yet still we do it! Jesus stands before us, ready and willing for us to hand our concerns to Him. It ought to be the easiest thing in the world to do. It is certainly easy to *say* the words, "Jesus, I give my worries and my cares to you." But the words are empty without actions to bring them meaning.

To live those words, you must believe that God is all-loving and that He wants you to be well. You must believe that God is all-powerful and that nothing is impossible to those who believe in Jehovah-rapha. You must believe that God can give you very specific instructions and that He does so when you are willing to ask for them.

Satan is crafty and more often than not, you may find yourself picking back up the worries you have given to the Lord. When that happens, don't beat yourself up. Forgive yourself and turn your cares over to God one more time. God understands. He cares for you and waits lovingly to help.

O God, I come to You overwhelmed with my worries. I have many concerns and there are many decisions to make. I feel depleted, God, and I feel afraid. Lord, the truth is that there are days when I just want to crawl in bed and pull the covers over my head and hide. For what seems like the zillionth time, I give my cares to You, God. Each time I give them to You, I find myself taking them back. Teach me to keep giving them to You and to trust that You are showing me the path You want me to follow for my healing. In the name of Your Son, Christ Jesus, my Savior and my Redeemer, I pray, Amen.

Day 293

Some trust in chariots, and some in horses: but we will remember the name of the Lord our God. (Psalm 20:7 KJV)

In a few brief words, the Psalmist graphically describes the arrogance of men who choose to exalt themselves over God.

How sad it is when people misplace their trust. In the days of David some trusted the fastest chariot or the fastest horse. They felt that their safety rested on the power of their "tools." David warned against putting trust in things which have the appearance of power rather than in the Lord God Almighty.

Our situation is no different today. We now have very sophisticated technological tools, and their capacity and power is astounding. In the health arena we have machines that see inside our bodies, instruments that can make incisions with lasers, and drugs powerful enough to kill deadly bacteria.

But beware of putting all of your trust in any of these tools – whether they be drugs, treatments, or surgeries. Power does not lie in our inventions; the only true power lies in the Lord God Almighty.

This does not mean to refuse to use them any more than David was to reject chariots or horses. After all, they are useful tools and many are life-saving ones. The issue is how to use them and when to use them. Most people make the decision to follow a certain medical treatment and *then* pray to God for a successful outcome. Ask God's advice *first*, not last.

On a wider scale, we need more people to pray for a new direction for science. We need to pray for more and more godly scientists, who will ask God *first* how they should explore and who will seek guidance in each step as they create. Bringing God into the creative process insures that we benefit our world instead of harm and destroy it. Your prayers can make a difference for our world and for our children's world.

Almighty God, I pray for all the scientists, inventors, and technicians. Touch them, Lord, so that they desire to work with You and in harmony with Your will and plan for us as a people. Give me the courage to speak out where I see our future compromised by harmful practices. Give me the strength to stop following the opinions of others blindly and instead to ask Your advice and to make Your answer my final one. In the name of Your Son, Jesus Christ, my Savior and my Redeemer, I pray, Amen.

Day 294

With God we will gain the victory, and he will trample down our enemies. (Psalm 60:12 NIV)

As long as you remain faithful to God, you will be victorious because God is the Lord of Lords, the Holy of Holies, the Mightiest of the Mighty.

There are often many times in the course of your illness when you have thoughts of despair and defeat. Usually these come at times when you are in pain or are filled with bone-wearying fatigue. Your brain is sluggish and you just don't care any more. These are the times when satan is draining your energy, blinding you to the glory of God's healing power, and deafening your ears to the voice of the Holy Spirit.

Put on some music that sings praises to the Lord and reach for the Holy Scriptures. Speak out loud the declarations and covenants of the Lord God Almighty. Say as vigorously as you can, "With God I will gain the victory and He will trample down my enemies." Turn to Ephesians and read Chapter 6 verses 10 through 18.

Finally, be strong in the Lord and in his mighty power. Put on the full armor of God so that you can take your stand against the devil's schemes. For our struggle . . . is against the powers of this dark world and against the spiritual forces of evil in the heavenly realms. . . . Stand firm then, with the belt of truth buckled around your waist, with the breastplate of righteousness in place, and with your feet fitted with the readiness that comes from the gospel of peace. In addition to all this, take up the shield of faith, with which you can extinguish all the flaming arrows of the evil one. Take the helmet of salvation and the sword of the Spirit, which is the word of God. And pray in the Spirit on all occasions with all kinds of prayers and requests. (NIV)

Feel God's strength pour into you. Feel God's protection surround you. Know that, as long as you stand firm in the Lord, satan must flee from you. Illness must leave your body. Claim God's healing power.

Almighty God, with You I gain the victory. I rest in Your power and accept Your protection, strength, and healing. In the name of Your Son, Christ Jesus, who bore my infirmities on the Cross, I pray, Amen.

Day 295

He sent his word and healed them, and delivered them from their destructions. Oh that men would praise the Lord for his goodness, and for his wonderful works to the children of men! And let them sacrifice the sacrifices of thanksgiving, and declare his works with rejoicing. (Psalm 107:20-22 KJV)

Quicken thou me according to thy word. . . . This is my comfort in my affliction: for thy word hath quickened me. (Psalm 119:25, 50 KJV)

God's Word heals. "To quicken" means to be made alive. The Psalmist is saying "Make me alive and vital according to Your Word, God. This is my comfort in my affliction, for Your Word brings me to life."

God's Word in the Holy Scriptures is inspired by the Holy Spirit and it shows you God's overall plan for you as His beloved child. It reveals to you how God works in your life and how God wants you to act and to live. It contains God's promises to you as well as God's commands.

Immerse yourself in God's Word and ask the Holy Spirit to reveal to you particular passages that are most relevant for you for that day. The Holy Scriptures are meant to lift you up, to strengthen you, and to bring you into closer communion with the Lord God Almighty. They are to make you more alive and more vital in your service to God.

God "sent His Word and (it) healed them," Psalm 107 says. This is not just a promise *from* God; it is a reality *of* God. God sent His Word and you *are* healed. It is done. It means little to believe that God *can* heal *someone else* unless you believe that God *is* healing *you*. Believe that God's Word applies to you personally.

God's Word says that Jehovah-rapha is the God who heals you (Exodus 15:26). God's Word says that "God anointed Jesus of Nazareth with the Holy Spirit and power, and . . . he went around doing good and healing all who were under the power of the devil, because God was with him" (Acts 10:38). God's Word says that "by His stripes we are healed" (Isaiah 53:5).

Stand on the Word of God and receive your healing.

Almighty God, You sent Your Word to heal me and deliver me from my destruction. I praise You for Your goodness and for Your wonderful works. I rejoice and give You thanks. I receive Your healing, Jehovah-rapha, and I praise Your Holy Name. Make me alive and vital, Lord. Quicken me according to Your Word. In Jesus' name, I pray, Amen.

Day 296

This day I call heaven and earth as witnesses against you that I have set before you life and death, blessings and curses. Now choose life, so that you and your children may live and that you may love the Lord your God, listen to his voice, and hold fast to him. For the Lord is your life, and he will give you many years in the land he swore to give to your fathers, Abraham, Isaac and Jacob. (Deuteronomy 30:19-20 NIV)

God sets before you free will. He gives you the power to choose what you want – life or death, blessings or curses. And He urges you to choose Him, to choose life.

This Scripture tells us what flows from choosing life: you will live, love the Lord your God, listen to His voice, and hold fast to Him. God is very aware that every moment in the day presents you with choices. Most are tiny choices, but they are choices nevertheless. When you choose life, you proclaim your love of God. And when you choose life, you must depend on God's guidance by listening to His voice.

Each morning when you wake up, say "thank you" to God and consciously choose life for the new day. If you feel sick, this can sometimes be difficult. There are some mornings when you wake up tired before the day has even begun. The hours that stretch before you seem long, and fatigue leads you into feelings of despair.

It is at these moments that it is all the more important to choose life. Remember, when God is in your cheering section, who can defeat you? The Lord *is* your life so to choose life is to choose God.

When you feel sick, the little choices for life are often as meaningful as big ones. Which herbs to take today for your recovery? Which healing remedy to use? Which foods to eat for your optimum nutrition? Which activities to engage in? Listen to God's voice and He will guide you.

Almighty God, I boldly proclaim that I choose life. I choose life, God! I shout it with all of my might. I love You, my Creator. I turn to You and listen for Your voice. Show me the path You want me to follow and I will walk it. I hold fast to You, O God, my Strength and my Salvation. You are Jehovah-rapha, my Healer. Help me to fulfill Your mission and Your purpose for me on this earth. Hold me in Your loving arms. In the name of Your Son Jesus Christ, my Savior and my Redeemer, I pray, Amen.

Day 297

So do not worry or be anxious about tomorrow, for tomorrow will have worries and anxieties of its own. Sufficient for each day is its own trouble. (Matthew 6:34 AMP)

Worry is actually the voice of the devil whispering in your head. Worrying and being anxious put you in partnership with him instead of with Jehovah-rapha. Once you begin worrying, it takes on a life of its own, and there seems to be no end to it. What if this? What if that? Maybe this. Maybe that. Should I do this? Or should I do that?

Worry has many physical consequences. It drains you and depletes your energy. It puts a great strain on your immune system and, thus, interferes with your ability to fight infection and disease. It creates imbalance in your body down to the cellular level.

When you feel sick, you are in a very vulnerable position, and worries seem to multiply if you do not stay grounded in your faith. Because of the way our culture has developed, most of us have become very dependent on believing that modern medicine is the solution to all our health problems.

Holy Scripture tells us that there is a place and a time for everything, so there is a place and a time for modern medicine. However, when we feel sick, our first thought should be to go to God for guidance. We should be willing to be open to consider His own remedies, which He spread over the planet in extraordinary profusion. Herbs, essential oils, and natural substances are part of God's great blanket of healing.

When you first notice a symptom, don't use your energy worrying about it. Take it to God in prayer. If you are told to seek a medical professional, do it. Or if you are told to go to the natural world for your healing, do it. You may be told the exact herb to take, just as Isaiah was told to put a fig poultice on Hezekiah. If not, ask which natural health professional to go to see. Or do some research on your own.

The more you learn the more useful you can be as God's partner. And the more you know, the less you will worry.

Almighty God, I admit it – I'm worried. And I know that this worry is based on fear and that fear doesn't come from You. Here it is, God – my whole bag of worries. Take them all. Flood me with Your power so that I will be strong in my faith. Keep my feet on Your healing path and keep me focused on this moment right now. Remind me that You are in charge of my life and You hold all my tomorrows in Your loving hand. In the name of Your Son, Jesus Christ, I pray, Amen.

Day 298

Now a man named Ananias, together with his wife Sapphira, also sold a piece of property. With his wife's full knowledge he kept back part of the money for himself, but brought the rest and put it at the apostles' feet. Then Peter said, "Ananias, how is it that Satan has so filled your heart that you have lied to the Holy Spirit and have kept for yourself some of the money you received for the land? Didn't it belong to you before it was sold? And after it was sold, wasn't the money at your disposal? What made you think of doing such a thing? You have not lied to men but to God." When Ananias heard this, he fell down and died. And great fear seized all who heard what had happened. Then the young men came forward, wrapped up his body, and carried him out and buried him. (Acts 5:1-6 NIV)

This is a very powerful illustration of the fact that guilt kills. Terror and extreme fear also kill. You can't carry guilt around for long without its affecting your whole being. It will eat at you slowly but surely. In addition to the mental and emotional stress, there is a real impact on the functioning of your immune system and on the organs of your body. Terror stresses your adrenals to their maximum limits, and sometimes the pressure put on them is too much to sustain.

Some people mistakenly believe that God killed Ananias for lying to the church. But read this Scripture again. It says that, when Ananias heard the truth spoken and saw his deeds revealed, "he fell down and died," not that God killed him. When Peter confronted Ananias' wife, he told her what happened to her husband and predicted that the same thing would happen to her. "At that moment she fell down at his feet and died." She was slain by both her terror and her guilt.

What secrets are you hiding? Do not be deceived by the evil one into thinking that they are hidden either from God or from the cells in your body. The stress of keeping these secrets is affecting you every minute of the day and night – no matter how strong you think you might be. Sooner or later the truth will come to light and you will have a very heavy price to pay.

Confess your sins and make atonement for them. Only then can you ask for healing with a clean heart.

Almighty God, I confess that I have sinned. Give me the courage to atone for my mistakes and to make the best restitution that I can. Forgive me, Lord. Thank You for cleansing me and thank You for healing me. In the name of Your Son Jesus Christ, I pray, Amen.

Day 299

He who dwells in the shelter of the Most High will rest in the shadow of the Almighty. I will say of the Lord, "He is my refuge and my fortress, my God, in whom I trust." Surely he will save you from the fowler's snare and from the deadly pestilence. He will cover you with his feathers, and under his wings you will find refuge; his faithfulness will be your shield and rampart. You will not fear the terror of night, nor the arrow that flies by day, nor the pestilence that stalks in the darkness, nor the plague that destroys at midday. A thousand may fall at your side, ten thousand at your right hand, but it will not come near you. You will only observe with your eyes and see the punishment of the wicked. If you make the Most High your dwelling – even the Lord, who is my refuge – then no harm will befall you, no disaster will come near your tent. For he will command his angels concerning you to guard you in all your ways; they will lift you up in their hands, so that you will not strike your foot against a stone. You will tread upon the lion and the cobra; you will trample the great lion and the serpent. "Because he loves me," says the Lord, "I will rescue him; I will protect him, for he acknowledges my name. He will call upon me, and I will answer him; I will be with him in trouble, I will deliver him and honor him. With long life will I satisfy him and show him my salvation." (Psalm 91:1-16 NIV)

No pestilence, no plague, no terror, no arrow of the enemy – *nothing* can harm you when you dwell faithfully in the shadow of the Almighty. God commands his angels to guard you and protect you. Though ten thousand may fall from the illness around you, *you* do not have to fall if you hold to the Word of God. See the angels of the Lord surrounding you and lifting you up. See them ministering to you as God's special healing team.

Notice that your protection and deliverance are conditional. You must love the Lord, acknowledge His name, and call upon Him. You must declare Him as the Lord God Almighty. If you believe in your heart that you will never be well, you have determined that your illness is stronger than the power of the Lord, and you have exalted it and the evil one to a position higher than the Lord. Be single-minded in your belief in the will and the power of God. Call upon Him and obey His instructions exactly. If you do these things, Jehovah-rapha promises to deliver you.

Wonderful Jehovah-rapha, I love You, I acknowledge You, and I call upon You. Send Your angels to lift me up. Deliver me, Lord. Show me your salvation and satisfy me with long life. In Jesus' name, Amen.

Day 300

"Have faith in God," Jesus answered. "I tell you the truth, if anyone says to this mountain, 'Go, throw yourself into the sea,' and does not doubt in his heart but believes that what he says will happen, it will be done for him." (Mark 11:22-23 NIV)

When you feel sick or have been injured, your health problem seems like a mountain. A BIG mountain. Jesus told us not to worry about mountains in our path because, if we would have faith, we could accomplish anything.

It is interesting that in this Scripture, Jesus tells us to talk to the mountain, saying, "Go throw yourself into the sea." Once again in Scripture we are shown how important *words* are – not only God's Holy Word but also our own. Through them we voice either our authority over the situations in our life or our fears and helplessness to them.

First, you must learn about your body and how it works. As you comprehend the mechanisms of your disease or illness, you understand what has gone wrong and what is needed to bring your body functions back into proper balance and operation. Once you know that information, then speak with authority to your illness, and command it to operate according to God's design and plan for it.

For example, suppose you have been diagnosed with osteoporosis, a condition that occurs when bones lose their minerals and normal density. Include in your prayer words to this effect, "In the name of Jesus, I command my bones and the organs of my body to return to their proper function. I command my digestive system to assimilate properly the calcium, magnesium, boron, and other minerals which I am supplying to my body. I command my parathyroid glands to regulate my calcium levels properly. I command the osteoblast cells to wake up and to build new bone cells to make my bones strong and healthy. I command my body pH to return to normal and my kidneys to function healthily."

Make your words specific and authoritative. Speak in faith and visualize everything that you are saying as happening just as you speak the words. Finally, command the evil one to leave your body and enforce God's Word on every cell. Claim the healing power of Jehovah-rapha.

Almighty God, as Your Son commanded me, I speak to the mountain of my illness to be transformed. I command satan to leave me, and I command every cell in my body to function according to Your Divine plan. You are the God who heals me and I stand on Your Holy Word. In Jesus' name, I pray, Amen.

Day 301

Nicodemus brought a mixture of myrrh and aloes, about seventy-five pounds. Taking Jesus' body, the two of them wrapped it, with the spices, in strips of linen. This was in accordance with Jewish burial customs. (John 19:39-40 NIV)

The use of herbs and spices was quite common in the time of Jesus. We see here a reference to aloes being used to anoint the body of Christ prior to His burial. One of the most well known plants, the aloe has been used for thousands of years for many beneficial purposes.

The part of the plant that is used is the gel from the leaves. It contains an agent that relieves pain, beginning to work as soon as it is placed on a wound or burn. Aloe helps to repair tissue rapidly because it stimulates the normal growth of living cells.

It is extremely effective for burns, the most effective application being simply to cut off a leaf, slitting it open length-wise, and then laying it on the burned area with the exposed gel against the burn. The aloe gel is also used to soothe and heal sore nipples of nursing mothers. It stimulates circulation in areas where there are wounds. It is very useful either to prevent or to remove infection.

When applied externally, it helps to remove dead layers of skin, and it also moisturizes and improves skin tone. For this reason it is used in many cosmetic preparations. Before using any product with aloe added, check all the other ingredients in the preparation, and make sure it contains only pure, organic contents. God created the aloe to be an extremely effective penetrating healing substance which moves quickly through all the layers of the skin. If the product you are using contains chemicals, synthetic substances, and toxic materials, these harmful and unhealthy additives will also penetrate deeply into your body.

Aloe vera juice may be consumed in liquid form to help with constipation and to expel pinworms. It increases stomach activity and may be useful for stomach repair. The components of the aloe plant cause contraction of muscle tissue, such as the uterus and the colon, so it should not be used by women who are pregnant.

Our Creator has given us a gift to be treasured in the little aloe plant. Be sure to grow one in your home and use it wisely for your healing.

Dear God, thank You for the wonderful little aloe plant. How grateful I am for all its many benefits. I will learn about its therapeutic properties and will use it wisely for my healing. In Jesus' name, I pray, Amen.

Day 302

The eye is the lamp of the body. If your eyes are good, your whole body will be full of light. But if your eyes are bad, your whole body will be full of darkness. If then the light within you is darkness, how great is that darkness! (Matthew 6:22-23 NIV)

How do you perceive your own soul and how do you perceive the world around you? As Jesus warned, our experience depends on the way that we look at ourselves and at life. If our perception is filled with the light of God's love, then our soul and our world will be filled with that light. However, if our perception is dark, distrustful, and laden with fear, then our soul and our world will be cloaked in darkness.

Your perception determines what you select to bring into your life. If you perceive yourself as unworthy of love, you are not likely to choose people to be in your life who will value and respect you. If you perceive the world to be filled with obstacles and disappointment, you are not likely to make choices for happiness.

Take an honest look at your perception of yourself. Do you love yourself? Do you respect yourself? Do you feel God's joy within you even during hard times? Do your family members and friends treat you with kindness, respect, and love? Do you feel fulfilled and valued? Do you love others? Do you feel loved? Do you feel safe? Do you trust God? Do you trust God enough to ask His guidance *and to follow it*, no matter what?

If the answer to any of these questions is no, then be courageous enough to go within, to find the hurts and the fears, and to make the changes you need to make. When you let go of the past and forgive yourself and others, you can look at the world with a new vision.

Even though Jesus was not talking about the quality of your eyesight, there is a connection between your perceptions and your eyesight. If it is painful spiritually and emotionally to look at the world, the body complies by helping you to see less and less. In order to be healed, you have to be willing to see clearly *internally* as well as to wish to see clearly *externally*.

Be willing to forgive yourself and others. Jesus repeatedly told those He healed that their sins were forgiven and to go their way, not making the same mistakes.

Wonderful Jehovah-rapha, cleanse me in my soul. Forgive me of my sins and help me to forgive myself and others. I want to see clearly, Lord, both in my heart and with my eyes. Thank You for healing me. In Jesus' name, I pray, Amen.

Day 303

Perseverance must finish its work so that you may be mature and complete, not lacking anything. If any of you lacks wisdom, he should ask God, who gives generously to all without finding fault, and it will be given to him. (James 1:4-5 NIV)

James, the oldest half-brother of Jesus, speaks of perseverance, maturity, and wisdom. Many people fail to be healed because they lack these essential qualities.

We are particularly immature when it comes to matters of our health. We often play the helpless victim to sickness by taking no responsibility for having allowed our bodies to become vulnerable. We advocate the germ theory which blames the invading organisms for our problems instead of the terrain theory which holds the condition of the host accountable for creating an environment amenable for the harmful organisms to thrive.

We usually trust human medical opinions totally instead of giving the final decision to the Great Physician concerning our treatment. We demand one pill or one simple treatment as a cure so that we don't have to make any changes in our lives.

James tells us the blunt truth: if you lack wisdom, ask God. If you want to know what to do about your health, ask the Creator who made your body. God will provide the answers for you, and you must be tough enough to persevere in carrying out every single instruction just as He gives it. Healing programs using God's herbs are usually just that – healing *programs*. You didn't get sick overnight and there is no magic pill that is going to heal you. You spent weeks, months, and often years neglecting and mistreating your body.

The Great Physician may lead you to a program combining many herbs and natural substances for your recovery. If so, God requires that you keep asking for daily advice on modifications to that program. He holds you to the test of perseverance to see if you remain faithful to Him and hold steadfast to the course. He may advise you to seek conventional medical treatment as well. If so, do it. The Great Physician gives generously and does not want you to lack anything.

Wonderful Jehovah-rapha, give me wisdom to hear You clearly and perseverance to finish the work You set before me. I know You want only the best for me and You will lead me step by step to my healing if I am willing to be obedient to Your voice. In Jesus' name, I pray, Amen.

Day 304

Seeing then that we have a great high priest, that is passed into the heavens, Jesus the Son of God, let us hold fast our profession. (Hebrews 4:14 KJV)

How good are you at "holding fast?" Jesus always kept His mission clearly focused in His mind and heart, and He held fast to His purpose without ever wavering.

Do you profess Jesus Christ as your Lord and Savior? Then hold fast to His instruction in the Great Commission to "obey everything I have commanded you" (Matthew 28:20).

Do you profess Jesus Christ as the one who "took up our infirmities and carried our diseases" (Matthew 8:17)? Then hold fast to the fact that this includes you. Jesus Christ your Savior took *your* infirmities and carried *your* diseases to the Cross. Profess this belief and hold fast to it.

Do you profess Jesus Christ who told you that "if you live in Me and My words remain in you and continue to live in your hearts, ask whatever you will, and it shall be done for you" (John 15:7)? Then do as your Savior instructs. Live in Him, walk according to God's will, and hold fast to the promise of your healing.

Do you profess Jesus Christ who said, "I assure you, if anyone steadfastly believes in Me, he will himself be able to do the things that I do; and he will do even greater things than these, because I go to the Father" (John 14:12)? Then let every thought and every action fulfill His words, and hold fast to your trust that Jesus spoke the truth.

It is easy to say words, to make a verbal profession of belief. The hard part is to *live* the words you speak. Holding fast is faith in action. It is belief manifested by doing. Hold fast to the promise of your healing. Hold fast to God's Holy Word. Hold fast to your belief that satan has been defeated. Hold fast to the sovereignty of the Lord God Almighty.

Wonderful Jehovah-rapha, I profess my faith that You are the God who heals me. I profess my faith in Your Son Jesus Christ who took my sins and infirmities to the Cross. I hold fast, O Lord. I look past my symptoms and focus on Your healing power. You are my Deliverer, Protector, and Healer. Thank You, God. Show me the path You want me to follow for my recovery and I will walk it. In the name of Your Son, Jesus Christ, I pray, Amen.

Day 305

Can a mother forget the baby at her breast and have no compassion on the child she has borne? Though she may forget, I will not forget you! See, I have engraved you on the palms of my hands. (Isaiah 49:15-16 NIV)

What more tender image is there than that of a mother nursing her infant? It is an image of supreme love, of protection, of nurturing, of caring. Most mothers fulfill the image presented here and love their children with a bond that is the strongest on earth. No one questions the sacrifices that a mother will make to provide for her child and to protect her young.

God tells us that a mother's love pales in comparison to the love He has for us. It is almost incomprehensible for a mother to forget her child. Nevertheless, God uses that as an illustration. "Though *she* may forget you, *I* will not forget you!" He promises. "I will never, ever forget you. See! Come and look! I have engraved you on the palms of my hands."

Stop to think for a moment what it means that God has engraved you on the palms of His hands. It means He has made you a part of Him. It means that it is His will that you never be separated from Him. It means that He wants you to experience everything that living in the presence of the Lord entails. It means that He is constantly making plans for you. In Jeremiah 29:11-14, God declares, "For I know the plans I have for you; plans to prosper you and not to harm you, plans to give you a hope and a future."

Even though we don't remember it, we all carry within us the sense of being that helpless, vulnerable infant. As adults, when we experience difficult challenges, we may find ourselves feeling the old feelings of helplessness. We may even move away from God. But He will never move away from us.

We have a parent who cannot let us down and whose love for us is so deep and so vast that we cannot comprehend it. This loving Father will never fail us.

Dear Heavenly Father, whether or not I had a loving, nurturing earthly parent is no longer an issue. What is important is that I now understand how much You love me as Your child. What is important is that I know in the depths of my being that You will not leave me and You will not fail me. You have engraved me in the palms of Your hands, and, therefore, You carry me with You always. Thank You, God, for being faithful to me. Hold me tightly in Your loving arms. In Jesus' name, I pray, Amen.

Day 306

Have you not put a hedge around him and his household and everything he has?
(Job 1:10 NIV)

The story of Job as traditionally interpreted is quite unsettling. It tells of a good man who followed God, and yet God apparently turned him over to satan and all kinds of awful things happened to him. Let's take another look at the lessons from Job.

Satan complains to God about Job, "Have you not put a hedge around him and his household and everything he has?" Imagine a hedge of protection around you, your family, and everything you have. What was Job like inside that wall? Was he sick? No, he was healthy within God's hedge of protection. Were his family members sick? No, they were healthy within God's hedge of protection. Here again we see evidence of God's will for us.

What happened to the wall? The traditional interpretation is that God removed it. But look at the Scripture. God said to satan, "Everything Job has is in your hands." Job had already put chinks in the wall himself by continually offering sacrifices to God in behalf of the improper behavior of his children. Instead of having faith in his offering, he kept making the sacrifices repeatedly, revealing that he was now fear-based instead of faith-based. Job later admits that everything he feared came upon him. We know that, when we operate from fear, we have succumbed to satan's lies.

What has happened to your own wall of protection? Have you, or those from whom you are descended, removed it? With choice after choice, have you removed your protective wall one brick at a time? Job finally said, "Teach me, and I will hold my tongue; and cause me to understand wherein I have erred" (Job 6:24). You must do the same.

No matter what you may have done in the past, God wants to redeem you. He still wants to work His healing power on you. Your course is ever the same – to stand faithfully on God's Word and in trust in Jehovah-rapha, the God who heals you.

Almighty God, I have strayed from Your path. Forgive my sins and restore Your hedge of protection around me. Guide me so that I do not weaken that hedge again but instead work with You to keep it strong. Thank You for Your mercy on me and Your tender love. In the name of Your Son, Jesus Christ, I pray, Amen.

Day 307

For the Lord God is a sun and shield: the Lord will give grace and glory: no good thing will he withhold from them that walk uprightly. O Lord of hosts, blessed is the man that trusteth in thee. (Psalm 84:11-12 KJV)

Holy Scripture tells us that God will withhold no good thing from us if we are willing to walk uprightly and to be obedient to His instructions.

Too often when people feel sick, they fail to comply with God's direction so they stand outside the shield of the Lord instead of under it.

When we ask for guidance for our healing, most of the time we are told to use God's remedies. This presents a major problem for many people. They say, "If God won't give me a miracle, then I won't do it His way. I want a quick fix and I'm determined to get it. If it means having a body part removed, then I'll do it. I just want an immediate solution that interferes as little as possible with my life as I choose to live it."

Man's drugs are poisons. Each medicine is tested for its effective dose (ED) and its lethal dose (LD), going to market only when the ED is lower than the LD and being limited to prescription use because of its potential for damage. Even when used according to the directions, the large majority of drugs can cause death. Most of man's drugs suppress symptoms and, thus, allow the body relief in order to do its own healing.

God's remedies are totally different since their function and purpose are totally opposite. God's "medicine" is actually concentrated food; these herbs and plants do not suppress symptoms but instead nourish, support, and heal the cells and tissue that are not functioning properly. They are therapeutic in their wholeness *when used in the manner and for the purpose that God ordained.* We are expected to learn about them and to understand the effect that The Great Physician designed them to have so that we can apply them properly and safely in our recovery program. Isolating and extracting individual components may be useful; however, that process sometimes carries a significant risk with a negative result.

Declare God as your sun and shield and ask Him for guidance for your healing. Have the maturity to accept your responsibility for your part in this process and to walk uprightly before Him. Be courageous enough to obey Him and allow Him to bless you with every good gift.

Wonderful Jehovah-rapha, help me to stop looking for the easy way out. Be my sun and shield. I strive to walk uprightly on the path that You set before me. I am blessed by Your abundant grace and good gifts. Thank You for healing me, Lord. In Jesus' name, I pray, Amen.

Day 308

He called his twelve disciples to him and gave them authority to drive out evil spirits and to heal every disease and sickness. (Matthew 10:1 NIV)

Once again we see the scene of Jesus passing on to His followers His dual mission of preaching the gospel and healing the people. Once again we see Jesus giving His disciples authority over satan and evil spirits as well as the power to heal every disease. Notice that no sickness is beyond the power of healing by the disciples. Not a single one.

Why is the emphasis on healing important? Because God was making the Garden accessible to us again. God never stopped loving us and He wants every one of His children to live as He intends. He wants us to live whole and complete standing before Him as Adam did before he chose to know evil.

God never removes from us the right of free will. He always allows us to choose partnership with satan instead of with Him. But through the sacrifice of the body of Jesus Christ, God offered the wholeness of the Garden to us once again while we are still in physical form. Jesus tells us of that over and over again. "Your faith has made you whole," He said to one person after another.

Don't let satan keep you from being healed. Jesus gives us the authority to reclaim our bodies. Jesus gives us the authority to cast satan out. Jesus bore not only our sins on the Cross but also our sicknesses. It is written! Hallelujah! How blessed we are!

Claim the healing of Christ this moment. Enforce the Word on every cell of your body. Remember that Jehovah-rapha is the God "who gives life to the dead and calls things that are not as though they were" (Romans 4:17).

Thank You, God, for healing me. I declare my willingness to follow Your Son Jesus Christ and to carry on His mission. I see Him walk up to me, lay His hands upon me, and restore me. I see Him give me power and authority over sickness just as He gave power and authority to His followers two thousand years ago. In His name, I command satan to leave my body. In His name, I command every organ, gland, tissue, and cell to function normally according to Your Divine plan. I stand on the Word which says "By His stripes I am healed." With grateful thanks in Jesus' name, I pray, Amen.

Day 309

This is the word that came to Jeremiah from the Lord: "Stand at the gate of the Lord's house and there proclaim this message: 'Hear the word of the Lord, all you people of Judah who come through these gates to worship the Lord. This is what the Lord Almighty, the God of Israel, says: Reform your ways and your actions, and I will let you live in this place. Do not trust in deceptive words and say, "This is the temple of the Lord, the temple of the Lord, the temple of the Lord!" If you really change your ways and your actions and deal with each other justly, if you do not oppress the alien, the fatherless or the widow and do not shed innocent blood in this place, and if you do not follow other gods to your own harm, then I will let you live in this place, in the land I gave your forefathers for ever and ever. But look, you are trusting in deceptive words that are worthless. Will you steal and murder, commit adultery and perjury, burn incense to Baal and follow other gods you have not known, and then come and stand before me in this house, which bears my Name, and say, "We are safe" – safe to do all these detestable things?" Has this house, which bears my Name, become a den of robbers to you? But I have been watching! declares the Lord.' "
(Jeremiah 7:1-8 NIV)

God's people were in serious peril. They did as they pleased and then thought that they could return to the Temple of Jerusalem for protection. Through Jeremiah, God tells His people that they are going to be held responsible for what they do. They will not receive protection if they have failed to live according to God's Word and direction.

Those who feel sick need to pay heed to this message of Jeremiah. You cannot go running for the protection of God's wings if you have ignored His direction in your healing process. You cannot make assumptions that you should have a certain treatment and then go crying for help if it doesn't work out the way you planned. God is always watching. He knows when you place anything before Him. He wants your trust to be in Him and Him alone. He wants to be the One to whom you go for advice and counsel. He wants to be the One who tells you what path to follow for your healing – whether through medical treatment, herbs, essential oils, chiropractic, laying on of hands, etc. He exhorts us to listen to Him. He urges us to place Him first in our lives. He promises that, if we do, He will fulfill the promises of His Word.

Almighty Lord, I turn from deceptive words and I reform my ways. You and You alone are my God, my protector, and my healer. Lead me, Lord, according to Your plan for my life. In Jesus' name, I pray, Amen.

Day 310

He was despised and rejected by men, a man of sorrows, and familiar with suffering. . . .
Surely he took up our infirmities and carried our sorrows. . . . But he was pierced for our
transgressions, he was crushed for our iniquities; the punishment that brought us peace
was upon him, and by his wounds we are healed. (Isaiah 53:3-5 NIV)

Here is a passage that is often used to convince us that Jesus died on the Cross for our souls but not for our bodies.

Let's take a closer look at the words in Hebrew. The passage actually reads:

He was despised and rejected by men, a man of <u>makob</u> and familiar with
<u>choli</u>. . . . Surely he took up our <u>choli</u> and carried our <u>makob</u>.

The word *makob* is translated "pain" throughout the Old Testament, and the word *choli* is translated "sickness" or "disease." Therefore, the passage reads as follows:

He was despised and rejected by men, a man of pain, and familiar with sickness/
disease. . . . Surely he took up our sickness/disease and carried our pains.

Yes, Jesus died for our sins and our souls. But He took more to the Cross. We see this underscored in the words of the apostle Matthew, who in Matthew 8:16-17 wrote, "He . . . healed all that were sick: that it might be fulfilled which was spoken by Esaias the prophet, saying, 'Himself took our infirmities, and bore our sicknesses.' " The translation from the Greek in the Gospel of Matthew came through much more accurately and clearly.

Take your illness, your disease, your pain, your sins, and your emotional wounds, and hand them over to Jesus. Lay them at the foot of the Cross. Now turn your eyes away from the Cross and toward your Resurrected Lord, sitting at the right hand of the Father. You are free!

Dear God, each day I understand better the sacrifice that Your Son Jesus Christ made for
me. Replace my fears with faith, my doubt with belief. I come to You, willing to be made
whole in every aspect of my being – my soul, my mind, my emotions, and my body. I am
healed, Jehovah-rapha by Your mighty hand and by the blood of Your Son Jesus Christ.
Amen.

Day 311

Now, Lord, consider their threats and enable your servants to speak your word with great boldness. Stretch out your hand to heal and perform miraculous signs and wonders through the name of your holy servant Jesus. After they prayed, the place where they were meeting was shaken. And they were all filled with the Holy Spirit and spoke the word of God boldly. (Acts 4:29-31 NIV)

It is interesting that in The New International Version this section of Scripture is subtitled "The Believers' Prayer." Think about that for a moment. This is a prayer of those who believe in the Father, Son, and Holy Spirit. What does it say? First, it acknowledges the supreme sovereignty of Jehovah, the mighty I AM. "Sovereign Lord, you made the heaven and the earth and the sea, and everything in them." Next, it quotes Scripture of David and speaks of those who conspired against Jesus. Then it makes certain requests of God.

What do the believers ask for? They ask for two things. They ask God to give them boldness to speak His Word, and they ask for God to stretch out His hand and to heal. Here again we see the dual purpose and the dual mission revealed.

We are no different from the first believers. We have the same spiritual needs and the same physical needs. The evil one often tries to convince us that times are different now and that the signs and wonders that applied to the early church do not apply to us today. But Jesus is the same yesterday, today, and tomorrow. The Lord God Jehovah is the same God with the same will and the same power. So there is no reason why we should not pray the same prayer of the believers and expect the same results. Pray it right now.

Mighty Lord, I am a believer. I am a believer just like the believers who lived two thousand years ago, so I pray the prayer of believers as it is recorded in Your Holy Scripture: Sovereign Lord, You made the heaven and the earth and the sea and everything in them. You spoke by the Holy Spirit through the mouth of your servant, our father David: Why do the nations rage and the peoples plot in vain? The kings of the earth take their stand and the rulers gather together against the Lord and against his Anointed One. Enable me, Your servant, to speak Your Word with great boldness. Stretch out Your hand to heal and perform miraculous signs and wonders through the name of Your Holy servant Jesus. In Jesus' name, I pray, Amen.

Day 312

On a Sabbath Jesus was teaching in one of the synagogues, and a woman was there who had been crippled by a spirit for eighteen years. She was bent over and could not straighten up at all. When Jesus saw her, he called her forward and said to her, "Woman, you are set free from your infirmity." Then he put his hands on her, and immediately she straightened up and praised God. . . . The Lord answered him, "You hypocrites! Doesn't each of you on the Sabbath untie his ox or donkey from the stall and lead it out to give it water? Then should not this woman, a daughter of Abraham, whom Satan has kept bound for eighteen long years, be set free on the Sabbath day from what bound her?"
(Luke 13:10-13, 15-16 NIV)

A woman had been crippled by a spirit for eighteen long years. Jesus saw her and called her to Him. What did He do? He did what He was sent by the Father to do for all of us: He set her at liberty. "Woman," He said, "you are set free from your infirmity."

Satan wants to bind all of us. We are his target, and he seeks to control us by making us weak and helpless. He binds us through finding our inner vulnerabilities and weaknesses – through our anger, our guilt, our shame, our fear, our grief, our loneliness. He convinces us to focus on our losses and to spend our days seeking revenge or crying with sorrow and regret.

He also binds us by misleading us and getting us to make unwise choices leading to actions that are harmful to ourselves or others. He persuades us to gorge ourselves on synthetic, genetically engineered, irradiated, pesticide-laden foods, and then so distorts our thinking that we blame God for our resulting illness. He whispers to us that we can wait one more day before we begin a nutritious diet, exercise program, and healthy lifestyle. One more day follows one more day until we run out of days.

Jesus came to liberate the captives. Like this woman, He calls us to Him. "Come over here," He is calling to you. "Come over here. I can see you are hurting. I can see you are bound. Come here and let me help you." He smiles and you are blessed by His love, compassion, and healing.

Almighty Heavenly Father, thank You for breaking my chains and lifting my burdens. I accept Your power and authority in my life. I accept Your Son Jesus Christ as my Risen Savior, who has set me free. Thank You for loving me and healing me. In Jesus' name, I pray, Amen.

Day 313

From that time on Jesus began to explain to his disciples that he must go to Jerusalem and suffer many things at the hands of the elders, chief priests and teachers of the law, and that he must be killed and on the third day be raised to life. Peter took him aside and began to rebuke him. "Never, Lord!" he said. "This shall never happen to you!" Jesus turned and said to Peter, "Get behind me, Satan! You are a stumbling block to me; you do not have in mind the things of God, but the things of men." (Matthew 16:21-23 NIV)

Satan uses fear to manipulate and entrap us and to divert us from living according to God's will. In this passage in Matthew we see how Jesus handles satan's use of fear to subvert God's will. Jesus knows His purpose; He knows that He has come to redeem mankind and that He is the atonement. He knows that He must suffer an earthly death in order to accomplish God's will for man's salvation.

We also know that Jesus loves Peter. He has already told Peter that he (Peter) is blessed and that he will become the foundation of the new church. So when Peter voices his fear and resistance to God's will, Jesus delivers some sharp and harsh words. "Get behind me, satan!" Jesus recognizes that the words of fear that Peter speaks are coming from satan, who is using fear to attempt to turn Jesus from fulfilling the will of God.

Just as Jesus was very clear about His purpose, you have to be clear that it is God's will that you, as His child, be healthy. Sickness is not useful to God, but sickness is very useful to satan. It saps you of your physical strength and diminishes your vitality. But more than that, it usually becomes fertile ground for fearful thoughts. You detail your symptoms as they manifest, and, as you focus on them, they grow. The more they grow, the more fearful you become. It becomes a vicious cycle.

Stop giving satan your power. Learn to recognize the voice of satan whenever you hear it, just as Jesus did. Be harsh with satan. Tell him to get away from you. Choose God's protection and God's love. Make a choice to fulfill God's will and God's purpose for your life.

Almighty God, when I hear whispers of fear, help me to recognize the voice of satan in them. Give me strength to look to You and Your Holy Word. Help me to give each symptom to You. Guide me in the path for my healing that You direct for me. Show me the way. I focus on You, Your Holy Word, and Your constant guidance. In the name of the Father, Son, and Holy Spirit, I pray, Amen.

Day 314

And in him you too are being built together to become a dwelling in which God lives by his Spirit. (Ephesians 2:22 NIV)

You are the habitation of the Lord. God and His Holy Spirit dwell in you. Since your body is the earthly vessel, the earthly home, of this precious Holy Spirit, it is your responsibility to take care of it. Your body is a Holy temple and must be treated as such.

Pay attention to your body and treat it with care and kindness. How many things each day do you do to be kind to your body? How much time do you give to creating a healthy environment for your body? Some actions are really simple and take only moments. For example, while you are working, take a minute – sixty little seconds – to stop and breathe deeply. You may choose to look at the sky or just close your eyes and inhale slowly and fully. As you do so, thank God for your life and for healing you – body and soul. Take one of these prayer moments every thirty minutes and see how vitalizing it can be.

Other things take more time and more commitment. Spending time exercising your body requires commitment, especially if you have a sedentary lifestyle. Walking is perhaps the ideal exercise because it also allows you to renew yourself spiritually at the same time. While you are walking, notice nature around you – whether it is the sky above, a flower struggling through a crack in the sidewalk, or the trees that surround you. Find something each day and say "thank you" to God.

Preparing healthy meals with as much organic produce as possible takes time, effort, and sometimes financial sacrifice. And another part of healing nutrition is adding herbs to your diet. Check out some books from the library. Find a health food store where the people are knowledgeable.

Learn as much as you can about God's remedies for us. These are God's gifts and He expects us to use them. Honor your Holy temple and provide it with respect, attention, and loving care.

Dear God, You have given me this body as a precious temple of the Holy Spirit – as Your habitation. Help me to care for it with love, nourishing it physically and spiritually. Sometimes I feel too tired, Lord, to do the things I know I should do. And sometimes I just seem too busy with the trivia of life. Remind me of Your priorities, Lord, and keep me focused on the things that are truly important so that I can join in full partnership with You for my healing. Thank you. In Jesus' name, I pray, Amen.

Day 315

I am the Lord thy God, which have brought thee out of the land of Egypt, out the house of bondage. Thou shalt have no other gods before me. (Exodus 20:2-3 KJV)

When we feel sick, most of us turn first to the medical system. We go for a diagnosis, for relief, and for a cure.

We are usually frightened and often weakened by our illness so that calm thinking is difficult. We are presented with test results and given treatment options. Usually we are told what results to expect. Often we are even told how long we will live if certain things are done or not done.

When confronted with this system of medicine, it is very easy to forget the first and most important commandment: Thou shalt have no other gods before me. What is God saying to us? He is telling us to follow only Him with absolute obedience. He is forbidding us to follow anyone else blindly for *any* reason. He is telling us to turn to Him and only Him for the answers for our life.

No doctor is God, and his opinion is only that – an opinion. Remember this if you get a chilling diagnosis and prognosis. Accept no doctor's verdict about your condition as Divine truth. He has told you the best that he knows. However, the knowledge available to him is miniscule compared to the knowledge of the Great I AM.

Only God really knows what is needed for your healing. Go to God. Ask Him for guidance in each step of the process of your healing. Ask Him if you need medical advice. Ask Him which doctor is the right one for you. Ask Him which treatment, if any, you should follow.

Listen to God's voice and follow His guidance. He wants you to be well and will tell you exactly what to do.

Dear merciful Lord, it is sometimes hard for me to stand firm in my faith when I hear a doctor tell me that awful things will happen to me and when he holds up my medical tests as proof. I feel so scared. I know that You see beyond the appearance of things and that Your reality is the only true one. But, God, I admit that I get caught up in the appearance presented by my symptoms and my medical tests, and medical opinions. Help me, God. Strengthen my faith. Tell me what You want me to do. You are Divine truth. You know the exact path for me to follow. Show me the way and I will obey. In Jesus' name, I pray, Amen.

Day 316

And he was withdrawn from them about a stone's cast, and kneeled down, and prayed. Saying, "Father, if thou be willing, remove this cup from me: nevertheless not my will, but thine, be done." And there appeared an angel unto him from heaven, strengthening him. And being in an agony he prayed more earnestly: and his sweat was as it were great drops of blood falling down to the ground. And when he rose up from prayer, and was come to his disciples, he found them sleeping for sorrow. And said unto them, "Why sleep ye? rise and pray, lest ye enter into temptation." (Luke 22:41-46 KJV)

Jesus is our model, our perfect example of how to handle life, so let us look at what happened in the Garden of Gethsemane. Knowing what lay before Him, Jesus was filled with extreme emotional turmoil. He prayed to the Father, *"if thou be willing,* remove this cup from me: nevertheless *not my will, but thine,* be done." He was asking if there was another way within God's will to overcome the evil one. During this time of Jesus' agony, God did not abandon His Precious Son but sent an angel from heaven to strengthen Him.

Remember that Jesus never once asked God if it were God's will for Him to heal the sick. Not one single time. Why? Because He knew it was God's will that people be healed and made well. He knew that disease and infirmity is not the will of the Father.

Like Jesus in Gethsemane, we, too, are sometimes distressed and filled with emotional turmoil. We, too, know what it is to have a sleepless night. Most often we spend it tossing and turning – or medicating ourselves into oblivion. Jesus shows us the way to handle it, however. Pray. Pray earnestly. Be careful of using the words, "if it be thy will." It is written that God is your Healer so use the qualifying phrase "if it be thy will" only for guidance in knowing the method of healing rather than for the ultimate result of the healing itself.

And if you don't feel calmer or more at peace, pray *more* earnestly. You will be given strength, guidance, and support. God will send angels to sit with you through the night and will provide the Holy Spirit to reveal the answers to your problems. Pray, believe, and remain steadfast. Your Savior has overcome the world.

Merciful Father, give me strength to handle the difficult situations in my life. I know you want me to be well. Give me guidance to show me the path that is Your will for me. I will walk it, Lord. In Jesus' name, I pray, Amen.

Day 317

Christ redeemed us from the curse of the law by becoming a curse for us, for it is written: "Cursed is everyone who is hung on a tree." He redeemed us in order that the blessing given to Abraham might come to the Gentiles through Christ Jesus, so that by faith we might receive the promise of the Spirit. (Galatians 3:13-14 NIV)

We were created with the breath of life of the Almighty Lord, and we were given every good thing according to God's will for us. God's will was made perfect in the Garden of Eden as it was in heaven. However, just as was true in heaven, He allowed his creations on earth the right to free will. God wanted His children to love Him, worship Him, and honor Him not because they had to do so but because they chose to do so.

Adam and Eve wanted to know evil, however; so they disobeyed the instructions of the Lord. Thus, the curse fell upon them and every one of their descendants. The Old Testament details the establishment of laws to control the effects of evil, and it told stories of life under the curse, during which time God never gave up totally on His beloved creation.

God's ultimate solution was to send His Son Jesus Christ to redeem us from the curse of the law. He was made the curse for us and He was made sin for us (2 Corinthians 5:21). He bore our sins (1 Peter 2:24) and He bore our sicknesses (Matthew 8:17). Our redemption was full and complete – both body and soul. No power over us was left to satan either at the spiritual level, the mental level, or the physical level. Forevermore there was to be no more curse (Revelation 22:3) for those who believe in Jesus Christ.

Believe God's Word that this is true. Live your faith. The curse can have no power over you unless you allow it. Sickness cannot remain in your body unless you allow it. The evil one cannot control your life unless you allow him. You are redeemed. As the beloved child of God, you have been given a personal Savior who calls you by name and who asks that you follow Him. Accept Him into your heart and glorify Him in your body.

Dear God, thank You for sending Your Son Jesus Christ to redeem me from the curse of the law so that by faith I may receive the promise of the Spirit. Whereas in Adam I sin, in Jesus Christ I am saved. Whereas in Adam I was cursed, in Jesus Christ I am redeemed. Whereas in Adam, I am subject to sickness and disease, in Jesus Christ I am healed. I rejoice in the salvation of the new covenant, and I offer myself to You in service according to Your will for my life. In Jesus' name, I pray, Amen.

Day 318

But you will receive power when the Holy Spirit comes on you; and you will be my witnesses in Jerusalem, and in all Judea and Samaria, and to the ends of the earth. (Acts 1:8 NIV)

We are all called to be witnesses for Christ. Just as Jesus repeatedly sent His followers out with the dual mission to spread His message of love and healing, we are likewise called to tell the entire world about His act of redemption – of soul and of body.

In order to do this Jesus has given us power – power through the Holy Spirit. The Greek word used for "power" is *dynamis*, which means power, ability, and miracle. As believers in Christ, you are to be a dynamic, forceful, active witness.

"For John baptized with water, but in a few days you will be baptized with the Holy Spirit," Jesus said. When the power of the Holy Spirit fills us, we are changed forever. We cannot remain victims. No longer does satan have any authority over us.

Satan cannot rule in our hearts or actions again unless we let him nor can he claim our bodies through disease unless we allow him to stay. The power of God, of Jesus Christ, and of the Holy Spirit is our shield and our means of transformation.

Take some time today to invite the Holy Spirit to fill you. Feel the Holy Spirit's presence. Feel the power of transformation within you. Ask Jesus Christ to lay His hands on you and to cleanse and heal you at every level of your being – your soul, your mind, your emotions, and your body.

Ask Jehovah-rapha, The Great Physician, for His healing grace and for His guidance concerning any actions you need to take at the physical level for your healing. Listen quietly. Then bathed in the power of the Holy Spirit, take action.

And witness to others of the miracle that is happening in your life through the grace of God.

Wonderful Jehovah-rapha, too often I look at my infirmities and allow myself to feel helpless and frail. I know that isn't what You want for me. So today I stand strong through the power of the Holy Spirit which You have sent to be with me always. I want to be a witness for You. I want all who see me to see Your love and healing shining through. Guide me, God, in the path You want me to follow. In the name of Your Son, Jesus Christ, I pray, Amen.

Day 319

And let us consider how we may spur one another on toward love and good deeds. Let us not give up meeting together, as some are in the habit of doing, but let us encourage one another – and all the more as you see the Day approaching. (Hebrews 10:24-25 NIV)

We have seen the huge proliferation of support groups that have sprung up for people who have specific illnesses and diseases. People can go for emotional support, for information, and for advice. Almost all of these groups have an underlying belief that conventional medical treatment is the only reasonable method for healing. That is fine for those who share those beliefs.

You may wish to form a "God First in Healing" support group for people who believe that God should direct all decisions for healing. A "God First in Healing" group is centered and grounded in prayer. It is one where people come to spur one another on during the days when it is difficult to wait on the Lord and to provide encouragement when satan's whispers of doubt creep in.

It is a group where people share information and ideas, not only about conventional treatment possibilities but also on the numerous alternative treatment methods. Instead of following only established medical treatments, members allow God to reveal each person's own individual healing pathway. Those who are attracted to this group are also open to allowing God to suggest some of His own remedies be included in people's healing and recovery.

We need each other. We need to pray with and for each other. Jesus told us that where two or more were gathered, He would be in their midst. Where else would Jesus want more to be than in the midst of those earnestly seeking liberty from their infirmities? Join together and discover the power of mutual love and caring.

Wonderful Jehovah-rapha, help me to find other people who are on their own path to recovery. I need support and encouragement from others who understand my concerns and my doubts and who can share in my ups and my downs. What a joy it is to have special people to pray with me and for me. I am lifted and revitalized by those who are walking the walk to recovery just as I am. In the name of Your Son, Jesus Christ, I pray, Amen.

Day 320

In Joppa there was a disciple named Tabitha (which, when translated, is Dorcas), who was always doing good and helping the poor. About that time she became sick and died, and her body was washed and placed in an upstairs room. Lydda was near Joppa; so when the disciples heard that Peter was in Lydda, they sent two men to him and urged him, "Please come at once!" Peter went with them, and when he arrived he was taken upstairs to the room. All the widows stood around him, crying and showing him the robes and other clothing that Dorcas had made while she was still with them. Peter sent them all out of the room; then he got down on his knees and prayed. Turning toward the dead woman, he said, "Tabitha, get up." She opened her eyes, and seeing Peter she sat up. He took her by the hand and helped her to her feet. Then he called the believers and the widows and presented her to them alive. (Acts 9:36-41 NIV)

Here we have an amazing story. A woman named Tabitha (also called Dorcas) "who was always doing good and helping the poor" and who was a good servant of the Lord, became ill and died. We aren't told any details about what happened to her. All we know is that she was cut short in a productive time of her life.

Peter was summoned, and, when he got to Joppa, he found Dorcas, lying in preparation for burial. Sending everybody out of the room, he got down on his knees, and prayed. The breath of life returned to Dorcas and she got up, healed and well.

When we feel sick, we often feel our life force ebbing from us. Some of us may have had a doctor give us a death sentence. But no human being is God. It is the Lord God Almighty who has the ultimate power of life and death. Do not hand your life over to satan. Hand your fears of dying before your days are fulfilled over to God.

The power that Peter tapped is the same today as it was two thousand years ago. Call upon God, listen to His instructions for your healing, and follow them exactly. Then know that God has plans for you and that they are for your good and your future.

Almighty merciful Father, I admit that I am afraid of dying before I fulfill Your mission and purpose for me. Remove my fear, O Lord. Guide my steps so that I walk in partnership with You and do not get distracted by the evil one. Raise me up, Lord, and keep me in Your loving care. In Jesus' name, I pray, Amen.

Day 321

For you have been born again, not of perishable seed, but of imperishable, through the living and enduring word of God. For, "All men are like grass and all their glory is like the flowers of the field; the grass withers and the flowers fall, but the word of the Lord stands forever." And this is the word that was preached to you. (1 Peter 1:23-25 NIV)

As a Christian, you have been born again. What a comfort and a joy that is. What does Peter say we have been born as? Imperishable seed. Imperishable because it flows from the eternal Word of God. No matter what happens to us, we cannot die. Our body will eventually die but the soul that is *us* will never die. We have been saved and redeemed through the atonement of Jesus Christ for our sins.

What is it that makes us imperishable seed? The Word of God. The living and enduring Word of God. Deep within us we must plant the seed of the Word of God, and we have to nurture it so that it will take hold and root.

Just as we plant the seed of the Word about love and eternal life, we must also plant the seed of the Word about faith, healing, and our spiritual life. The words of Jesus make powerful seeds. "Your faith has healed you. Go in peace and be freed from your suffering" (Mark 5:34). "You are set free from your infirmity" (Luke 13:12). "I am willing. Be clean" (Luke 5:13). "If you have faith as small as a mustard seed, you can say to this mountain, 'Move from here to there' and it will move. Nothing will be impossible for you" (Matthew 17:20-21). Plant these seeds of Jesus' words deeply in your heart and in your soul and in your body.

Now you must use your faith. You must believe that these words are true. And you must live expecting them to be fulfilled. If you focus on your symptoms instead of on your faith, you will be doing the same thing as a foolish farmer who goes out every day and digs up his seed to see if they are growing yet. What kind of yield will he have?

Be like the wise farmer and trust that the seed is growing within you. Ask the Holy Spirit for guidance to know how best to nourish it each day. You will be told the exact steps that you are to take in the healing process.

Wonderful Jehovah-rapha, I am Your imperishable seed. And I have the seed of Your Word within me. I plant the seed of faith that You are Jehovah-rapha, the God who heals me. Show me how You want me to nurture this seed so that it may manifest in my life and in my recovery. In Jesus' name, I pray, Amen.

Day 322

Their fruit will serve for food and their leaves for healing. (Ezekiel 47:12 NIV)

Have you ever thought about the staggering abundance of herbs that exist on our beautiful planet Earth? Do you believe they are the result of an accidental process – or do you believe that each plant was created with specific intent for a specific purpose by a Loving Creator?

What makes herbs so special? We know that they are as much of God's creation as we are, and, because of that fact, they are filled with God's blessed energy. They are vibrantly alive and each one sings its own song of praise to God. This song can actually be felt as a kind of vibrational energy.

Nature is filled with God's energy. Pick a tree you like and hug it. Put your arms around it and let your whole body lean into the tree trunk. Let your heart and your abdomen rest against the tree. Breathe deeply, close your eyes, and let every cell in your body feel the energy of the tree. It is Holy energy. Draw it in to your body.

If you have access to a growing herb, pick it and place it gently and respectfully in your hand. It might be a wild onion or some parsley or some sage. Cup your other hand over the plant, close your eyes, and let every cell in your body feel the energy of that herb. Focus on God's creation and give thanks for the plant in your hand.

In Ezekiel we are told that the leaves of the fruit trees were specifically created for our health and healing. God's herbs – and the essential oils within these herbs – are intended to be used to restore balance to our bodies. Every time we use herbs internally or externally, we bathe our cells in the Holy energy of God. When we pray for their effective use, we welcome the Holy Spirit at every level of our being. Learn about these precious treasures given by your loving, compassionate Heavenly Father. Use them wisely for the purpose they were intended and say, "Thank You."

O, wonderful Creator, I bow in awe to the glory and majesty of Your magnificent Creation. Thank You for the plants which You declared to me to be for food, and thank You for herbs and essential oils which You provided for my health and healing. Lead me, O God, to a greater understanding of how Your herbs work according to Your plan for my healing. Give me the perseverance to learn all I can about them, and give me the guidance to use them for my best and highest good. In Jesus' name, I pray, Amen.

Day 323

For the thing which I greatly feared is come upon me, and that which I was afraid of is come unto me. (Job 3:25 KJV)

It is a fascinating phenomenon that we draw to ourselves those things to which we give our focus and attention. When we live in a state of fear, we often find that we have more things about which to be frightened. Our alarm grows and grows as life seems more and more threatening.

A medical diagnosis of a physical problem generally carries with it a prognosis – or a likely result of the progression of the disease. Sometimes the prognosis is blindness, being crippled, or even dying. Have you received a medical report of similar magnitude? If so, now what do you do?

Your main challenge is to remain grounded in God's Word and to keep your focus on the power of Jehovah-rapha. God does not send you fear and despair; He sends you strength and healing. The key is to monitor your thoughts. "Whatever is true, whatever is noble, whatever is right, . . . think about such things" (Philippians 4:8). Watch the words you speak because you create your world with your words. Pay attention to what you say today. Do you want to live the literal meaning of your words? When you say, "My back is killing me," do you really want to live that experience? When you say, "I'll never be able to walk again," is that what you want? Express your current situation in terms of what you are experiencing for the moment. Be very careful when you use the powerful statement of "I am." Change statements about your health such as "I am tired" to "I feel tired."

Follow the pattern of Christ Jesus who never gave any power to fears about the obstacles put before Him. He was very clear that with God nothing was impossible. Jesus never forgot His mission – to deliver God's message of love and to heal God's children. People who focus on their purpose are less likely to get sidetracked by fear. Determine God's mission for your life and keep your mind focused on it. If fears come to your mind, recognize that those thoughts are from satan, and tell him to get behind you and to go away. Jehovah-rapha is the God of all that is good and positive.

Almighty God, I can relate to Job when he said that the things he feared ended up happening to him. Help me, God, from falling into the same trap. You do not bring me these fears; satan does. Keep me focused on Your Divine purpose for my life. In Jesus' name, I pray, Amen.

Day 324

Your word, O Lord, is eternal; it stands firm in the heavens. Your faithfulness continues through all generations; you established the earth, and it endures. Your laws endure to this day, for all things serve you. If your law had not been my delight, I would have perished in my affliction. I will never forget your precepts, for by them you have preserved my life. (Psalm 119:89-93 NIV)

In the beginning was the Word, and the Word was with God, and the Word was God. He was with God in the beginning. Through him all things were made; without him nothing was made that has been made. In him was life, and that life was the light of men. The light shines in the darkness, but the darkness has not understood it. (John 1:1-5 NIV)

As ye have therefore received Christ Jesus the Lord, so walk ye in him: Rooted and built up in him, and established in the faith, as ye have been taught, abounding therein with thanksgiving. (Colossians 2:6-7 KJV)

Sometimes we forget that God is eternal. Christ Jesus is eternal. And the Word is eternal. It always was, is now, and ever shall be. The Word is truth and life and light. God's will is revealed in His Word and it has never changed from the beginning.

Without the Word we cannot survive. It is our blueprint for living and the scaffolding upon which we build our lives. It is the source of our strength and the focus of our very being. We cannot fail when we obey God's Word and implement it in our lives.

Walk in Christ Jesus. Hand Him your doubts and your unbelief so that you may be rooted and built up in Him. Jesus warned that those who did not put His words and teachings into practice would be like a house built on sand that would be washed away when the storms come.

Jesus spent His life doing the eternal will of the Father. He healed everyone who came to Him, and He sent His disciples out to heal everyone who would receive them. Accept the will of the Father for you to be healed. Ask for His deliverance from your affliction and give Him thanks.

Wonderful Jehovah-rapha, I serve You and find delight in Your Word. I will never forget your precepts, for by them you have preserved my life. I stand rooted in You and my Savior Christ Jesus. In Jesus' name, I pray, Amen.

Day 325

Jesus left there and went to his hometown, accompanied by his disciples. When the Sabbath came, he began to teach in the synagogue, and many who heard him were amazed. "Where did this man get these things?" they asked. "What's this wisdom that has been given him, that he even does miracles! Isn't this the carpenter? Isn't this Mary's son and the brother of James, Joseph, Judas and Simon? Aren't his sisters here with us?" And they took offense at him. Jesus said to them, "Only in his hometown, among his relatives and in his own house is a prophet without honor." He could not do any miracles there, except lay his hands on a few sick people and heal them. And he was amazed at their lack of faith. (Mark 6:1-6 NIV)

The hometown people of Nazareth believed that they knew who Jesus was – a carpenter, a son of Mary and Joseph, and a brother. They didn't notice anything unusual about Him when He was growing up, and they were comfortable with Him. Now here He was going around teaching, preaching, expressing ideas that astounded them, and even doing miracles. What had happened to the person they thought they knew? They were angry – but mostly they were afraid.

They would have to change in order to be with Him. Their fear and lack of faith held them back. The result was that Jesus could not do any miracles there, and He was able to perform only a few healings.

Don't be discouraged if some – or even all – your friends and family do not support you in walking a God-directed path to recovery. You will be talking a different talk and walking a different walk. They are used to the "old" you, and they will say, "But you are taking your life in your own hands." They often cannot understand that for the first time you are taking responsibility for your health and giving your life totally to the care and guidance of God. This approach is frightening to those who believe that there is only one way to healing.

Learn to discern with whom to discuss your health situation and with whom it is best to be silent. Do not try to convince anyone to accept what you are doing. Instead, seek out those who *can* support you in following God's guidance. Hold to your faith and give Jesus full honor in *your* house.

Wonderful Jehovah-rapha, bring people into my life to support me in my healing journey. Give me courage to keep my house a place that gives full honor to Your Son. Give me strength to follow Your guidance for the healing of my temple. In Jesus' name, I pray, Amen.

Day 326

These are rebellious people, deceitful children, children unwilling to listen to the Lord's instruction. They say to the seers, "See no more visions!" and to the prophets, "Give us no more visions of what is right! Tell us pleasant things, prophesy illusions. Leave this way, get off this path, and stop confronting us with the Holy One of Israel!" . . . This is what the Sovereign Lord, the Holy One of Israel says: "In repentance and rest is your salvation, in quietness and trust is your strength, but you would have none of it. You said, 'No, we will flee on horses.' Therefore you will flee! You said, 'We will ride off on swift horses.' Therefore your pursuers will be swift!" . . . Yet the Lord longs to be gracious to you; he rises to show you compassion. For the Lord is a God of justice. Blessed are all who wait for him! (Isaiah 30:9-11, 15-16, 18 NIV)

Why is it that we think we have better answers than God? Over and over again God offers solutions to our problems but we are sure we know a better way. Often God's answers seem impossible or ridiculous – or even stupid. With an army in hot pursuit, God told his people that their strength was in "quietness and trust." But no, they relied on the appearance of the situation, trusted in their horses and fled in fear. The only result was that their pursuers were as swift as they were.

God is constantly having to deal with human beings who are stubborn and rebellious. We become filled with arrogance, and we are convinced that we are the creators of knowledge and truth. This is especially true in the medical field and in issues relating to our health. We are "unwilling to listen to the Lord's instruction."

We tell God that He doesn't have any place in the study of scientific "facts." We place our faith in scientific theories and forget that they are theories and not God's truth. We foolishly tell God that we will "leave His way and get off His path because we are tired of being confronted with the Holy One of Israel!"

God is a patient God. He is filled with compassion for us and He wants to heal us. Sometimes He uses the methods we have discovered and invented. But other times He tells us "in quietness and trust is your strength." Don't tell God, "I will have none of it." Say instead, "yes, Lord, I hear You and I will obey."

Almighty God, thank You for being patient with me. I have been rebellious and I am sorry. I want to be healed, and I am willing to listen to You and to follow Your instructions. Guide me, O compassionate Lord, and I will be obedient. In the name of Your Son, Jesus Christ, Amen.

Day 327

Therefore the Lord himself shall give you a sign; Behold, a virgin shall conceive, and bear a son, and shall call his name Immanuel. Butter and honey shall he eat, that he may know to refuse the evil and choose the good. (Isaiah 7:14-15 KJV)

Butter. Here is another food that we have been told is very unhealthy for us to eat. Again, let us turn to the Scriptures. Isaiah tells us that the Messiah will eat butter and honey. Why? So that He will know how to *choose the good* and to refuse the evil. Isn't that an interesting statement? Think about it for a moment and meditate on it.

Our health – or lack of it – is in large part due to the consequences of choices we have made. Years and years of unwise food consumption eventually takes its toll on our organs, and we become ill. Certainly Isaiah is not suggesting a diet of nothing *but* butter and honey; however, he is clearly stating that butter and honey are classified as good things.

The latest scientific reports seem to be confirming Isaiah. We humans invented margarine with the intention that it be an improvement over natural butter, but now it appears that margarine creates health problems that are worse than the ones we thought butter caused. Being a saturated fatty acid, butter does contain cholesterol. However, it is digested by the human body in such a way that generally does not raise the levels of harmful fats in the blood. Eaten in moderation, it is indeed a good food.

Remember, too, that the butter discussed in the Holy Scriptures was made from wholesome, raw milk from healthy cows. Amazingly, even today bacterial counts allowed for raw milk is far *lower* than that for pasteurized milk.

Should you eat butter? Don't make any assumptions; instead, go in prayer and ask God what you should do. Meditate until you receive clear answers through the Holy Spirit about the advisability of butter in your diet at this particular point in your healing. Then follow all the guidance that you are given.

Wonderful Jehovah-rapha, too often I follow the opinions of men instead of asking You what decisions I should make in my life. Then when things go wrong, I turn to You. Help me, Lord, to go to You first. All I need to do is to take the time to ask – and yet I too often find excuses for not doing so. I want to be well, God. Instruct me about the foods that You want me to eat. Help me to work in full partnership with You, my God who heals me. In the name of Your Son, Jesus Christ, I pray, Amen.

Day 328

Let not your heart be troubled: ye believe in God, believe also in me. (John 14:1 KJV)

Stop worrying. Trust God. Trust Jesus. Six simple words get to the heart of Christian faith.

What is trust all about? The first part of trust is believing. It is believing that God *can* do what He says He *will* do. And it is believing that God *does* do what He says He *will* do. This level of trust is totally spiritual, and most Christians generally profess to have this faith.

The second part of trust is action. Beliefs are meaningless unless they are manifested in action. Trusting in God means asking God's direction in your daily activities and listening for His answers *before* proceeding. This is especially true when it comes to your health.

Let's take a simple example. Suppose you have an ordinary headache. How many times do you reach for a bottle of painkiller without ever asking God what is the healthiest course of action for you to take? Now let's move to something much more difficult. How many times do you follow medical opinions for serious problems without asking The Great Physician for His instructions as well?

Having received the best medical advice you can get, lay down your own opinions – and the opinions of others – at the feet of Jesus so that you can hear God's voice clearly. Lay down your own logic – and that of others – which has only the narrow view of a human being.

Open yourself up to allow God's perfect wisdom to be revealed to you. Then follow exactly what you receive from Jehovah-rapha. This is the way to eliminate worry and fear from your life. This is belief in action. This is trust made reality.

Jehovah-rapha, I confess that my mind wanders to all my symptoms and my illness too often in the day, and I find myself worrying about what I see and what I feel in my body. God, fill me with the words of Your Son who exhorted me to stop worrying, to believe in You, and to believe in Him. God, just for today I declare my trust in You and in Your Son Jesus Christ. Just for today I will LIVE my trust in You and in Your Son Jesus Christ. You are Jehovah-rapha, the God who heals me. Your Son healed ALL who came to Him; and He said, "Your faith has made you whole." I believe. I trust. Thank You, God. In Jesus' name, I pray, Amen.

Day 329

Going on from that place, he went into their synagogue, and a man with a shriveled hand was there. Looking for a reason to accuse Jesus, they asked him, "Is it lawful to heal on the Sabbath?" He said to them, "If any of you has a sheep and it falls into a pit on the Sabbath, will you not take hold of it and lift it out? How much more valuable is a man than a sheep! Therefore it is lawful to do good on the Sabbath." Then he said to the man, "Stretch out your hand." So he stretched it out and it was completely restored, just as sound as the other. (Matthew 12:9-13 NIV)

This story from Matthew emphasizes the importance that God places on saving His people – and on healing them. When Jesus is challenged with the question of the legality of healing on the Sabbath, He gives an illustration of a shepherd saving a sheep that has fallen into a pit on the Sabbath Day. "How much more valuable is a person than a sheep!" He exclaims.

Standing before Him on a Sabbath day is a man with a withered hand. Jesus demonstrates that the real issue doesn't have to do with rabbinical law; it has to do with the importance that God places on meeting the needs of His children. The Son of God is very clear that it is always God's will for His children to be rescued. Notice that Jesus includes healing as one aspect of deliverance.

In this particular instance, how does Jesus perform the healing? He tells the man to take action. This is an action of faith in advance of any manifestation of healing. "Stretch out your hand," He says. The man believed, followed the instruction that he was given, and was healed.

God is your Good Shepherd. He cares for you and wants to rescue you from the pit of sickness and disease. No matter what, no matter when. He sent His Son to bear your infirmities on the Cross. He sent the Holy Spirit as the beacon of truth to guide you and to reveal to you what action you are to take. Over and over again He tells you that He has a plan for you and that it is a plan for good. Jehovah watches over you as a shepherd guards his sheep, protecting, healing, and saving you.

Wonderful Jehovah-rapha, I am one of the little sheep in your flock who has fallen into the pit and needs Your rescue. I call to You and place my total trust and belief in You. Reveal to me today the actions You want me to take and I will do them. Thank You for healing and restoring me. In the name of Your Son, Jesus Christ, my Savior and my Redeemer. Amen.

Day 330

Of all the animals that live on land, these are the ones you may eat: You may eat any animal that has a split hoof completely divided and that chews the cud. . . . Of all the creatures living in the water of the seas and the streams, you may eat any that have fins and scales. (Leviticus 11:2-3, 9 NIV)

Since proper nutrition is an important key to health, God's Word is filled with guidance about what is healthy to eat. We are told that the herbs and plants are to be for food. And we are given instructions with regard to land animals, water animals, birds, and insects.

As Christians, it is still appropriate that we study and follow the instructions about food that were given in the Old Testament. They are very relevant to us today, and now we know the reason why that is true. The animals that do not fall into the "clean" category have a common characteristic: they have a high tolerance for toxins in their system. Most of them are scavengers. Unfortunately, some foods are included that many of us find extremely tasty: for example, oysters, lobster, pork, shrimp, and catfish.

When God created our world, He needed a clean-up crew that would eat garbage and still be able to survive. They would be walking, swimming, and flying garbage-recycling plants. So, He created pigs as part of his land clean-up crew, vultures to feed on dead carcasses, and catfish and shellfish to keep oceans, rivers, and lakes clean. The systems of all these animals are able to sustain a high level of bacteria, viruses, and parasites without themselves dying.

It is hazardous to eat food prepared from animals that have a high toxin level in their system because, by doing so, we risk infection. It is well known that a large proportion of food poisoning in humans comes after we eat pork or shellfish. We have violated God's health law when we eat them.

As you walk on your path to your healing, pay attention to the foods you eat. You will find that, if you obey God's food guidelines, you will greatly assist your healing process.

Blessed Creator, thank You for providing guidelines in Your Holy Word to tell me which foods are healthiest for me to eat. I confess that I love some of the items You have told me are hazardous. Speak to me, O God, and teach me the foods that are best for me to eat as part of my recovery. I will do my part in providing my body the best nutrition I can. In Jesus' name, I pray, Amen.

Day 331

Then I heard the voice of the Lord saying, "Whom shall I send? And who will go for us?" And I said, "Here am I. Send me." (Isaiah 6:8 NIV)

God needs willing helpers. Those of us who feel sick and are hurting are called to be special ambassadors of Christ to help others who are experiencing the same suffering. Take the time every day to pray for others who are ill or injured.

There are many people who do not know where to turn and who have never heard of the healing power of God. There are those who believe in God but who feel unworthy of being healed. There are others who are too weak to act in their own behalf. And there are the saddest ones of all – those who feel alone, abandoned, and afraid.

Through your own suffering you have a special calling. Everyday pray for others who are ill. Here is a prayer which you may use, or you may prefer one of your own. Before you begin, select a male or a female and pray appropriately:

Merciful God, there is someone today who is sick, hurting, and afraid. I don't know who this person is, Lord, but You do. You can see her now. I humbly ask that You send a special angel to be with this person, God. You know her fears, her pain, her fatigue. Speak to her in a way that she can hear You and help her to find the guidance that she needs. Lift her, comfort her, and touch her with Your healing hand. If she does not know Your Son, Jesus Christ, I pray that someone will come to share the good news with her – that Your Son has already redeemed her, soul and body. In Jesus' name, I pray, Amen.

After you finish praying, sit quietly for a moment, visualizing in your mind an angel ministering to this person and caring for her (or him). Remember our Lord's words that, as you have done for the least of these, you have done it also for Him. By helping others, you bring greater healing into your own life as well.

Merciful Lord, help me to help others who are hurting. I want to be a good ambassador for Your Son Jesus Christ and to fulfill His command to go into all the world spreading His message. Sometimes when I am really down, I suddenly feel lifted – and I often think that somewhere someone is praying for me. I want to pass it on, Lord, and to become part of the chain of Your love. In Jesus' name, I pray, Amen.

Day 332

Jesus replied, "No one who puts his hand to the plow and looks back is fit for service in the kingdom of God." (Luke 9:62 NIV)

Not that I have already obtained all this, or have already been made perfect, but I press on to take hold of that for which Christ Jesus took hold of me. Brothers, I do not consider myself yet to have taken hold of it. But one thing I do: Forgetting what is behind and straining toward what is ahead, I press on toward the goal to win the prize for which God has called me heavenward in Christ Jesus. (Philippians 3:12-14 NIV)

Too many people waste their lives living in the past. They are consumed by resentment for wrongs done to them, by grief over losses and traumas, and by regret for mistakes and errors. They live with the words, "if only" on their lips and spend endless hours and days reliving events that have long since passed.

This kind of behavior is fertile ground for the evil one. He loves to keep you mired in unresolved issues of the past because it is one of the best ways to prevent you from engaging in living in the present. You cannot be here, fully present today in your body and soul, when you are focused on yesterday.

When you are constantly looking behind you, you can't see where you are, and you will drive blindly into the future. The failure to connect with the current moment creates a spiritual imbalance that leads to a mental and physiological imbalance. Illness often results.

Are you living in the past? Pay attention to your thoughts, and actually write down issues that concern something that happened in the past but still occupy your attention. Turn each situation over to God. Ask for forgiveness for your part in the event. If you need to make atonement to someone, do it. Ask God to reveal to you what you can learn from the situation. Then move on!

Paul says that he forgets what is behind and instead takes hold of Christ Jesus. Today is all we really have. Yesterday is gone. And tomorrow is always a day away. Christ Jesus offers us life abundant today, this moment. Live in Him and glorify His name.

Wonderful Jehovah-rapha, teach me to live in this moment. I let go of the past and connect fully to You in this glorious day that You have given me. Show me how to fulfill Your purpose for my life. Forgetting what is behind, I press on in Your service, standing on Your Word and following Your Son, Jesus Christ. In Jesus' name, I pray, Amen.

Day 333

There are six things the Lord hates, seven that are detestable to him: haughty eyes, a lying tongue, hands that shed innocent blood, a heart that devises wicked schemes, feet that are quick to rush into evil, a false witness who pours out lies and a man who stirs up dissension among brothers. (Proverbs 6:16-19 NIV)

When you get off the track internally, you have moved from being in alignment with God to being in alignment with satan. There is no middle ground. If you are not of God, you are being manipulated by the evil one.

Keeping yourself mentally and spiritually grounded and following God's will is vital to your physical good health. As soon as you become vulnerable to the evil one, your body is open for illness and disease to take hold.

What things make us particularly vulnerable? Of course, there are many, but these verses in Proverbs list several. Arrogance, lying, killing innocent people, evil actions, and causing dissension. Isn't it interesting that lying and evil actions are both listed in two different ways?

How do these relate to your health problems? They are often the source of them because they are all satan's seeds. If they find fertile soil within you, then they can grow into illness. Once you have a health problem, if you continue to cultivate these qualities, you will have a very hard time getting well.

Arrogance particularly locks you into illness because it leads you to assume you know what actions you should take. These assumptions are often wrong, yet you are so sure they are right that you never ask God what His opinion is. Before you take action, pray and ask for guidance.

Jesus always connected the forgiveness of sins with His healing. Always. Thank God for sending His Son to bear your sins and your infirmities on the Cross. Lay down your weaknesses and your failures at the feet of the Resurrected One, and ask the Lord God Almighty to forgive you. Allow Him to wash you clean and to heal you.

Merciful Lord, I have done many things that I wish I had not done, and I have failed to do many things which I know I should have done. Forgive me, Heavenly Father. Wash me clean. Heal my spirit and my mind as well as my body. I give myself to You completely and I put myself-totally in Your loving care. In the name of Your Son, I pray, Jesus Christ, Amen.

Day 334

That the Lord Jesus the same night in which he was betrayed took bread: And when he had given thanks, he brake it, and said, "Take, eat: this is my body, which is broken for you: this do in remembrance of me." After the same manner also he took the cup, when he had supped, saying, "This cup is the new testament in my blood: this do ye, as oft as ye drink it, in remembrance of me." (1 Corinthians 11:23-25 KJV)

Jesus established the ordinance that we call The Lord's Supper. Sharing it with others is a very special time for Christians, for it brings us close to each other and to our Lord Jesus Christ.

Notice that we partake of both bread and wine. Why two items? If Jesus wanted us to remember Him, we would need only one. Perhaps two items were important because there were two parts to His mission and there were two parts to His sacrificial death. It is written that Jesus bore our sins *and* our infirmities on the Cross. Jesus knew that, and, therefore, He gave us The Lord's Supper to remind us.

". . . he . . . took bread. And when he had given thanks, he brake it, and said, 'Take, eat: this is my body, which is broken for you.' " He took the infirmities of our body to the Cross. We eat the bread in remembrance of His body which was broken for us. We eat the bread in remembrance that "his life may be revealed in our mortal body" (2 Corinthians 4:11). We are to live fully and healthily in this body in complete service to the Lord God Almighty.

Will our mortal bodies live forever? Of course not. When we have fulfilled our days, we know, as faithful believers in Jesus Christ, that we will one day meet our Savior face to face in God's heavenly kingdom in the place He has prepared for us.

When Jesus took the cup, He said, "This . . . is the new testament in my blood." The wine represented Jesus' death for our eternal souls. It is His sacrifice on the Cross for our sins and transgressions. Though our bodies will die, our souls will have eternal life.

Celebrate the Lord's Supper with special thanksgiving, knowing that Jesus was the perfect Atonement for you – body and soul.

Almighty God, thank You for the sacrifice of Your Son Jesus Christ, who died on the Cross for me. For me. He bore my sins and He bore my infirmities. I eat the bread and am not afraid to live, fulfilling Your purpose for me on this earth. And I drink the cup and am not afraid to die, passing into life eternal. In Jesus' name, I pray, Amen.

Day 335

Let the sea resound, and everything in it, the world, and all who live in it. Let the rivers clap their hands, let the mountains sing together for joy; let them sing before the Lord. (Psalm 98:7-9 NIV)

What a beautiful picture of all the earth singing before the Lord. All creation sings to its Maker. God created everything to be filled with its own kind of energy. Every single thing that exists is comprised of atoms, and those atoms have electrons that whirl around and around a nucleus. They are motion that never stops as long as that object exists.

So the mountains do indeed sing with their own music, their own vibration, their own energy. Our Creator designed much of that energy to be healing for us. It is interesting that essential oils are one way that we can tap into that healing energy. The Holy Scriptures are filled with references to the use of essential oils. Jesus was given frankincense and myrrh at His birth; His feet were bathed with spikenard during His days of ministry; and His body was wrapped in cloths dipped in myrrh after His crucifixion.

In the lovely passage from Psalms we see the trees of the mountains singing together. Juniper has been used for centuries for urinary tract infections and for kidney and bladder problems. Birch has been used to strengthen bones and relieve bone and muscle pain. Cedarwood has been used by the American Indians for its purifying action on problems such as acne and skin diseases. Spruce has been used to restore the glandular system, including the pineal, thymus, and adrenal glands. Fir has been used for bronchial problems and respiratory complaints.

Essential oils have many regenerating, detoxifying, and oxygenating qualities. Their molecules are able to pass through cell walls quickly, and some even can pass the blood brain barrier which may make them useful to people with brain disorders such as Alzheimer's and Parkinson's disease. Because the vibrational energy of essential oils is higher than the human body, they lift the energy within us and thus help to restore health to us.

Learn about the therapeutic value of essential oils, and ask the Holy Spirit if they would be useful in daily anointing for your healing.

Great Creator, thank You for Your Divine energy. Guide me in learning about natural substances such as essential oils. Show me which ones can be most useful in my healing. You have provided so many healing remedies to me in nature, O Lord. Help me to use them wisely. In the name of Jesus Christ, my Savior and my Redeemer, I pray, Amen.

Day 336

Now on his way to Jerusalem, Jesus traveled along the border between Samaria and Galilee. As he was going into a village, ten men who had leprosy met him. They stood at a distance and called out in a loud voice, "Jesus, Master, have pity on us!" When he saw them, he said, "Go, show yourselves to the priests." And as they went, they were cleansed. One of them, when he saw he was healed, came back, praising God in a loud voice. He threw himself at Jesus' feet and thanked him – and he was a Samaritan. Jesus asked, "Were not all ten cleansed? Where are the other nine? Was no one found to return and give praise to God except this foreigner?" Then he said to him, "Rise and go; your faith has made you well." (Luke 17:11-19 NIV)

All ten men are cleansed of leprosy, but *pay attention to this:* only one man was pronounced well by Jesus. Doesn't this seem to be strange? Jesus had healed them all at the same time and in the same way. The only reason that the Samaritan came back was that he recognized that his healing had been accomplished and he wanted to say "thank you." But only this one man was considered by Jesus to be well!

Sick people today play out this Scripture over and over, particularly in our society. We confuse the disappearance of symptoms with being well. Being well is returning to the wholeness of body, mind, emotions, and soul that God intended. It means far more than not having lesions of leprosy on your body or a consumptive cough or a growing tumor. It includes those things, but it is far more than those things.

It is particularly easy today to go for the "quick fix." We buy into the illusion that, if we can make a symptom go away, we have solved the problem. We want to make no changes in our choices or behavior, and we take no responsibility for the consequences of our actions. To follow this pattern we guarantee that we will be sick again, perhaps with the same problem but more often with a more serious one. And we are too foolish to see the connection. In fact, we usually insist that there is none.

Do you want to feel better momentarily? Or do you want to be truly well? Adopt an attitude of gratitude that will keep you close to God. It will keep you receptive to hearing God's will for you, and it will keep you willing to follow that guidance with active choices for healing in your life.

Gracious God, I am grateful for each step in my healing. Thank You, God, thank You. I declare my faith in You, Jehovah-rapha. I am willing to follow Your guidance and to make whatever changes You want me to make. In the name of Your Son, Jesus Christ, I pray, Amen.

Day 337

But thanks be to God, which giveth us the victory through our Lord Jesus Christ. There-fore, my beloved brethren, be ye stedfast, unmoveable, always abounding in the work of the Lord, forasmuch as ye know that your labour is not in vain in the Lord. (1 Corinthians 15:57-58 KJV)

Be steadfast and unmovable. Don't let anything distract you away from God's purpose for your life. Don't let anything push you out of God's will for you. Check in with God a zillion times a day to make sure that you are "abounding in *His* work."

What if you feel sick or infirm? You are still a child of God, and you still must be about His business. No labor for the Lord is in vain. Living to the fullest and to the limit of your capacity for each moment, whatever it might be, is to glorify God.

Sense the exhilaration in these words of Paul. We have been given victory through our Lord Jesus Christ. We have been given victory over *everything*. Eventually our mortal body will die, but even death cannot claim us because our eternal souls will live forever with God.

No matter what physical situation you are in, keep your eyes on the victory of the Resurrected Christ. No matter what physical situation you are in, give thanks to God for His Word that nothing is too hard for Him. No matter what physical situation you are in, remain steadfast and unmovable in believing His promises to you. No matter what physical situation are you are in, abound in His work.

Witness for Him. Let everyone you meet feel the Lord's love and light radiate within you. Let everyone you meet see the Lord working in you and through you. Let everyone you meet be filled with awe at seeing the power of the Lord at work.

Don't compare who you are or what you are doing with anyone else. You are unique. There is only one person with your particular mission and your particular path. Satan may attack you, but the victory is God's if you will claim it. God can create something beautiful out of every situation. Trust Him. Be unmovable.

Almighty God, thank You. You give me victory over every obstacle through Your Son Jesus Christ. Help me to be steadfast and unmovable, always abounding in Your work. Let me be a witness for Your glory and Your power and Your goodness. In the name of Your Son, Jesus Christ, I pray, Amen.

Day 338

No temptation has seized you except what is common to man. And God is faithful; he will not let you be tempted beyond what you can bear. But when you are tempted, he will also provide a way out so that you can stand up under it. (1 Corinthians 10:13 NIV)

The evil one whispers to us frequently and persistently, many of his temptations relating to some lifestyle choice which will negatively affect our health. We must stand firm and remember that God always provides us a way out so that we do not have to succumb to poor choices.

The whispers come so softly and subtly. "It's too cold to take a walk today." "There's no time for lunch today." "There is no time to rest this Sunday." "You'd better skip your morning prayer time because you overslept." The little arrows come one by one.

There are many temptations which come to us, but one to which we can all relate are food temptations. Our health is a reflection in large part of the foods we eat. The whispers of the evil one convince us to gorge ourselves on either high-calorie foods lacking in nutrition or highly processed foods almost devoid of nutrients.

How do we handle these temptations? First, put on the armor of the Lord, including the "shield of faith, with which you can extinguish all the flaming arrows of the evil one" (Ephesians 6:16).

Second, ask God for His protection and for His guidance to show you the way out.

Third, ask your friends and your family for help. Tell them what your health goals are and what lifestyle choices you are making. Don't insist that they adopt your plan for themselves. Simply ask that they support and encourage you. If they want to eat foods which you consider to be unhealthy, don't criticize them for doing so. Just say "no thank you" and allow them to do as they wish.

Stand firm on the path that Jehovah-rapha shows you.

Wonderful Jehovah-rapha, I am grateful that You are faithful to me. I am tempted often, God. I get tired and I get busy and I get distracted. And then it is easy to find an excuse not to do the things that I should and to do the things that I know I shouldn't do. Help me stand up to the arrows of the evil one, God. I want to be a full partner with You in my recovery. Show me the way out so that I can stand firm and not stray from the path You want me to follow. In the name of Your Son, Jesus Christ, I pray, Amen.

Day 339

Let them praise his name with dancing and make music to him with tambourine and harp. (Psalm 149:3 NIV)

Then man goes out to his work, to his labor until evening. (Psalm 104:23 NIV)

Human beings were not created to sit still all day long behind desks or the wheel of an automobile. Our bodies were made to walk, run, bend, turn, stretch, and dance. Movement was meant to be such an integral part of our lives that the concept of "exercise" would be puzzling. Unfortunately for the large majority of adults and children in this country, we now have to schedule periods of exercise into our sedentary lives in order to maintain good health.

Every system of the body needs movement in order to function normally. Circulation of the blood accelerates; breathing increases; lymphatic fluid moves; the glands and organs are stimulated and massaged. Toxins are flushed from our tissues; fat is burned instead of stored; and cells bustle with life and activity. The bowels work regularly; muscles are toned; and weight is normalized. Movement affects not only our physical self but also our emotional self. Many people who are depressed find that their spirits are lifted and normalized simply by taking regular walks. Endorphins flow and soon they are humming as they walk along.

If you feel ill, ask God if you are to begin a program to move your body. If you are currently unable to walk, blink your eyes, pucker your lips, and move whatever body parts that you can. It is best to begin slowly, increasing activity each day. "No pain, no gain" is a foolhardy philosophy. Movement should be pleasurable, and you can increase your stamina by extending yourself without reaching a point of pain. If you aren't smiling and praising God while you are exercising, consider doing something else! Offer your exercise to the Lord and rejoice! Dancing is a marvelous way to move your body. It connects body and spirit together, and is a delightful way to connect to other people and to God.

Wonderful Jehovah-rapha, I have been too sedentary for too long. I praise Your name in dancing and moving my body. I especially love taking a walk when I can look at the sky, the trees, and all the handiworks of nature that You generously gave to us. Through movement and work I stimulate all the systems of my body to function better, and I glorify Your name through my exercise. In Jesus' name, I pray, Amen.

Day 340

By wisdom a house is built, and through understanding it is established; through knowledge its rooms are filled with rare and beautiful treasures. (Proverbs 24:3-4 NIV)

When you have a health condition, one of the essential ingredients to being a partner with God for your healing is to seek knowledge about it. There are two major facets of learning. The first concerns the way that your body works. Always look for common links between your various health conditions. For example, suppose your triglyceride level is high and your blood sugar level is at the high end of the normal range. In this case, one possible link is a malfunctioning pancreas.

The second aspect of study concerns God's remedies for human health problems. God designed your body. No human is ever likely to understand the way that it functions as thoroughly as God does. Don't forget that fact when you receive emphatic opinions, especially ones of doom, from human beings. God also created plants and He considered them to be so critical to the well-being of people that one of the two first instructions He gave to man was to order that plants be used for food.

Some people believe that the plants evolved, that later man evolved, and that it just happens that plants taste good as food and meet a good many of the needs of people. The Holy Scripture tells us that God designed plants specifically for our healing. "Their fruit will serve for food and their leaves for healing" (Ezekiel 47:12).

Therefore, search for God's remedies. To fail to do so is to ignore God's instruction. It is to follow the assumption that all man-made remedies are superior to God's remedies. Of course, many of man's medicines are beneficial and useful, but to label God's remedies as old-fashioned or out-moded is pure folly. Scripture said long ago, "My people perish for lack of knowledge" (Hosea 4:6). Why are we so stubborn in refusing to allow God's leadership? Open your mind and heart to the glory of God's creation and to the use of God's remedies – essential oils and herbs – for your healing where you are guided to do so.

Almighty God, help me to build a strong temple for Your glory. Give me wisdom to seek Your advice and guidance for every step I take on my path to recovery. Show me the way to find books, teachers, and instruction so that I may expand my understanding of my body and my health conditions. Thank You for sending Your Son, who bore my illnesses on the Cross and who has redeemed me, soul and body. In Jesus' name, I pray, Amen.

Day 341

Refrain from anger, and turn from wrath: do not fret – it leads only to evil. (Psalm 37:8 NIV)

This Psalm isn't telling us never to allow the feeling of anger. When it is functioning normally, anger is a human emotion that tells us that we have been violated in some way. To suppress it is unhealthy.

However, anger is supposed to be a momentary warning sign, like a yellow light. It flashes, we notice it, we make a decision about it, and then we release it. It's all a fairly rapid process. Once we feel our anger, it is up to us to make a wise choice in how to handle it. Choosing to lash out in wrath at others either verbally or physically leads only to our being controlled by the evil one. On the other hand, choosing to use our anger to strengthen our boundaries and make our position clear to the other person means that we have decided to follow our sovereign Lord.

Most of us have a hard time letting go of anger. The longer we hold onto it, the stronger it gets. Some people direct their anger outward at others, and some people turn their anger inward toward themselves. Both choices lead only to pain and suffering. Letting go of anger is hard because you must do two things: you must take sole responsibility for having nurtured it, and you must then make a conscious decision not to continue carrying it. You must face the hurt and the sorrow that lies underneath it.

Perhaps the hardest anger to deal with is anger toward God. Many of us are angry with God, particularly for events that happened in our past. We are angry because we feel that God failed to protect us and let us down. This anger stands in the way of trust and faith. Look into your heart. God already knows what is there. If you are ready to be free of it, be courageous enough to acknowledge your anger and offer it to Him. Let Him fill you with His healing love.

Merciful Father, I have misused my anger. I have held onto old hurts and kept anger alive. Most of all, God, I have felt angry with You. I feel ashamed to admit it but it is true. The child inside of me is angry with You and sometimes is also afraid to trust You. Help me, Lord, to heal the wounds of this child. I stand before You as an adult, not as this child of long ago. I take full responsibility for my decisions. I choose a new life with You, Lord. Cleanse me of all anger. Fill me with Your healing love. In the name of Your Son, Jesus Christ, my Savior and my Redeemer, I pray, Amen.

Day 342

Let the redeemed of the Lord say so, whom he hath redeemed from the hand of the enemy.
(Psalm 107:2 KJV)

The central message of God's Holy Scripture is that God loves you and has redeemed you fully. You are His beloved child and He wants you safely in His care. Do you believe this in the innermost places of your heart? If so, then declare your faith, and proclaim the victory that has been won for you.

Let all the words of your mouth reflect your belief that Jehovah-rapha is the God who is healing you. Speak according to the example of Jesus Christ, who repeatedly instructed His followers to do as He did. "You can have what you say," He told us in Mark 11:23; therefore, let your words declare God's solutions instead of satan's problems.

We have been redeemed from the hand of the enemy. It has already been done. Satan has no authority over us unless we give it to him. None.

Nevertheless, satan is persistent, and, as the father of lies, he is always ready to take advantage of our weak places. Whenever he can get us to be fearful, he claims a victory. Whenever he can get us to use careless words of death (such as "I'm dying for a drink of soda."), he claims a victory. Whenever he can get us to speak of our symptoms and pains instead of our trust in God's healing path for our recovery, he claims a victory.

When you are overwhelmed by the appearance of illness, stand up and say boldly, "I am redeemed by the blood of Jesus Christ. I am redeemed! And by His stripes I am healed. Satan, you have no power over me and you must leave my body. Body, I declare that you are healed in the name of Jesus Christ, who bore my infirmities on the Cross. I know that my Redeemer lives, and because He lives, I have life abundantly."

Almighty God, You have redeemed me from the hand of the enemy, and I sing my grateful praises! You are the great Jehovah-rapha, and in You I place my total trust. Let the words of my mouth reflect my full faith that You are healing me, and help me to be aware of the times when I sabotage my healing through careless, "faith-less" words. You sent Your Son Jesus Christ to show me the way and to overcome the evil one forever. Thank You, Lord, for delivering me. In Jesus' name, I pray, Amen.

Day 343

All Scripture is God-breathed and is useful for teaching, rebuking, correcting and training in righteousness, so that the man of God may be thoroughly equipped for every good work. (2 Timothy 3:16-17 NIV)

What is our best teacher and the best source for help, for encouragement, for examples? The Holy Scripture. God wants us to use His Holy Word as our guide because it marks the way for us.

In this letter written to Timothy, Paul describes Holy Scripture as "God-breathed." Isn't that a beautiful way to express the fact that it is divinely inspired? Yes, it was written by human beings and reflects their biases and limitations. Yet, in spite of that, God's voice rings out clear and true.

It is so important to turn to God's Word when you feel ill or have been injured. It is your beacon, lighting the way for you. It will teach you God's truth and God's good news – that He is the God who heals you and that Jesus Christ bore your sins and infirmities on the Cross for you.

It will also instruct, correct, and train you. It will teach you how to pray. It will teach you how to live. It will teach you healthy foods to eat. It will teach you how to ask for healing. It will teach you the importance of asking the Holy Spirit for guidance. It will teach you how to trust.

It will train you by example. It is filled with illustrations of men and women who sought God – as well as those who rejected God. It will show you the lessons of Jonah, Job, Hezekiah, and Ezekiel. It will show you the example of His Son Jesus Christ.

It will even rebuke you. It will show you the consequences of your actions. It will show you the results of failing to forgive others. It will show you the results of immoral physical activities on your body. It will show you the results of tempting God by willfully doing something harmful to your body and then asking for protection and healing.

The Holy Scripture is the teacher of the church and it is your teacher personally. Turn to God's Word. Hear the Lord God Almighty speak to you.

Dear God, thank You for giving me Your Holy Word as my teacher and my guide. Today I take the time to explore Your Word and to ponder on its meaning for me in my life. Guide me to the lessons in it that will be most helpful for me today. Thank You. In Jesus' name, I pray, Amen.

Day 344

He replied, "I saw Satan fall like lightning from heaven. I have given you authority to trample on snakes and scorpions and to overcome all the power of the enemy; nothing will harm you. However, do not rejoice that the spirits submit to you, but rejoice that your names are written in heaven." (Luke 10:18-20 NIV)

Jesus is eternal. He was with the Father from before the beginning. Here in Luke we hear Jesus telling us that He was there when satan was cast out from heaven. When we feel overwhelmed by challenges and when it seems that we are thwarted at every turn, remember these words of Holy Scripture.

Jesus was present before satan and Jesus was present after satan. Satan was only an angel. He was never divine and never will be so – even though what he seeks is our worship, or at the very least, our fear.

Now look at the next words, "I have given you authority to trample on snakes and scorpions and to overcome all the power of the enemy; nothing will harm you." To whom is He talking? In this text He is talking to the seventy-two missionaries He sent out to do two things – to heal the sick and preach the gospel that the kingdom of God is near. Are these special people, learned people, extraordinary people? No. They are "just folks," like you.

"I have given you authority," He says. What does this mean? It means that you can use the name of Jesus just as though He were here in the flesh. It means that you can call on Him anytime to act in accordance with the will of God.

What do you have authority over? Satan. You are to have authority to trample on the evil one and to overcome anything the evil one sends your way. That includes trials and tribulations. That includes injustices and disasters. That includes sickness and disease.

Claim the authority that Christ has given to you. Speak the dominion of the Lord God Almighty over your disease. Command it in the name of Jesus to leave you. Proclaim the healing of Jehovah-rapha.

Almighty God, it is written that Your Son Jesus Christ has given me authority to overcome all the power of the enemy. No power is stronger than Yours. Nothing will harm me. I command satan out of my presence. I command disease out of my life. I stand on Your Holy Word. Thank You, Lord. In Jesus' name, I pray, Amen.

Day 345

He who is loose and slack in his work is brother to him who is a destroyer and he who does not use his endeavors to heal himself is brother to him who commits suicide. (Proverbs 18:9 AMP)

This is a verse that forces you to take a second look. Most versions of the Bible don't include the second half of it which reads, "and he who does not use his endeavors to heal himself is brother to him who commits suicide." This part of the verse appears in the Greek translation of the Old Testament called *The Septuagint,* and The Amplified Bible includes it in its translation.

God wants us to be well. He does not want us to lie down and die – or to let illnesses "take their course" until they kill us.

What God intends is for us to join in full partnership with Him for our recovery. God is the source of all our healing, and we must turn to Him *first* and to those things which he has provided for us in the natural world. We must seek His direction and guidance in each step of our healing process and follow exactly what we are told to do.

When guidance tells you to seek out a doctor or a health care practitioner, find one who will pray with you. Find one who is open to using natural substances whenever possible instead of limiting his recommendations only to man-made substances. Find one who is willing to tell you *all* the options available for your healing – and not only pharmaceutical or surgical ones.

Find one who, as Dr. Robert Mendelsohn writes in *Confessions of a Medical Heretic,* truly practices the statement in the Hippocratic oath that says: "First, do no harm." Find one who is willing to support you in following your best understanding of God's plan for your healing.

Make sure that you place The Great Physician first in your heart, your soul, your life, and your healing program.

Almighty God, you are The Great Physician. You are the God who heals me. I take responsibility for my health and for working in partnership with You to find the pathway to wellness which You have ordained for me. Help me to keep my focus clear and Your truth firm within me in my discussions with medical personnel. Help me to choose the right natural substances, and guide me to the right methods to be used for my healing. With grateful thanks I pray in Jesus' name, I pray, Amen.

Day 346

As the Father has loved me, so have I loved you. Now remain in my love. If you obey my commands, you will remain in my love, just as I have obeyed my Father's commands and remain in his love. I have told you this so that my joy may be in you and that your joy may be complete. My command is this: Love each other as I have loved you. (John 15:9-12 NIV)

To remain in Jesus' love is a very effective way to accelerate your healing. Envision Jesus walking toward you. As you approach Him, you feel His enormous love embrace You. He smiles and then puts His hands on your head, creating waves of healing love throughout your whole being. Next He touches every part of your body that needs healing. As His hands touch you, you feel the warmth penetrate deeply within.

Hold the sensation as long as you can. Hear Jesus say, "Remain in my love. Remain in my love." Do you feel a sense of peace and a complete trust for Him? If so, allow yourself to open your heart and expose your deepest emotions to Him. Some may seem too powerful for you to examine without human assistance, and, if that is the case, see Jesus gently tuck them back inside until you seek counseling from a minister or other professional.

If you feel secure enough to continue, then select one of your emotions that is particularly painful to you. It may be guilt; it may be shame; it may be anger; it may be grief; it may be terror. Pick it up and review all the events surrounding it. Let yourself feel the emotions. Remind yourself of the loving arms of Jesus holding you and supporting you.

After you have acknowledged the pain and the hurt, decide if you want to carry it around for awhile longer. If you do, put it back in your heart. If not, hand it to Jesus and say, "Jesus, I give this hurt to you. Take it now. Fill the place where it was with your love and your joy."

Remember, Jesus wants you to have *joy!* Instead of holes or empty places inside where the old hurt used to be, you have Jesus' healing love and abiding joy locked deeply within. Rest in the peace of your Savior.

Dear God, in the name of Your Son Jesus I come today asking You to help me to follow the commands of Jesus and to remain in His love. There are many days, God, that I don't feel the joy that Jesus speaks of. And I don't feel His peace. I know that, when that happens, I have strayed from Your presence. Enfold me in Your love, God. Fill me with Your healing power. Transform the old pain I carry and help me to release it from my body and my soul. In Jesus' name, I pray, Amen.

Day 347

His divine power has given us everything we need for life and godliness through our knowledge of him who called us by his own glory and goodness. Through these he has given us his very great and precious promises, so that through them you may participate in the divine nature and escape the corruption in the world caused by evil desires. (2 Peter 1:3-4 NIV)

God's Word tells us that God has already given us everything we need for life. It has *already* been given. It is ours through God's Son, God's covenants, and God's Word. What is the purpose of the Word? "So that through it you may participate in the Divine nature."

Let your mind comprehend what it means to "participate in the Divine nature." Remember that God created us in the beginning as beings imbued with Divine nature. God created us in the likeness and image of Himself because He wanted our company. With each element of creation He spoke it into being with His Word and then declared it to be good.

Does the Divine nature and God's likeness and image include sickness and disease? Of course not. Does it represent God's will for us? Of course not. If we really believed it was Divine nature for us to be ill and God's will for us to be sick, we would not race to the doctor to be healed. We would not build hospitals and medical schools and laboratories. To use any of those things if we really believe God wants us to be sick would be to flaunt God's will just as rebelliously as Adam and Eve did when they ate of the fruit of the knowledge of good and evil. Sickness is clearly the tool of the devil which destroys God's life force within us and saps our strength and vitality.

Rejoice in the promises of God's Word. Rejoice in the desire of God to give you every good thing. Affirm your faith in Christ Jesus who bore your sins and infirmities on the Cross of Calvary and who redeemed you forever. Let your life be a witness to God's glory and grace and healing power.

Divine God, You have given me everything I need for life. You have sent Your Word and Your Son Jesus Christ to proclaim Your great and precious promises, and through them I am called to participate in Your Divine nature. Help me to reject the corruption in the world caused by evil desires, and protect me from attacks of the evil one. Keep me focused on Your goodness and glory and healing power. In Jesus' name, I pray, Amen.

Day 348

Then you will call, and the Lord will answer; you will cry for help, and he will say: "Here I am." (Isaiah 58:9 NIV)

What do you when you need to be healed? "Then you will call and the Lord will answer; you will cry for help and He will say, 'Here I am.'" No matter what your situation is, the Lord God Almighty is there for you. God is always Jehovah-rapha, the God who heals you.

Remember that you are a partner with God in your recovery. If the appearance is that you aren't being healed, it is wise to review what you have been doing. Take a look at your spiritual habits. Make sure you put on your shield of armor against the evil one each morning and each evening. Take time to read the Holy Scriptures each day and to fill your mind, heart, soul, and body with God's Word. Pray constantly throughout the day, especially offering prayers of gratitude and joy.

Check to make sure that you are not making assumptions about what you should do about your health without first getting guidance from the Holy Spirit. Your assumptions may seem reasonable, but remember, "there are things that seem right to a man but in the end they lead to death."

Be sure not to rush God. It can be frustrating to wait on the Lord, but that is often what we are asked to do. This is not a passive waiting, but an active waiting. As you wait, focus on a positive outcome by "calling things that are not as though they were."

Also follow God's health laws and take all the actions you are guided to make. Be aware that there may still be a piece of your health "puzzle" missing. Keep asking for guidance and revelation knowledge from the Holy Spirit for what to do. Keep exploring options and expanding your knowledge. Be alert for all forms of direction which God sends to you.

Lastly, remember that you are not a failure. God is a faithful God. What He requires is that you remain steadfast and faithful to Him.

Almighty God, help me to release my expectations about my healing and to wait on You and Your timing. I am doing my best to follow your health laws and to walk closely with You. If there is something I am not doing as You want me to do, show me. I trust in You, God. I know that You are Jehovah-rapha. Thank You for healing me. I praise Your Holy name that You always answer my call for help and say, "Here I am." In Jesus' name, I pray, Amen.

Day 349

Dear friends, do not believe every spirit, but test the spirits to see whether they are from God, because many false prophets have gone out into the world. This is how you can recognize the Spirit of God: Every spirit that acknowledges that Jesus Christ has come in the flesh is from God, but every spirit that does not acknowledge Jesus is not from God. (1 John 4:1-3 NIV)

Do not put out the Spirit's fire; do not treat prophecies with contempt. Test everything. Hold on to the good. Avoid every kind of evil. (1 Thessalonians 5:19-22 NIV)

Walking the path of obedience to God depends on going in prayer, listening to His voice, and following the instructions we are given. But can we trust everything that we "hear"? How can we tell the difference between God's voice and satan's voice?

This problem was well understood by the early Christians. The Apostle John in 1 John 4:1 tells us to "test the spirits to see whether they are from God" and the Apostle Paul warns us to "test everything." Why? Because when you pray for advice and counsel, you want to make sure that the evil one is not already perched on your shoulder ready to whisper his lies and deceptions in your ear.

There are times when you feel absolutely sure that you are connected truly and clearly to God. Learn to recognize the sense of clarity and confidence that you have at those times. There is actually a certain Holy energy that you feel. Divine energy can come only from God so you want to learn to recognize that inner sense and "knowing."

Be sure to put on the armor of the Lord just as instructed in Ephesians 6:10-18. Go in prayer to God. Command satan to leave you. Call on the blood of Jesus which has redeemed you. Pray in the name of Christ Jesus who defeated satan.

If you are still not sure about the source of the instructions you have received, ask a brother or sister in Christ to pray with you. Surround yourselves with the power of the Lord God Almighty and His mighty angels.

Almighty God, in the name of Jesus I command satan to leave me. I stand in the blood that Jesus shed for me and seek Your truth, O Lord. Reveal to me exactly what You want me to do for my healing and recovery. In the name of Your Son, Jesus Christ, I pray, Amen.

Day 350

The Lord said to Gideon, "You have too many men for me to deliver Midian into their hands. In order that Israel may not boast against me that her own strength has saved her, announce now to the people, 'Anyone who trembles with fear may turn back and leave Mount Gilead.' " So twenty-two thousand men left, while ten thousand remained.
(Judges 7:2-3 NIV)

Imagine Gideon's shock when God told him that his army was too big! How could his army be too big since it was still very small compared to the army of the enemy? Pay close attention to what God said to Gideon for His reason for wanting Gideon to have a much smaller army composed only of those strong in their faith: He did not want the people of Israel to boast to God that they had saved themselves. He wanted them to be clear that He and He alone was their deliverer.

We have much the same situation when we feel sick. We have been invaded by the evil one. To fight him we have developed an impressive array of weapons in conventional medical treatment – drugs, surgery, and radiation, to name a few. We have become quite boastful of our discoveries, inventions, and manipulations of chemicals. There is nothing wrong with our having these things as long as we remember that they are man-made and not God-made and, therefore, are subject to certain limitations.

Not one medical treatment heals because healing comes from *life* – and it is *the living body* which heals. We forget that fact and too often exalt these medical treatments to the level of God. We put our faith in them without even asking God whether we should use them in our own particular situation. We utilize them without seeking God's advice or exploring God's remedies. When they work, we credit them with our recovery, and when they don't, we often blame God.

God does not want us to boast that we have saved ourselves or healed ourselves through our own treatments alone. *"I* am the God who heals you," He declares. Join in partnership with Him as your *first* resort and not as your *last* resort. Stand with Him in faith.

Wonderful Jehovah-rapha, I affirm that it is You and You alone who heals me. You are the source of all life, and it is Your touch that causes my body to come into balance, wholeness, and proper function. Thank You for Your healing herbs and essential oils and for human treatments which assist in the healing process. Guide me according to Your path for my healing. In Jesus' name, I pray, Amen.

Day 351

And pray in the Spirit on all occasions with all kinds of prayers and requests.
(Ephesians 6:18 NIV)

Prayer is a powerful essential in every Christian's life. Paul tells us here to pray about *everything*. Pray on *all* occasions. Pray with *all* kinds of prayers and requests. God *wants* you to come to Him with your concerns.

Do you believe Paul is correct? If so, then praying about the recovery of your health is critical and needs to be a part of every element in your healing. Should it not be an important part of every consultation you have with a health care professional? Doctors depend greatly on test results to "prove" your health reality, and standard treatments are used which have been developed to deal with the symptoms of the identified condition. These treatments are the options the doctor has available but there are other options from other arenas as well. There are always numerous natural health options available for any health condition a person may have.

Why is it that we have allowed conventional medical care to exclude God? Why is it that most doctors believe it would be inappropriate and unprofessional to pray with you? Some cannot handle your questioning their judgment and authority. If you do not do what they want you to do, they do not want you as their patient.

By the grace of God, there are now some medical professionals who are willing to pray in the Spirit with those patients who desire it. Seek them out. Ask all your doctors to pray with you for guidance. All of you need specific guidance from the Lord for your particular health condition. Accepting any person's opinion and undergoing any standard treatment based on that opinion can lead to disastrous results in the end if God is not also consulted in the process. God is your authority and your healer. Let Him be the judge of the way He wants you to be healed.

If you cannot find a doctor willing to pray with you and willing to be open to whatever God directs (even if it is something other than what he has in mind), then take some time after your medical appointments to go to God in prayer yourself. But how powerful it is to pray together with your doctor for your healing and for God's guidance in your care!

Almighty God, I will gather the courage to ask my doctor to pray with me for Your Holy guidance for my healing. I want to know Your path for my healing – and only Yours. Show me the way. In Jesus' name, I pray, Amen.

Day 352

Then little children were brought to Jesus for him to place his hands on them and pray for them. But the disciples rebuked those who brought them. Jesus said, "Let the little children come to me, and do not hinder them, for the kingdom of heaven belongs to such as these." When he had placed his hands on them, he went on from there. (Matthew 19:13-15 NIV)

Jesus valued children. He liked to have them around and scolded His disciples from keeping the little ones away from Him. Children teach us many important lessons. One that is especially vital to our health is to appreciate play. Good old-fashioned fun. Play involves laughter, joy, and delight but it is more than that. Play stimulates our creative qualities and encourages us to expand our spirit.

If you feel sick, it is vital that you bring play into your life. One of the best and most obvious ways to do that is to be around the play experts – young children, of course. If you do not have young children of your own and are able, "adopt" a child for a "play day" occasionally. Whether it is for an hour or two, an afternoon, or an entire day, spend time with children, playing games, reading, walking in the park, talking. Being with them will fill your heart with joy and will awaken you to the simple delights of a very young soul. Not only will you be helping yourself, but you will be a godsend to grateful parents who can have a little time to meet their own needs. There are children everywhere who will bloom with your attention and love.

If you don't feel well enough to supervise a young one, go to a park and watch the children there. Smile and laugh along with them. Join them in your mind if you aren't able to join them with your body. Another way to make contact is by being a pen pal to a child. You can write short notes and stories and send little trinkets from time to time, such as a new barrette or a toy car. In return, your child can draw pictures for you or share a flower or a pebble he found just for you.

Be creative in thinking up a way to bring the play of children into your life. There is much healing in a child's smile and there are many lessons to learn from seeing a small hand reach for yours.

Wonderful Jehovah-rapha, help me to discover the child inside myself who likes to play. Help me to look at the world with the delight of young eyes and to sparkle with joy. There is so much healing in laughter. Bring me a child who loves jokes, Lord. In the name of Your Son, Jesus Christ, I pray, Amen.

Day 353

So Peter was kept in prison, but the church was earnestly praying to God for him. The night before Herod was to bring him to trial, Peter was sleeping between two soldiers, bound with two chains, and sentries stood guard at the entrance. Suddenly an angel of the Lord appeared and a light shone in the cell. He struck Peter on the side and woke him up. "Quick, get up!" he said, and the chains fell off Peter's wrists. ... Peter followed him out of the prison, but he had no idea that what the angel was doing was really happening; he thought he was seeing a vision. . . . When they had walked the length of one street, suddenly the angel left him. Then Peter came to himself and said, "Now I know without a doubt that the Lord sent his angel and rescued me from Herod's clutches and from everything the Jewish people were anticipating." When this had dawned on him, he went to the house of Mary the mother of John . . . where many people had gathered and were praying. Peter knocked at the outer entrance, and a servant girl named Rhoda came to answer the door. When she recognized Peter's voice, she was so overjoyed she ran back without opening it and exclaimed, "Peter is at the door!" "You're out of your mind," they told her. When she kept insisting that it was so, they said, "It must be his angel." But Peter kept on knocking, and when they opened the door and saw him, they were astonished. (Acts 12:5-7, 9-16 NIV)

Why was Rhoda the only one who accepted from the beginning that Peter had returned to them? Perhaps she was the only one who had prayed for his rescue truly believing in her heart that the Lord could accomplish it. All the Christians were "earnestly praying" yet they were apparently going through the motions without having absolute faith in God's power of deliverance.

How do you pray for your healing? Like the Christians at Mary's house with faint hope rather than strong faith? Or like Rhoda, with real belief in your heart? When you see the first evidence of the impossible in your body, do you say, "I must be out of my mind," and dismiss it? If so, your healing may slip away through your fingers. Pray without doubt, knowing that with God all things are possible.

Wonderful Jehovah-rapha, cleanse me of all doubt which is brought by the evil one to undermine my belief in You. Lord, I am overwhelmed by Your mighty power to deliver me. Let me be single-minded in my trust and faith in You and Your healing desire and grace. By the stripes of Your Son Jesus Christ, I have been healed. In His name, I pray, Amen.

Day 354

Who of you by worrying can add a single hour to his life? (Matthew 6:27 NIV)

"Who of you by worrying can add a single hour to his life?" Jesus asks. God our Father has determined how long He wants us to live and no matter what we do, we cannot add one hour to our life beyond the will of the Father. Worrying, planning, and manipulating is useless. We do not have full control over our lives and we must recognize that.

Even though we cannot add one hour to our life, we surely have the power to shorten it through our actions. And satan will gladly help us as much as he can. Is this part of God's will for us? No, but He gives us the free will to make our own choices. Our early destruction of our temple is the result of satan and often of our own will as well.

How do we shorten our lives through our own will? Primarily in two ways. One is by disobeying God's health laws. Take the time to study them and to learn what God has told us about keeping our temple strong.

Another is by making assumptions based on our own beliefs, understanding, and desire. What about you? Are you ignoring symptoms, hoping they will just go away? Are you trying to meditate yourself into a reality of your own creation? Are you trying to will yourself well? Are you forging ahead with a treatment based on human judgment just because you think you "ought" to or because someone says you "have" to do it?

The solution is so simple. Take absolutely everything to God in prayer, and then *listen* and follow the guidance your receive. You cannot be filled with both trust and obsessive worry at the same time. Whenever you feel the worry start to creep in, turn it over to God immediately. He can change any circumstance the evil one has thrown at you.

Your heavenly Father has a plan for you and it is a plan for your good. Trust Him and walk in faith.

Almighty God, I confess I worry too much about my illness. I admit that I want it to go away instantaneously by the touch of Your hand. However, I surrender now, Lord, to Your will for my healing and for the particular way You choose for me to return to health. I will do it Your way, God. Let me hear clearly what path You want me to follow. In the name of Your Son, Jesus Christ, my Savior and my Redeemer, I pray, Amen.

Day 355

No, in all these things we are more than conquerors through him who loved us. For I am convinced that neither death nor life, neither angels nor demons, neither the present nor the future, nor any powers, neither height nor depth, nor anything else in all creation, will be able to separate us from the love of God that is in Christ Jesus our Lord. (Romans 8:37-39 NIV)

God is love. God loves *you* – more than you can possibly comprehend. Can you take this truth into the very core of your being? Can you absorb it fully? Love is Holy because it is the essence of God. Yet sadly, it is often elusive to many people.

We think of love as an emotion, as something we feel. Yet it is much more than a feeling. Love is defined and expressed much more by action than by feelings. It is far easier to *say* "I love you" than it is to *live* "I love you." And therein lies the key to the reason that many people do not trust love. They have been betrayed once too often by people who claimed to love them. So they withdraw inside and put up a protective wall to shield themselves.

Illness often follows because we need love like flowers need water. Our health depends on the constant flow of giving and receiving love, like a great circle of Divine smiles. Love is Holy energy, healing energy, connecting energy.

Look deeply within your heart. Do you allow God's love to flow freely to you? Or do you feel unworthy? Do you remember times from long ago when you felt alone and abandoned and still carry those feelings? Do you fear being betrayed? These emotions are all blocks to God's love. In order to be well physically, you will need to face these inner conflicts and to heal them.

Hear Paul tell you that nothing, absolutely nothing, can stand in the way of God's love for you. He loved you so much that He sent His Son to redeem you completely. He sent His Son to forgive your sins and to heal your body. He sent His Son for you.

Merciful God, I have wounds of the heart. You are the God of love and today I allow myself to be open to Your love so that it can flow through my soul and my body. I allow myself to believe that there is no power that can separate me from Your awesome love. I feel tears of joy as I allow Your love to heal my soul, my mind, my emotions, and my body. In Jesus' name, I pray, Amen.

Day 356

When Jesus had called the Twelve together, he gave them power and authority to drive out all demons and to cure diseases, and he sent them out to preach the kingdom of God and to heal the sick. (Luke 9:1-2 NIV)

Jesus came to redeem us from the sin of Adam. He also came to show us how to live in a way pleasing to God. In this passage in Luke we see Jesus setting up His church and teaching His followers what they were supposed to do. He wanted them to carry on the dual mission that He Himself had.

What was that dual mission? To preach the kingdom of God and to heal the sick. Two things, both working in tandem with each other. Healing wasn't to be an afterthought or something to be done if there was time. Healing was on an equal footing with preaching. This was the way Jesus wanted His church to act. How many churches today do as much healing as they do preaching?

Notice that Jesus gave His disciples power and authority to do the healing that He commanded. He came to free us from satan, and He gave power and authority to His followers so that the work of satan could no longer stand in the face of the Redeemer. Our salvation was complete and whole and included our entire being – both soul and body.

Do you believe in this dual mission today? You have to decide if you think that what Jesus taught was just for those who lived two thousand years ago or if you think that what Jesus taught is valid for you right now. Was the power and authority given by Jesus just for the disciples or for the members of the first century? No, it is given to you through the Cross.

You have been redeemed. When you walk to Jesus and say, "I believe," then all power is available to you. Jesus still calls you today to follow Him and to follow His commandments. Preach the gospel *and* heal the sick. God wants you – soul *and* body, whole before Him.

Almighty God, I am grateful that Your Son Jesus Christ gave me more than hopes and dreams – He gave me power and authority. Therefore, in the name of Jesus Christ, I claim the power and authority to command satan to leave my body. Satan cannot have me. I have been redeemed, Father, by the blood of Your Precious Son. I am saved – body and soul. I am healed – body and soul. I am Yours, God – body and soul. In the name of Your Son, Jesus Christ, I pray, Amen.

Day 357

For this reason, since the day we heard about you, we have not stopped praying for you and asking God to fill you with the knowledge of his will through all spiritual wisdom and understanding. (Colossians 1:9 NIV)

How much happier our lives would be if we would surround ourselves with people who would pray for us and ask God to fill us with the knowledge of His will through all spiritual wisdom and understanding. Here is a major key to our healing. Find such friends and hold them close.

You need intercessory prayer. You need others to pray for you. Voices lifted up to heaven in your behalf are vital for the health of your body – as well as your soul. Studies have shown that people who are prayed for heal more rapidly and need less medication than people who are not prayed for. And the person being prayed for doesn't even have to be aware of the prayers in their behalf.

There are many, many tools and ways to healing. You need revelation knowledge of which ones are right for you. Is it God's herbs? Is it essential oils? Is it homeopathic medicines? Is it conventional medical treatment? Is it chiro-practic care? Is it exercise? Is it nutritional support? Or is it a combination of one or more or all – plus, of course, prayer and faith? The answers will come through the spiritual wisdom and understanding which Paul describes.

Seek out friends who will pray with you and for you. Find a church where people believe in the healing that Jesus taught. Find a church where people believe that Jesus took your infirmities – as well as your sins – to the Cross. Ask these people to pray for your recovery. Ask them to pray that God will fill you with knowledge of His will for the particular path you are to follow for your recovery.

There is great power, comfort, and strength in the loving prayers of brothers and sisters in Christ who pray believing that Jehovah-rapha is healing you.

Gracious Lord, I am grateful for the wonderful people who are praying for my recovery and who are praying for Your spiritual wisdom and understanding of the healing path that You want me to take. Thank You, Lord, for bringing these people into my life. Thank You for their caring, their concern, and their love. And, Lord, today somewhere someone is sick and hurting and feeling alone. I offer this prayer to You in their behalf that You will show them the way to their healing. In Jesus' name, I pray, Amen.

Day 358

The earth is satisfied with the fruit of thy works. He causeth the grass to grow for the cattle, and the herb for the service of man: that he may bring forth food out of the earth. (Psalm 104:13-14 KJV)

The Psalms were written to expound the glory of the Lord God Almighty and in the process many health truths are shared with us. This Psalm reveals to us one of the fundamental laws of nutrition – the source of nutrients for us is found in the plants.

Let's take a look at the chain of nutrients. What do plants need in order to live? Minerals, water, and sunlight. The plants take in these elements and process them. Their leaves, flowers, stems, and roots then become loaded with a myriad of substances necessary for our nutrition and for our healing. Herbs are plants that have dense amounts of healing nutrients, and essential oils are the lifeblood of the plants. Consequently, they are applied and consumed in much smaller quantities than "ordinary" foods. For example, we usually eat smaller servings of garlic than we do of string beans, and we apply tiny amounts of dill essential oil compared to the amount we would use as a seasoning.

What most people don't know is that plants are our best source of minerals. God created the plants to be able to take the minerals from the soil and package them in a way in which the human body can digest and assimilate them. We can eat the rock and the soil directly (which is the source of many mineral supplements today); however, when we consume them in that form we assimilate very little of it. Our bodies were not designed to digest rock.

Most of us may choose to eat some meat and fish, and the Scriptures provide guidelines for us to do so in the healthiest way. However, if we rely on animal products as the major component of our diet, we are depending on second-hand food for our own nutrition. God intended that we get the majority of our nutrition firsthand from the plants. The plants, herbs, and essential oils are truly "for the service of man."

Almighty Lord, You created this glorious world in which I live. I have taken so much of it for granted and have too often failed to give proper value to the plants which You provided in such abundance. As I learn more about the way that my body works, I appreciate the function of plants in filling my body's needs for nutrients. I will choose to eat appropriate amounts of fruits and vegetables for my health. And how grateful I am for the herbs and essential oils which You gave for my service. In Jesus' name, I pray, Amen.

Day 359

As he went along, he saw a man blind from birth. His disciples asked him, "Rabbi, who sinned, this man or his parents, that he was born blind?" "Neither this man nor his parents sinned," said Jesus, "but this happened so that the work of the God might be displayed in his life. As long as it is day, we must do the work of him who sent me. Night is coming, when no one can work. While I am in the world, I am the light of the world." Having said this, he spit on the ground, made some mud with the saliva, and put it on the man's eyes. "Go," he told him, "wash in the Pool Siloam" (this word means Sent). So the man went and washed, and came home seeing. (John 9:1-7 NIV)

The disciples assumed that the only cause of illness and infirmities was sin by either the person or the person's parents. They accepted the fact that illness comes from the evil one – but they assumed that either the blind man or his parents were at fault. Sometimes satan attacks us when we have done nothing "wrong." A car hurtles across a median and hits us even though we were obeying all the rules of good driving. The accident is still satan's handiwork even though we ourselves were not at fault.

In this story from John, Jesus said that neither the man nor his parents had sinned. Notice that He did not say that God had made the man blind. What He did say was, "This happened so that the work of God might be displayed in his life." And He immediately restored the man's sight. What is the work that God displayed? His healing. His healing! If the work of God to be displayed was the man's blindness and the man's acceptance of his blindness, then Jesus would never had healed him. Jesus never once worked contrary to the will of God. In fact, He made a point of saying that He had come to do the will of God and the will of God only.

How wonderful it is to know that the point of this story is to illustrate that God's work and God's glory are be revealed through His healing!

Dear God, I come to You with my illness. Sometimes I, too, ask the question, "What did I do wrong?" Lord, I offer myself to You. Reveal Your glory to the world through my healing. I witness for You now and I will witness for You forever. Let me proclaim to all who see Your mighty hand at work healing me, "This is the work of Jehovah-rapha being displayed in my life." Thank You, God. In Jesus' name, I pray, Amen.

Day 360

God did extraordinary miracles through Paul, so that even handkerchiefs and aprons that had touched him were taken to the sick, and their illnesses were cured and the evil spirits left them. (Acts 19:11-12 NIV)

Some healings are true miracles. We are told in this passage of Holy Scripture that "God did extraordinary miracles through Paul." The glory of God is truly awesome: here was a person who had persecuted and killed many Christians and who later came to do extraordinary miracles.

What is a miracle? It is a way that God uses to say, "I am here. I am the Lord God Almighty." It is an event that is so contrary to what people believe "ought" to happen that all who witness it recognize that something awesome has happened. Notice that the writer of Acts does not say that Paul did the miracles. *God* did the miracles by using Paul as His instrument.

What were these miracles? Paul touched handkerchiefs and aprons, which were taken to sick people and the people recovered. Certainly, touching pieces of cloth is not a usual way for healings to occur.

How were the healings of the sick manifested? By having their illnesses cured and evil spirits leave them. The healings were complete. The people were set free from their infirmities and bondage.

Today many people who say they want to be healed are really looking for a miracle. They may get one. However, God never promises you an instantaneous, miraculous recovery.

Since God is interested in having His children walk with Him in full partnership, one way He accomplishes that is to grant healing as a part of a journey, as a part of a process. This allows you time to understand your part in your illness and to accomplish your own changes within to bring yourself into alignment with God's healing power.

Let God be God, and get out of His business. Allow Him to be Jehovah-rapha, the God who heals you according to His Divine plan.

Dear God, I am filled with awe at Your mighty power. You are the God who heals me and I will accept whatever way You choose to accomplish it. I trust that You know the perfect path for my healing and I will walk it with You. Thank You for sending Your Son as my example and as my Savior and my Redeemer. In Jesus' name, I pray, Amen.

Day 361

This is the confidence we have in approaching God: that if we ask anything according to his will, he hears us. And if we know that he hears us – whatever we ask – we know that we have what we asked of him. (1 John 5:14-15 NIV)

If we ask anything according to His will, God hears us. And if we know that He hears us, we know that we have whatever it is that we asked of Him. Why? Because we have already established that what we are asking is according to His will. It is only when we ask for things outside of God's will that we get into trouble.

It all sounds simple, but, of course, we know from bitter experience that it is not. Satan seeks to get us off the track. He uses our vulnerabilities and weaknesses against us, and he deceives us into believing certain things are God's will when that is in fact not true. And he also deceives us into believing other things are *not* God's will when in fact they *are*. This is the reason that prayer and meditation are so important. We have to ask God for His direction in all the small questions of our life – as well as the large ones.

You need to get clear in your mind that it is God's will for you to be well. The prayer, "God, please heal me if it is your will" is a weak prayer because it is doubt-filled. Jesus repeatedly and consistently healed every single person who came to Him. It had to be God's will for all to be healed because he healed them all and never left one single person sick.

What isn't clear about God's will is the *way* He chooses for your healing to be manifested. Don't succumb to satan's tricks and make assumptions about God's path for your healing. Don't assume you "should" do anything. Ask before each decision. Then you will be sure to be in alignment with God's will.

When you are in harmony with God's will, you know that He has already done what you ask. Therefore, focus on living each day taking action according to your guidance. Regardless of the symptoms you may still feel, live with peace in your heart and joy radiating for all to see. Live your life in faith, knowing that nothing is too hard for God and that He has the perfect plan for your highest good.

Wonderful Jehovah-rapha, I have confidence in You. It is written that You hear anything I ask that is according to Your will. Help me to be patient, Lord, while You work Your perfect will in my healing. Reveal Your guidance to me, and I will obey. Thank You. In Jesus' name, I pray, Amen.

Day 362

You are free to eat from any tree in the garden, but you must not eat from the tree of the knowledge of good and evil, for when you eat of it you will surely die. (Genesis 2:16-17 NIV)

Many people believe that everything that happens in the universe is caused by God. When bad things happen to good people, they believe that God caused the tragedy, accident, or illness for some reason known only to the Almighty and that when they get to heaven they will understand.

The problem with this philosophy is that God's Word clearly states that He allows all His children to have free will. He even allows His angels to have free will. After satan rebelled against God, he was banished from heaven, taking *one-third* of the angels with him. The evil one and his minions stalk the earth creating disaster in their wake and making every attempt to get us to do likewise. This is not God at work, but the devil at work. When illness strikes, don't blame God for it. Look to the evil one and the ways you have been either vulnerable or cooperative.

God doesn't want His children to be puppets, incapable of doing anything that He doesn't control. He wants us to be *real*. He wants us to worship Him because we truly choose to give our hearts to Him and not because He forces us to pay homage to Him. Obedience is a major act of worship and through it we voluntarily offer our free will back to God and ask Him to direct and use it to His glory.

Are you angry with God for your illness? Are you angry with God for some trauma or tragedy in your past? God understands your hurt and He is waiting for you to come to Him. Offer your resentment, grief, and regret to Him. Ask God's forgiveness for blaming Him. Then allow His peace to fill and cover you and to wash you clean.

Remember that no matter what the evil one may do, God can create good from any situation. Ask God to reveal to you what you can learn from your current circumstances. Ask Him to strengthen you and to protect you. The evil one can *never* be victorious in the life of one who believes in, trust, and obediently follows Jehovah and Christ Jesus.

Almighty God, things have happened to me that weren't fair and that hurt me terribly. Forgive me, God, for blaming You and holding You accountable for them. Please transform their effect and bring something good out of this situation. Show me what I can learn so that I will not repeat this pattern again. In Jesus' name, I pray, Amen.

Day 363

Now on his way to Jerusalem, Jesus traveled along the border between Samaria and Galilee. As he was going into a village, ten men who had leprosy met him. They stood at a distance and called out in a loud voice, "Jesus, Master, have pity on us!" When he saw them, he said, "Go, show yourselves to the priests." And as they went, they were cleansed. One of them, when he saw he was healed, came back, praising God in a loud voice. He threw himself at Jesus' feet and thanked him – and he was a Samaritan. Jesus asked, "Were not all ten cleansed? Where are the other nine? Was no one found to return and give praise to God except this foreigner?" Then he said to him, "Rise and go; your faith has made you well." (Luke 17:11-19 NIV)

Of the many lessons in this story, let us focus on two additional ones. The first is that healing is often a process. The ten lepers asked for cleansing, and Jesus gave it to them, telling them to go to the priests. They were not healed at the moment that Jesus spoke, but they were healed *as they went on their way.* When they got to the priests, they were well, and, according to Levitical law, their healing was confirmed officially. Sometimes we are given recovery as the product of a journey to wellness rather than as the result of an instantaneous miracle. It may be slower and it certainly requires more faith, but is it less of a healing?

The second lesson is to be grateful. We are told here that only one man came back and said, "Thank you." And he was the only one who Jesus declared to be well. What about you? How many little miracles of healing occur in your life every day? Is your cough better today than yesterday? Have you said thank you? Or are you waiting until you are totally well?

View your recovery from the perspective of constant gratitude. Offer your thanks no matter what the appearance is about the state of your healing. Remember, Jesus said "thank you" to God for hearing Him before He ever called Lazarus forth from the grave. Right now, say out loud, "Thank You, God, for healing me." Claim His healing power.

Merciful God, I come with a grateful heart saying, "Thank You, thank You." It is written that You are the God who heals me and that my faith makes me well. So I stand joyously on Your Word, Jehovah-rapha. I hear Your Son say directly to me, "Rise and go; your faith has made you well." God, I will sing my song of thanksgiving to You glorifying Your name as long as I live. In Jesus' name, I pray, Amen.

Day 364

Trust in the Lord with all thine heart; and lean not unto thine own understanding. In all thy ways acknowledge him, and he shall direct thy paths. (Proverbs 3:5-6 KJV)

Do you trust God with your life? The answer would seem to be obvious. But is it? It is amazing how many people do not include God in the process of making their health decisions. They pray to God for health – but praying is talking *to* God, not listening to what God has to say.

Scripture warns us not to "lean on *our* own understanding." Medical tests, medical opinions, scientific facts – all these are part of *our* understanding. They are informative input based on the knowledge and the mind of man. Sometimes the information seems to be irrevocable fact, but remember that scientific "facts" have changed constantly through the centuries (and still change today) as human beings learn more and more.

God doesn't have any opinions. God has – and is – Divine truth. God knows everything there is to know about your body. In fact, there are things He knows about your body that no human being will ever understand fully. Therefore, we are told not to base our decisions *solely* on man's knowledge but to seek the Lord. Take your health issues to God in prayer, quieten your mind, and be open to hear God.

If you will let Him, God can give you *very specific* advice about the best way for *you* to receive the healing He desires. He wants to share this knowledge with you. He wants to direct you to the path that is right for you. You must listen on a daily basis, because the specific Divine instructions may change as you follow God's path.

Remain faithful to God's voice. You may hear that you are to apply certain essential oils, take certain herbs, use certain medications, have certain medical procedures, go to church elders for healing prayer, or receive healing through your own prayer and faith. Or you may be given a combination of these pathways to healing.

Just listen. Make sure you receive the voice of God and only the voice of God. Then act boldly no matter what anyone else says.

Almighty God, teach me listen to Your voice. As I gather information from my family, friends, and health advisors, give me strength to rely ultimately on Your Holy guidance. Sometimes I feel afraid when Your voice and their advice don't agree. Help me to hear You clearly. Then give me the courage to trust You as Moses and Noah did before me, and help me to walk the path You instruct me to walk. In Jesus' name I pray, Amen.

Day 365

For, lo, the winter is past, the rain is over and gone; the flowers appear on the earth; the time of the singing of birds is come, and the voice of the turtle is heard in our land; the fig tree putteth forth her green figs, and the vines with the tender grape give a good smell. Arise, my love, my fair one, and come away. (Song of Solomon 2:11-13 KJV)

Times of illness can seem like times of desolation. This beautiful Song of Solomon beckons you forward into the present and away from the past. Leave behind the winter of old beliefs that held you prisoner. Leave behind the rains of doubt that kept you trapped in your illness.

God calls to you, "Come away, my beloved child. Come away. I have new life for you. I am the source of all life and I give it to you again." Stand before your Creator and look with fresh, new eyes as you feel new birth within you.

Fill your heart and your soul with His Holy Word, and remember that, as you think, so are you. You will know the truth that God is not the author of illness and disease. The truth that Jehovah-rapha is the God who heals you shall set you free. Trust in the Lord with all your heart and lean not unto your own understanding. In all your ways acknowledge Him, and He shall direct your path.

Is there anything too hard for God? He sent His Son Christ Jesus to take your infirmities and bear your sicknesses. Jesus tells you that it will be done to you according to your faith. He also tells you that nothing shall be impossible to you. Hear Him say, "Whatever you ask for in prayer, believe that you have received it and it will be yours."

Your body is a temple of the Holy Spirit, who is in you, and it is to be honored and respected. Do not conform any longer to the patterns, traditions, and conventions of this world, but be transformed by the renewing of your mind.

Behold, the Lord God Almighty makes all things new. That means you, His beloved child. Have patience so that after you have done the will of God, you may receive the promise. God knows the plans He has for you – plans to prosper you and not to harm you, plans to give you hope and a future. Call upon Him. Seek Him and He will find you and will bring you back from captivity into His living glory.

O, Lord, my God, I stand on Your Word, leaving the winter of my past beliefs behind me. I come with a new heart and a new spirit. Take my life, Lord, and use it for Your Holy purpose and for Your glory. You are the God who heals me. Thank You, Lord. In Jesus' name, I pray, Amen.

Supplementary Resources

<u>Correspondence Course</u>
Biblical Nutrition Principles
    Carolina Natural Health Institute, Inc.
    2703 East Third Street,
    Greenville, NC 27858
    252-355-4665

This correspondence course is for those who would like to learn how to follow God's Word to be healthy. We examine the manufacturer's instructions for operating our car, so why don't we study God's Word for guidelines for our health? You will learn God's guidelines for health, especially in regard to grains, fat, meat, sweeteners, fruits, vegetables, spices, and beverages.

Other health correspondence courses are available to assist students in gathering the information they need to work in partnership with God in creating good health.

<u>Ezine – an Internet magazine</u>
The Christian Healer
    To subscribe: send a blank message to:
        TheChristianHealer-subscribe@egroups.com

This free Ezine is devoted to healing from the Christian perspective. Its missions are to raise the level of awareness of God's being the active Healer of all people, to demonstrate that human health is determined by the condition of the spirit/body/soul as one unified entity, to affirm the biblical teaching of prayer and anointing with essential healing oil as the most powerful healing modality, and to encourage Christians of all denominations to consider the establishment of healing ministries within their local assemblies.

Supplementary Resources

Church Workshop
The Power for Healing Workshop
   2395 New Milford School Road
   Rockford, IL 61109
   815-874-3358
   Email: Workshop@lynngroup.com

The Power for Healing Workshop is a ministry dedicated to helping churches re-establish themselves as spiritual healing centers. Workshop participants receive biblical grounding for the church's authority to become a Spiritual Healing Center for the sick and afflicted. This does not negate other healing modalities, but affirms God's will to use His church to heal His people.

Books:
A More Excellent Way
   By Pastor Henry Wright
   1999, Pleasant Valley Church, Inc., 1519 Pleasant Valley Road, Molena,
      GA 30258, 1-800-453-5775

Christ the Healer
   By F. F. Bosworth
   1973, Fleming H. Revell, a division of Baker Book House Co., Grand
      Rapids, Michigan 49516

What the Bible Says about Healthy Living
   By Rex Russell, MD
   1996, Regal Books, a division of Gospel Light, Ventura, CA

Carolina Natural Health Institute, Inc.

2703 E. Third Street
Greenville, NC 27858
Phone: 252-355-4665
Fax: 252-355-4599

Course 201 – Biblical Nutrition Principles ($75 plus $8.50 S&H)

Course 202 – Basic pH Health Principles ($95 plus $8.50 S&H)

Course 203 – Basic Nutrients ($85 plus $8.50 S&H)

Course 204 – Basic Herbology ($95 plus $8.50 S&H)

Package 205 Certified Natural Health Specialist ($330 plus $15 S&H)
Includes Courses 201, 202, 203, and 204

Course 250 – Basic Herbal Extracts ($195 plus $14 S&H)

Package 251 – Step by Step to Abundant Health ($515 plus $20 S&H)
Includes all five courses

NC residents add 6% sales tax.
VISA, MasterCard, Discover cards accepted

All courses are correspondence courses to be completed at the student's own pace of study. They are non-traditional courses (not meeting licensure requirements) because we have not sought and do not wish accreditation. As do many non-traditional teaching facilities, we award designations, not diplomas. We strive to provide every student with quality courses and an in-depth presentation of natural health material.

The Power For Healing Workshop

Put the power of spiritual healing to work in your church.
Three power-filled days that will change your life
and the lives of those you touch.

The Power for Healing Workshop will deepen your knowledge of God's will to heal body, spirit, and soul; equip you to be a healer of hurting people; enable you to begin healing ministries within your church; teach you to use the most powerful healing modality known to man; and give you hands-on training, working with our ministry team.

The Power For Healing Workshop is unlike any healing workshop you may have experienced. We are Bible-based (not church-based) ministry offering an absolutely fresh approach to the subject of spiritual healing. The training is intensive and deeply rewarding.

Today many churches are void of healing ministries. God tells us that He is our Healer, but few understand or believe it. Once you experience the power of Biblical healing, your life will be forever changed. People are hungry for spiritual healing, so it should come as no surprise that churches structured as Healing Centers are witnessing explosive growth.

Our ministry Team is grounded in Scripture. We know the power of prayer. We are experienced with the same therapeutic healing oils Jesus Christ taught His disciples to use. And we are ready to share this knowledge with you.

The curriculum covers six major topics including foundations for healing ministries, God's medicine chest, and hands-on healing. The fee includes a hardbound 377 page reference manual, a workshop manual, three full days of training, and much more.

Visit http://www.lynngroup.com/workshop.html online.
3295 New Milford School Road
Rockford, IL 61109
815-874-3358

The Christian Healer

The Christian Healer is a free, monthly Ezine
(a magazine sent by computer directly to your e-mail address)
devoted to healing from the Christian perspective.

God's lament that His people are destroyed for lack of knowledge (Hosea 4:6) has never been more true than it is today as it relates to sickness and health.

The mission of The Christian Healer is four-fold:

1. To raise the level of awareness of God as the active Healer of all people, answering prayer through Jesus Christ, our high priest.

2. To demonstrate that human health is determined by the condition of the spirit, body, and soul as one unified entity.

3. To affirm the Biblical teaching of prayer and anointing with healing oil as the most powerful modality known to man.

4. To encourage Christians of all denominations to consider the establishment of healing ministries within their local assemblies.

With God's Word as our authorization, Christian healing functions in ways that licensed, medical physicians cannot. With a reliance upon God (the Father), Jesus Christ (Mediator and High Priest), and prayer and anointing, Christian healing compliments traditional medical modalities and speeds all recovery.

The Ezine and The Power for Healing Workshop endeavor to spread the healing love and peace of Jesus Christ into every aspect of the Christian community. Our call is rooted and grounded in the love of God, the saving and healing power of Jesus Christ, the work of the Holy Spirit, and the teaching of Scripture.

To receive The Christian Healer online,
send a blank E-mail message to:
TheChristianHealer-subscribe@egroups.com

Healing

IN

His Wings

DAILY DEVOTIONS FOR HEALING

BY ANNE B. BUCHANAN

TO ORDER MORE COPIES,

Healing in His Wings --
Daily Devotions for Healing

Available from:
Carolina Natural Health Institute, Inc.
2703 E. Third St., Greenville, NC 27858
Phone: 252-355-4665   Fax: 252-355-4599